GENDERED DRUGS AND ME

Gender and Well-Being

Series Editors: Cristina Borderías, Professor of Contemporary History,
University of Barcelona, Spain and Bernard Harris, Professor of the History
of Social Policy, University of Southampton, UK

The aim of this series is to enhance our understanding of the relationship between
gender and well-being by addressing the following questions:

- How can we compare levels of well-being between women and men?
- Is it possible to develop new indicators which reflect a fuller understanding of
  the nature of well-being in the twenty-first century?
- How have women and men contributed to the improvement of individual
  well-being at different times and in different places?
- What role should institutions play in promoting and maintaining well-being?
- In what ways have different social movements contributed to the improvement
  of well-being over the last 300 years?

The volumes in this series are designed to provide rigorous social-scientific answers
to these questions. The series emerges from a series of symposia, organized as part
of COST Action 34 on 'Gender and Well-being: Work, Family and Public Policies'.
Participants were drawn from disciplines including economics, demography,
history, sociology, social policy and anthropology and they represent more than
20 European countries.

Gendered Drugs and Medicine
Historical and Socio-Cultural Perspectives

Edited by

TERESA ORTIZ-GÓMEZ
University of Granada, Spain

MARÍA JESÚS SANTESMASES
Consejo Superior de Investigaciones Científicas, Madrid, Spain

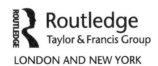

Routledge
Taylor & Francis Group

LONDON AND NEW YORK

First published 2014 by Ashgate Publishing

Published 2016 by Routledge
2 Park Square, Milton Park, Abingdon, Oxfordshire OX14 4RN
711 Third Avenue, New York, NY 10017, USA

First issued in paperback 2016

Routledge is an imprint of the Taylor & Francis Group, an informa business

British Library Cataloguing in Publication Data
A catalogue record for this book is available from the British Library

The Library of Congress has cataloged the printed edition as follows:
Ortiz, Teresa.
  Gendered drugs and medicine: historical and socio-cultural perspectives / by Teresa Ortiz-Gómez and María Jesús Santesmases.
    pages cm. -- (Gender and well-being)
  Includes bibliographical references and index.
  ISBN 978-1-4094-5404-5 (hardback: alk. paper)
  1. Medicine – History. 2. Social medicine. 3. Women in medicine – History. 4. Drugs – History. 5. Pharmaceutical industry. I. Santesmases, María Jesús. II. Title.

  RM301.55.O78 2014
  615.7--dc23

2013044882

ISBN 13: 978-1-138-27147-0 (pbk)
ISBN 13: 978-1-4094-5404-5 (hbk)

Contents

List of Figures

List of Tables

List of Contributors

Carrie Eisert, Princeton University, USA

Eugenia Gil-García, Universidad de Sevilla, Spain

Marta I. González García, Universidad de Oviedo, Spain

Agata Ignaciuk, Universidad de Granada, Spain

Ilana Löwy, CNRS, France

Alexandre Marchant, Institut des Sciences Sociales du Politique (ISP), CNRS, France

Carmen Meneses-Falcón, Universidad Pontificia de Comillas, Madrid, Spain

Teresa Ortiz-Gómez, Universidad de Granada, Spain

Esteban Rodríguez-Ocaña, Universidad de Granada, Spain

Nuria Romo-Avilés, Universidad de Granada, Spain

María Jesús Santesmases, Instituto de Filosofía, CSIC, Madrid, Spain

Heiko Stoff, Technische Universität Braunschweig, Germany

Ulrike Thoms, Otto-von-Guericke-Universität, Magdeburg, Germany

Jesper Vaczy Kragh, University of Copenhagen, Denmark

Acknowledgements

Every book holds a further story, one of people, institutions and funding. This book originated in the *Gendered Drug Standards: Historical and Socio-Anthropological Perspectives* workshop, held at the University of Granada in late November 2011. It was conceived as a step towards discussing the ways in which gender relations and gender values have shaped, and continue to shape, the research, production and consumption of drugs. A group of 30 scholars from different disciplines and countries joined in, and although not all are contributors to this volume, they took part in extensive discussions that enriched our approach, by placing gender at the core of our scholarships. The workshop was part of the European Science Foundation Research Networking Program, Standard Drugs and Drug Standards (ESF RNP DRUGS), which has also supported this book project. Additional funding was received from Spanish institutions: we would like to thank the *Ministerio de Ciencia e Innovación* and the *Instituto de la Mujer* for grants awarded for the Granada workshop and part of the editing process (*Ministerio de Ciencia e Innovación* A.C. HAR2011-14137-HIST and *Secretaría de Estado de Igualdad* A.C. 2011-0001-ACT-00006).

We are grateful to Lucía Artazcoz, María José Barral, Laura Cházaro, Angela Creager, Rafael Huertas, Carmen Meneses, Alfredo Menéndez, Consuelo Miqueo, Esteban Rodríguez Ocaña, Bettina Wahrig and Elizabeth Watkins for their constructive and pertinent comments on the first version of the manuscript. Special thanks go to Joanna Baines for her careful and insightful copyediting of the texts included in this book: she went beyond technical correction and committed herself to this project by patiently tackling the many queries that arose. For their inspiring encouragement and support, we are indebted to the series editors, Cristina Borderías and Bernard Harris.

Introduction

Teresa Ortiz-Gómez and María Jesús Santesmases

In the increasingly medicalised societies in which we live, drugs – whether prescribed by doctors or not – are part of a network of knowledge and practices on which multiple agents take effect. Gendered drugs as an articulating concept has a double genealogy: it focuses on drugs as material goods and objects within history and culture, and on the ways in which gender shapes objects and cultures, medical and scientific cultures included. The centrality of the object – drugs – is combined in the contributions to *Gendered Drugs and Medicine* with studies on gender and science for a historical and sociocultural study of drugs knowledge and practices, and of women as drug scientists, users, clinicians, consumers and, more generally, circulators.

Drugs have been included as agents in some histories of science and medicine, and in industrial histories of particular drugs and firms (among others, see Quirke and Slinn 2010; Simon and Gradmann 2010; Bonah et al. 2009; Rasmussen 2008; Tone and Watkins 2007; Bonah and Rasmussen 2005; Pieters 2005; Goodman and Walsh 2001; Bud 2008; Hobby 1985). More recently, the history of pharmaceutical research and development was the focus for the Networking Program, Standard Drugs and Drugs Standards (DRUGS), approved by the European Science Foundation and running from 2008 until 2013, to analyse standardisation in the development, regulation, marketing and use of modern pharmaceuticals (see, for example, Gaudillière and Thoms 2013; Gaudillière and Hess 2012; von Schwerin, Stoff and Wahrig 2013; Pieters and Snelders 2011; Santesmases and Gradmann 2011). The studies on gender and drugs in this book, even when relying in part on the existing historiography and recent sociological and anthropological approaches to medicines and addictive substances, focus on the role of gender in the construction of contemporary drugs cultures.

From Joan Scott to Judith Butler, gender has been defined and redefined by feminist scholars as a useful analytical tool for studying past and present social and power relations, social rules, and cultural symbols associated with women and men, the feminine and the masculine. Also useful for understanding subjectivities and personal and collective identities, gender has contributed to a recognition of the social character of bodily existence and the dialectical and non-hierarchical links between body and culture (Scott 1986; Butler 1999; Clarke 1998; Harding 1998; Fausto-Sterling 2000; Ettorre 2002). Recently, the concept of intersectionality has reinforced the need to explore relationships between gender, class and ethnicity, and has contributed to the conceptualisation of two key gender themes: diversity and agency – women as plural and changing social actors; and agents and victims – discriminating and discriminated against, users and researchers, passive recipients and activists (McCall 2005; Nash 2008; Ortiz and Ignaciuk 2012).

Since the mid 1980s, gender has been widely used in scholarly work, not only as a scientific category but also as a fashionable term. This success has unfortunately contributed to a neutralising and trivialising of its meaning, a distancing of the term from its challenging potential, reducing it to the level of an analytical variable rather than a feminist-situated research perspective (Jordanova 1993; Haraway 1995; Schiebinger 1989; Butler 1999; Riot-Sarcey and Salines 1999; Liu 1991; Whittle and Inhorn 2001; Löwy and Rouch 2003; Ortiz 2006). While 'gender differences' and 'gender bias' have become common biomedical technical terms, especially in the field of health statistics and studies on professional inequalities and doctor-patient relationships, gender has become a 'buzzword' (Wahrig 2013), frequently utilised in an ambiguous and depoliticised way. A great deal of medical and scientific research has contributed to this by denuding the term of its complex potential for understanding the social and cultural dimensions of any human issue. As Londa Schiebinger has recently emphasised, to mainstream gender analysis within knowledge production requires a consideration of gender in research design (Schiebinger 2010).

Along with gender, women have become a recognised research category within scientific inquiry. Women as agents in social, medical and scientific life and the genealogies they have constructed themselves, have probably received more acknowledgment than work incorporating a gender perspective (for some recent contributions, see Riska 2001; More, Fee and Perry 2009; Elston 2009; ETAN Expert Working Group 2000). By employing a gender perspective when studying the production, circulation and consumption of drugs in contemporary life styles, and by putting women at the centre of our research, we hope to demonstrate how the processes of the *culturalisation* of a drug and the *pharmaceuticalisation* of a culture, became mutually entwined (on pharmaceuticalisation, see Fraser, Valentine and Roberts 2009; Williams, Gabe and Davis 2008). The contributions to this book are intended to retrieve places – the household, the factory, the drugstore, the consulting room, public and private lives and spaces – and to retrieve times, stories and particular moments in history, historical trajectories and contemporary social lives of medicines and drugs (for gender and experimental sciences, see von Oertzen, Rentetzi and Watkins 2013). We endeavoured to interweave a type of object – drugs – and a conceptual and methodological category – gender. Drugs are considered here as healers and harmers, wonder substances and knowledge makers; objects that impact on social hierarchies, health practices and public policies. Gender is understood to be an analytical category which, together with race, ethnicity and class, enables scholars to make visible women's agency and representations of bodies and the sexes, as well as exploring how drugs have incorporated, reinforced and challenged gender rules, gender relations and social inequalities.

The chapters that follow discuss the classification of drugs – both as medicines and addictive substances – and consumers, on the basis of contemporary cultural dichotomies such as legal and illegal; addictive and non-addictive; personal choice and doctor-mediated prescription; disorder treatment or life-style choice. Cultures are composed by material agents, beyond the concepts that may contribute to understanding them. Drugs are discovered, created, and produced in laboratories, pilot plants and factories. Scientists, technicians, and the entire factory hierarchy take part in this manufacturing. Since the inception of the pharmaceutical drugs industry as we conceive it today, managerial decisions have impacted on manufacturing procedures, drugs research, and sales marketing. A whole space of the contemporary system of commodities production created the wonders of drugs action (see below).

Drugs in Historiography and Social Life

An *obsolete* definition of drug refers to a substance used in dyeing and, more generally, in chemical operations (Webster's Dictionary 1989). This definition retrieves a not so distant past when drugs were dyestuffs and chemicals in general, products used in chemical experiments. It was only during the late nineteenth and the beginning of the twentieth centuries that drugs obtained their healing character. The historiography displays a wide consensus regarding the beginning of the drugs era, of substances used to palliate or cure ailments, a therapeutic revolution in medicine when cure often followed diagnosis (Tone and Watkins 2007; Bonah and Rasmussen 2005; Quirke and Slinn 2010). The substances used, which would be evoked as agents of change in professional, social and cultural practices, were industrially produced, as John Lesch (2007) demonstrates in his study on the history of sulfa-drugs. So the factory, together with the chemical laboratory, became the space where a new style of living was literally manufactured (Quirke 2008; Pieters 2005). The therapeutic revolution followed the scientific and the industrial (Rosenberg 1977; Cunningham and Williams 1992), if we accept these terms as referring to historical periods rather than historically grounded conceptualisations. Throughout the historical trajectories of such revolutions, factories have not always been the settings for inventions or discoveries, but workshops and laboratories have been. The research setting of the laboratory – an academic space with its own cultures of authority, recognition and learning, often connected to a university – has contributed in modern times to the creation of new products, new substances to be used against pain, infection, and disease in general. As the economic history of innovation has repeatedly demonstrated, the collaboration between an industrial setting and a research laboratory has often been the most effective and well-known model of cooperative design for goods production – medicinal drugs included (Lesch 2007; Quirke 2008; Chauveau 1999 and 2006; Swann 1998; Santesmases 2011; for a brief discussion about industry and innovation, see Nelson 1986, also Cardwell 1994). The successful intersections between these two worlds, which have been studied in depth, have not only provided a pattern for the further production of innovations but also for the manner in which these patterns have been analysed. Links developed between the research laboratory and the factory contributed to contemporary health and wealth. The distribution of this wealth among wide populations in the West through welfare states following WWII provided medicine and other treatments for those whose health was under threat and contributed to the era of 'therapeutic plenty' (Green and Watkins 2012, 1; on welfare state policies, see the influential book by Skocpol, Evans and Rueschemeyer 1985).

Studies of early twentieth-century public health policies based on hygiene and vaccination campaigns offer an insightful array of analyses. What has been less explored is the intertwining after WWII of national health care systems, the extension of drugs as healers and the extent to which an increasing number of medicines overrun public policies. This would bring the role of public policies and the state back into contemporary cultures of medical drugs, where they are also agents within drug history (on public health see, among others, Rodríguez-Ocaña 2001; on regulation, see Daemmrich 2004). When considering the relation of state policies regarding medical care to those regarding drugs regulation, the private or public status of health care has been influential. Strong and early regulators, such as the US and Norwegian systems, have shown in quite different ways the extent to which public policies regarding drugs control, including manufacturing and prescription, have shaped drug consumption patterns (Lie 2014).

Inventors, producers, regulators and providers could hardly, however, account for the multiple agencies surrounding drug use in contemporary life culture. Drug use is provided with a protocol, a set of instructions resulting from randomised clinical trials – a contemporary method for drug testing agreed upon by practitioners, to be shown to drug regulators, such as the US Food and Drug Administration and the European Medicines Agency, administrations that have assessed the usefulness of every new drug put forward by the pharmaceutical industry since WWII (Daemmrich 2004; Marks 1997; Podolsky 2010; on clinical trials see Petryna 2009; on patents see Gaudillière 2008; Romero de Pablos 2011).

Once a particular drug has entered the market, a physician can prescribe it, or not; and that prescription is regulated so as the drug can be bought and sold either by prescription only or over the counter (for the US, Green and Watkins 2012). Children as consumers have not usually bought drugs, or procured prescriptions; by and large, adult women have done so, providing care at home under medical prescription, therefore age as well as gender has intervened in the procedure (see below). Drugs have thus enhanced medical authority and relocated consumers' agency – having shown patients to be untrained, uneducated citizens in search of, literally, prescription of a healing treatment in a cultural world of divided authorities, where medicine has achieved increasing social recognition and cultural agency to offer not only cure but scientific explanations of health and its disorders (on the cultures of diagnosis, Rosenberg 2002).

After WWII an additional agent played a part in the lives of drugs: an increasing network of international regulations. The World Health Organization, in its role as legitimator of national policies in regard to both health care and medicines, has become an agency where the knowledge and practices of medicine and drug prescription have been negotiated since WWII (see Borowy 2013), as has the European Medicines Agency in the European Union since 1995.

Taking substances, however, is not a new practice, characterising only contemporary societies and cultures. Scholars in anthropology and history have long documented substances to which people have attributed transformative powers, used in different cultures and times for a diverse range of purposes (van der Geest, Whyte and Hardon 1996; Gijswijt-Hofstra, Van Heteren and Tansey 2002). Since distant times and away from distant cultures, the meaning of 'taking a substance' has changed however, as have the sources and providers: from a woman healer to a male doctor; from a witch or magician – according to colonial terminology – to a pharmaceutical factory; from home to the consulting room and the clinic. Along such trajectories, drugs have also taken shape as illegal and legal, relating to the laws of their times and places. Addiction, habituation and changes in consciousness – the three activities attributed to drugs by Webster's Dictionary (1989) – have applied to both drugs and medicines, and have consistently shaped lifestyles and society at large.

Drugs either as medication or as substances included in a medication, when recognised by the pharmacopoeia and approved by national and international legal agreements, have not only been therapeutic. They have been used for a variety of other reasons, including disease prevention, as in the recent use of antibiotics to prevent prospective infections in surgery; to diagnose disease; and to create new anxieties such as antibiotic resistance and a wide range of adverse effects (Gradmann 2013; Coundrau and Kirk 2011; Timmermans and Berg 2003). On taking any of these substances, a person's metabolism is modified, and this is how biomedicine has been constructed: as a space of inquiry in which substances intervene, regulate, and modify the biochemical pathways of life phenomena (Green 2007). By defining and describing the metabolic action of a given substance, a standard human body has been established. And thus not only the drug has been standardised by the protocols and norms of manufacturing and prescribing, but also the human body: standardised so as to be able to characterise drugs and their action in human bodies. Ecks has proposed the term 'pharmaceutical citizenship', identifying citizenship as determined by access to pharmaceuticals and exploring how taking pharmaceuticals affects the citizen status (Ecks 2005, 241). This reciprocity between drugs and bodies has become one of the main subjects at the core of social and philosophical perspectives of bodies, care and drugs, an area to reflect on subjectivity and society (Mol 2002; Lock and Kaufert 2001; Preciado 2008).

Gender, Feminism and Drug Studies

The limited scholarship on gender and feminist approaches to the history and sociology of drugs and medicines has tended to focus on a narrow range of questions. The processes by which hormonal and psychotropic drugs have circulated and the role played by feminist activists and women's health movements in the processes of the design, acceptance or rejection of particular drugs have been well studied as we will show below. Women as producers, users and consumers of drugs has been an additional thematic area in which an emergent set of sources, from advertising and the media to oral history, are gaining prominence. It is in good part this body of work that inspired us to tackle the subject of this book as a collective endeavour.

Sex hormones, a product resulting in part from previous work on sex glands and the physiology and biochemistry of sex (Sengoopta 2006), began to be obtained and synthesised for commercialisation by the 1930s, in the Netherlands by Organon and in Germany by Schering. Nelly Oudshoorn (1994) has explained the far-reaching and rapid success of hormone treatments, the action and chemistry of which stabilised the idea of the woman's body as a cyclic and biologically-constrained body. Anne Fausto-Sterling (2000) has provided historical narratives of the many ways that sex hormones, even when given gendered names, can hardly be sexualised if we take into account the transformation of one into the other in the biochemical reactions taking place within human bodies (see also Oudshoorn 1994; Gaudillière 2005; Löwy 2006). Here we have an example, one of many, of how names and cultures of a particular time have shaped biological knowledge about woman for times to come.

Hormonal drugs have been interpreted as gendered products associated with the medicalisation and standardisation of the female body during the second half of the twentieth century, intervening in the regulation of normal processes and in women's identities and subjectivities (Watkins 1998; Marks 2001). These interventions have included menopause 'treatments' (Lock and Kaufert 2001); the suppression of menstruation without challenging femininity by the new contraceptive pill Seasonale or Season (Mamo and Fosket 2009; Kissling 2013); and attempts to control the height of healthy 'tall' girls (Rayner, Pyett and Astbury 2010). As medicalised mediators, hormones have been identified as agents in constructing the cultures of women's reproductive life (Roberts 2007). They have also been considered as ways of controlling and disciplining sexual and intersexual identities and personal subjectivities (Sanabria 2010 and 2013; Preciado 2008). Utilising the concept of 'gender asymmetry' in contraceptive research, Nelly Oudshoorn (2003, 6) has explained the difficulties of achieving a hormonal contraceptive for men as the result of research constraints and cultural questions linked to hegemonic ideas about masculinity and the onus of reproductive responsibility being on women.

Psychodrugs have been studied as 'mother's little helpers' (Pieters and Snelders 2007), and as genderised therapies that have prescribed gender 'from the couch' (Metzl 2003). Jonathan Metzl (2003) has demonstrated that the over-prescription of psychodrugs to women in the US between the 1950s and 1990s resulted from a perception of female disorders based upon gendered psychoanalytic representations of femaleness. The launching on the US pharmaceutical market of the anti-depressive Prozac in 1987 attracted a great deal of both public and academic discussion; Linda Blum and Nena Stracuzzi (2004) insightfully portrayed its effects in the disciplining of female bodies and through enhancing the productivity of elite women, contributing to a gendered social landscape in which women are regarded as particularly susceptible to medicalisation and psychodrug dependency.

Connections between feminism, women's health movements, and drugs have also received a certain amount of scholarly attention. In the late 1960s, the women's health movements arose in American and European countries in white middle-class feminist circles, as a response to gynaecological paternalism and an increasing medicalisation. Together with a promotion of self-help, cervical self-examinations, access to knowledge about the female body, and a claim for control over reproductive technologies and establishment of their own health care facilities, activists criticised medical consumerism and questioned the effects of contraceptive drugs and treatments on women bodies (Morgen 2002; Rosenbaum 2004; Löwy 2005; Seaman and Eldridge 2012).

The role and influence of feminist activists and women's health movements have been particularly studied in the case of the pill (Marks 2001; Sillies 2010), Depo Provera progesterone contraceptive shots (Kline 2010) and new contraceptive drugs such as emergency 'morning-after' pills and the subdermal implant Norplant (Watkins 2010; Prescott 2012). Authors agree that the issue of regulating contraception at the end of the twentieth century was an extremely complex one for women's health movements (see also chapter one of this book). A transition has taken place in feminist health activism towards further empowerment for women in decision-making regarding their own health and reproductive choices, by challenging medical authority and pharmaceutical industry interests that have maintained a rhetoric of women's vulnerability. Meanwhile, studies of clinical trials have focused on women (Junod and Marks 2002; Kline 2010) insisting there exists a gendered bias and equivocal assumptions of male and female health similarities and differences (Chilet Rosell et al. 2009 and 2010). Although such studies are regarded as a classical issue of feminist research, their conclusions and suggestions are having fewer consequences than expected on the ways in which clinical trials are conducted (Löwy 2005).

Long before any drug was referred to as such, many products, including cosmetics and food preparations, contributed to the wellbeing of those at the mercy of disorders, pain, disease and pregnancy. The entire medieval and modern historiography of women has been an insightful space of knowledge which has stimulated further studies, in history, and the sociology and anthropology of woman in history (Cabré and Ortiz 1999). Historians of medieval and early modern women have convincingly demonstrated the role played by recipes written and distributed by women as health providers, prior to the emergence of a male medical authority, the disciplinary structures and care administration of which achieved wide recognition (Cabré 2008; Leong 2008; Rankin 2007). The fragile border that would eventually separate the concept of recipes from that of prescribed medicines in later periods, most notably from the modern times onwards, suggests that the transition from one to the other took place under a fully genderised society that blew woman's role in care provision away when medicine emerged as an authoritative male professional space. Since the inception of this male authority in medical practice, recipe has remained a term for household practices (see also von Oertzen, Rentetzi and Watkins 2013) to be retrieved by 'the professional order' of the pharmacist as expert in following instructions from the pharmacopeia for particular mixtures prescribed by physicians before the industrial manufacturing of medicines (Gaudilliére 2008). Industrialisation changed gendered roles and reorganised a society based on gender classifications and qualifications, while the kitchen would remain a place in which technologies could be included, thus contributing to their social legitimisation throughout the Cold War era (Abir-Am and Outram 1987; Parr 2002; Oldenziel and Zachmann 2009).

Women in industrial production deserve more attention than they have thus far received. An exception to this is the participation of women in the origins of the contraceptive pill, as research promoters and trials participants. Margaret Sanger and Katherine D. McCormick provided the incentives for research to identify an oral contraceptive (Chesler 2007; Gordon 2002). Gregory Pincus developed the substance which would come to be the main component of the contraceptive pill and, together with Celso Ramón García and others, carried out the trials to test its activity in Puerto Rico. The women in Puerto Rico created their own environment by not fulfilling the expectations of the inventors (Marks 2001; Soto Laveaga 2009; Ramírez de Arellano and Seipp 1983), being neither patients nor trustworthy participants in testing a product that needed to be taken every day. Test success, however, is demonstrated by the entry to the market in 1960 of the first contraceptive pill, Enovid by Searle. Women have been fully active in the production of contraceptive methods and substances, and their perception of female bodies has influenced the way they have promoted birth control and, more relevantly for the subject of this book, the contraceptive substances themselves. These substances provided spaces of independence from men following sexual intercourse, enabling women to empower themselves. At the same time, the taking of sex hormones orally generated health risks identified very soon after their introduction, while the independence the pill afforded both women and men remained a powerful rationale for keeping pill consumption figures high, becoming a political tool for birth control (Watkins 1998; Tone 2001). While the pill has come to represent women's bodies, the process of pill invention, testing and manufacture displays a fully gendered drug trajectory. As a case of reflexive genderising, the history of the pill exhibits gendered agency in one of the most influential substances manufactured by contemporary society.

However, women as drugs users have seldom been researched. Sociologists Elizabeth Ettorre and Elianne Riska have employed an articulated gender perspective, which is creating a space for feminist research on women's health, medical authority, the pharmaceutical industry and the legal regulation of drug consumption (Ettorre and Riska 1995; Ettorre 2004; see also Curry and O'Brien 2006 and section three of this book).

A prospective agenda for studying gender and drugs from historical and socio-cultural perspectives is still pending. Subjects which deserve research and discussion include the impact of gender, ethnicity and class in the processes of designing, standardising and circulating drugs; how dominant ideas of masculinity and femininity influence and shape research, prescription and use of drugs (Wahrig 2013); and how pharmaceutical technologies manufacture gender-specific outcomes in lifestyles and social practices, altering life experiences such as reproduction, childbirth, menopause, sexual desire, depression and happiness. The processes of prescribing, selling, marketing and accepting or forbidding drugs either reinforce or challenge gender values and gender social relations, including social hierarchies and relationships between doctors and patients, prescribers and users. The roles assigned to women as patients and consumers of pharmaceuticals are permanently renegotiated. It is largely women who have bought – and still buy – the medicines consumed within the household, and they should therefore also be included as providers, the household itself a gendered space still lacking recognition alongside the hospital, the consulting room and the factory. The contribution of gendered medical practice to medicalisation and the higher drug consumption of women merits discussion, as does research into the differential effects drugs produce in women and men, or in particular groups of women and men. The participation and experiences of women in pharmaceutical research teams and medical practice, the lives and professional stories of women doctors, drug technicians and researchers, and the impact on these of gender relations and other hierarchies also deserve attention. These issues, among others, constitute the agenda at the origin of this book as a collective international project.

Gender approaches to the history and sociology of pharmaceuticals in the twentieth century have been undertaken in few publications. Although the role played by gender in drug history, marketing and clinical practices is difficult to deny, mobilising this approach has been a challenge, as the concepts of drugs and drug standardisation articulated in the historiography can hide, or at least contribute to excluding, gender and women's issues. Placing both women and gender at the core of research questions and analytical answers remains a challenge that the contributions that follow take up so as to participate in widening the space for gender studies.

This Volume as a Challenge to Drugs Studies

The specific approach to gender and pharmaceuticals at the origin of this collection was developed at two international scientific meetings: the workshop, *Gendered Drugs Standards. Historical and Socio-anthropological Perspectives*, held in Granada in November 2011, and the panel *Gender Standards in Drugs History: Crossing Boundaries*, at the 4th International European Society for the History of Science Conference, held in Barcelona in November 2010. These gatherings were held as part of the Research Networking Program of the European Science Foundation Standard Drugs and Drug Standards: A Comparative Historical Study of Pharmaceuticals in the 20th Century (hereafter DRUGS Network).

Gender was introduced in the early meetings of the DRUGS Network steering committee as a research category to be tackled within the network's workshops. The issues of gender and women were present in meetings of the DRUGS Network not specifically organised around gender and drugs. Themes such as breast cancer treatment, hormones and menopause, contraceptive marketing, and sperm and egg donation were addressed in workshops held in Berlin, in Zurich in 2012, and in Braunschweig 2011. This suggests that women and gender have been identified as such in a variety of works produced and communicated at the DRUGS meetings. It also suggests that the subject of women has not been a specific research theme, and that gender has not been employed as a fully productive and transversal analytical tool either in the DRUGS Network or in other programs and academic gatherings dedicated to the history of drugs, and social and cultural studies of pharmaceuticals and addictive substances.

The Granada Workshop was conceived as a step toward establishing gender as a category in the history and sociology of drugs, by placing therapy as a central object of enquiry within the agenda of the history of medicine and disease. The Granada workshop included researchers from eleven academic institutions based in eight different countries. Originating from many disciplines, including the history of science and medicine, the philosophy of science, the sociology of health, epidemiology, and the social anthropology of health and medicine, scholars brought together a range of different disciplinary and methodological approaches. We gathered with a common aim: to discuss the ways in which gender relations and gender values have shaped, and continue to shape, the research, production and consumption of drugs. The papers provided cultural, social and historical analyses concerning various international locations. From those contributions we have in this volume a set of ten chapters by authors from five countries.

This book is structured into three sections, reflecting the three aspects of the history and sociology of drugs in which gender approaches are relevant: the agency of women as researchers, producers and committed consumers; the cultural meanings embedded in contraceptives specifically designed for women; and the gendered representations and practices of drug users and addicts. As a collective project it displays landscapes of practices and of social life for a wider history of gender, drugs and medicine.

In Part I, women are especially prominent as consumers, producers, and even industrial and political targets: that is to say, as agents in a co-constructed history of drugs. Drugs develop agency by taking part in the shaping of the social and cultural life of contemporary gender and femaleness. Heiko Stoff studies the crucial role German housewife organisations played in the 1940s, in the prohibition of the food colourant butter yellow, which was subject to intense scientific scrutiny due to its carcinogenic nature. German women, however, remained silent for 30 years about oestrogens, another supposedly cancer-causing molecule. By following the debates surrounding the socialisation of these two drugs, this chapter illuminates German feminist movement practices and discourses during the twentieth century.

Marta González discusses the intervention of the pharmaceutical industry in the construction and definitions of female and male sexual desire in the search for a female Viagra. The new requirement of different models of sexual response for men and women and, consequently, of different ways of classifying their dysfunctions, far from revealing the true nature of sex differences, appear to be merely a consequence of attempts to extend the market of sex drugs to women by biomedicalising woman's sexual desire. The male pill, the development of which has been so intensively resisted (Oudshoorn 2003), is worth mentioning as a counter case that suggests drugs and their trajectories are fully genderised.

María Santesmases's chapter affords women agency in the history of Spanish antibiotics production and research. It places women at the centre of industrial drug production, in both the production line and the research laboratory, with the aim of reconstructing the history of early antibiotics production in Spain. Looking from a gender perspective at the similarities between the production of knowledge and the production of industrial drugs, Santesmases demonstrates the overlapping capacity of women as agents in the contemporary history of both research and industry.

Part II is centred on contraceptives, the impact of which on contemporary lifestyle and women's uses still merits further study. Not only national spaces but professional ones – including packaging, marketing, links with birth rates and population control, and the reconstruction of doctors and women as patients demanding prescription unrelated to disease – became cultures and practices studied by participants in the Granada workshop and in this collection.

In her chapter, Ilana Löwy examines the links between spermicides and microbicides. Spermicides were promoted and distributed by population experts who often failed to notice the sex and gender of their 'targets' – prospective woman users – while anti-HIV microbicides were championed by feminist activists attuned to women's specific plights. The history of contraception is a long and complex one, subject to local and national histories, standards and cultures, and to a varied set of agents. As Carrie Eisert demonstrates, being a daily regime to be integrated into women's lives, the very act of taking the pill became a subject of interest, research and innovation. Pill packages developed into representations of popular perceptions of women: women who were apt to forget to take the pill and were in need of supervision to ensure compliance. Doctor-patient relationships changed dramatically when women began to demand a contraceptive prescription when not suffering from any disorder. As is discussed by Agata Ignaciuk, Teresa Ortiz-Gómez and Esteban Rodríguez-Ocaña, during the 1960s and 1970s, Spanish doctors and their female patients shared an interest in oral contraceptives. The prohibition of the sale of contraceptive methods in Spain, which lasted until 1978, reflected a conservative discourse that was counteracted during the transition to democracy following Franco's death in 1975. The increased presence of women within medicine and gynaecology, and the establishment and expansion of family planning clinics, made favourable opinions of the pill visible. According to Ulrike Thoms, the 1961 launching on the market of the first contraceptive pill in West Germany, provoked fierce debates over morals and ethics, the nature of sexuality in general, and men and women's relationships in particular. The pill deeply challenged the professional identity of gynaecologists and the relationship between gynaecologists and women. Pharmaceutical companies assessed these changes, and adjusted their marketing strategies accordingly, establishing direct contact with women. Pills were displayed as part of a modern lifestyle, while the 'facts' of pure science and their claim to be the decisive experts limited discussion concerning the pill to male-dominated scientific circles, in which female consumers had no voice at all.

Part III tackles the question of addiction and the use of medicines and other drugs by consumers without medical supervision. These chapters pay particular attention to the gender inequalities in these processes, and to how these transgressions have taken different forms in women and men, in the past and the present. Gendered stereotypes of drug abusers and the social life of these stereotypes reveal similarly gendered social hierarchies and biopowers. Drug consumption and punishment participates in contemporary life, contributing to disciplining gendered dichotomies: women and men; female and male; health and disease; use and abuse; legal and illegal.

Jesper Vaczy Kragh studies the issue of gender and class in morphine addiction during the late nineteenth century. Having investigated German, French, and Danish sources, he argues that, contrary to the widely held notion that the majority of morphinists were women, morphinism was most frequently found in men, and more specifically, in male physicians, the most prominent demographic group among morphine addicts in this period. The medical profession had little to gain by drawing attention to addicted physicians and was, for a long time, uninterested in advocating strict regulations or laws which would criminalise drug users. Regulations enacted in the 1950s were based in class bias, being largely motivated by the spread of drug addiction to people of lower socioeconomic status.

Alexandre Marchant discusses the representation of drug abuse as a 'feminine vice' in France. Discussions about the 'new social plague' of drug abuse during the years 1969–1973 were influenced by stereotypes, despite the medical approach to addiction having changed. Debates on drug abuse were also utilised for a renewed staging of women's bodies, sites of liberation or decadence depending on the view of the agents and their cultural backgrounds.

In their chapter, Nuria Romo, Carmen Meneses and Eugenia Gil defend, emphasise that for harm-reducing policies in the field of drug dependency to be successful, a gender perspective must be included. They address contemporary relationships between young Spanish females and risk behaviours associated with the use of legal, but unprescribed drugs. Based on a questionnaire and discussion groups with a representative sample of Spanish male and female secondary school students, this chapter reveals the unexpected existence of groups of 'normal' female adolescents engaged in the most risky and almost illegal behaviours.

As a collective endeavour, this set of chapters demonstrates a complex trajectory for women and gender in drug history and social life. On one hand, these social and historical studies exhibit more agents than have been identified in the current historiography: women as well as men, drugs as well as doctors, and therapeutic regimes as well as prescriptions and consumption. On the other hand, they challenge previously accepted symmetrical narratives in drug history. The societies of the past and present explored in this collection interact to generate a corpus of knowledge that can help to bring women back into social and historical discourse. Gendered perspectives emerge whenever women are the subjects of research, whenever their active role is investigated and their representation analysed. Drugs have created new gendered spaces and hierarchies within societies and have contributed to maintaining and reinforcing a changing gendered social order: a fact insightfully demonstrated by the contributions here on the circulation of contraceptive knowledge and practices from the 1950s onwards. When a gender perspective is included in historical and social analyses of drug uses and production, as well as of advertising and wider public representations of drugs production and consumption, not only do women become visible, so do the boundaries between drug use and abuse. Medicalisation and legalisation of drugs is one of the foremost issues running through these chapters. Authority, medical practices and the law appear to have challenged every attempt to bring female agency into social practices and studies. The set of contributions to this book further challenge the public discourses and practices of authority, by showing women and gender in many spaces, physical as well as symbolic: in manufacturing and the circulating of drugs knowledge and practices in an increasingly medicalised culture; as users and abusers; and as producers and advocates for prospective producers and users. The entire iconography of contemporary culture is visualised here through multiple analyses of a medicalised, gendered society.

References

Abir-Am, P. G. and Outram D. (eds) (1987), *Uneasy Careers and Intimate Lives: Women in Science, 1789–1979* (New Brunswick, NJ: Rutgers University Press).

Blum, L. M. and Stracuzzi N. F. (2004), 'Gender in the Prozac Nation: Popular Discourse and Productive Femininity', *Gender and Society* 18:3, 269–86.

Bonah, C., Masutti, C., Rasmussen, A. and Simon, J. (eds) (2009) *Harmonizing Drugs: Standards in 20th-century Pharmaceutical History* (Paris: Glyphe).

Bonah, C. and Rasmussen, A. (eds) (2005), *Histoire et médicament aux 19e et 20e siècles* (Paris: Gliphe).

Borowy, I. (2012), 'Global Health and Development: Conceptualizing Health between Economic Growth and Environmental Sustainability', *Journal of the History of Medicine and Allied Sciences* 68:3, 451–85.

Bud, R. (2007), *Penicillin: Triumph and tragedy* (Oxford: Oxford University Press).

Butler, J. (1999), *Gender Trouble: Feminism and the Subversion of Identity* (New York: Routledge).

Cabré, M. (2008), 'Women or Healers? Household Practices and the Categories of Health Care in Late Medieval Iberia', *Bulletin of the History of Medicine* 82:1, 18–51.

Cabré, M. and Ortiz-Gómez, T. (1999), 'Mujeres y salud: prácticas y saberes. Presentación', *Dynamis* 19, 17–24.

Cardwell, D. S. L. (1994), *The Fontana History of Technology* (London: Fonatana).

Chauveau, S. (1999), L'invention pharmaceutique. La pharmacie française entre l'État et la société au XX° siècle (Paris: Sanofi-Synthélabo).

—————— (2006), 'L'essor des consommations médicales, l'innovation thérapeutique et sa diffusion', in Griset P. (ed.) *Georges Pompidou et la modernité. Les tensions de l'innovation 1962–1974* (Bruxelles: Peter Lang) pp. 275–90.

Chesler, E. (2007), *Woman of Valor: Margaret Sanger and the Birth Control Movement in America* (New York: Simon & Schuster Paperbacks).

Chilet Rosell, E. Ruiz Cantero, M. T. and Horga, J. F. (2009), 'Women's health and gender-based clinical trials on etoricoxib: methodological gender bias', *Journal Public Health* 31 (3): 434–5.

Chilet Rosell, E., Ruiz Cantero, M. T., Laguna-Goya, N. and De Andrés Rodriguez-Trelles, F. (2010), 'Recomendaciones para el estudio y evaluación de las diferencias de género en los ensayos clínicos de fármacos en España', *Medicina Clínica* 135:3, 130–34.

Clarke, A. (1998), *Disciplining Reproduction: Modernity, American Life Sciences and 'the Problems of Sex'* (Berkeley: University of California Press).

Condrau, F., & Kirk, R. G. (2011), 'Negotiating hospital infections: The debate between ecological balance and eradication strategies in British hospitals, 1947–1969', *Dynamis*, 31:2, 385–405.

Cunningham, A. and Williams, P. (eds) (1992), *The Laboratory Revolution in Medicine* (Cambridge: Cambridge University Press).

Curry, P. and O'Brien, M. (2006), 'The male heart and the female mind: A study in the gendering of antidepressants and cardiovascular drugs in advertisements in Irish medical publications', *Social Science and Medicine* 62:1, 1970–77.

Daemmrich, A. (2004), *Pharmacopolitics: Drug Regulation in the United States and Germany* (Chapel Hill/London: University of Carolina Press).

Ecks, S. (2005), 'Pharmaceutical Citizenship: Antidepressant Marketing and the Promise of Demarginalization in India', *Anthropology and Medicine* 12:3, 239–54.

Elston, M. A. (2009), *Women and Medicine: The Future* (London: Royal College of Physicians).

ETAN Expert Working Group (2000), *Promoting excellence through mainstreaming gender equality* (Brussel: European Commission).

Ettorre, E. (2004), 'Revisioning women and drug use: gender sensitivity, embodiment and reducing harm', *International, Journal of Drug Policy* 15, 327–35.

Ettorre, E. and Riska, E. (1995), *Gendered Moods: Psychotropics and Society* (London: Routledge).

Fausto-Sterling, A. (2000), *Sexing the Body: Gender Politics and the Construction of Sexuality* (New York: Basic Books).

Fraser, S., Valentine, K. and Roberts, C. (2009), 'Guest Introduction: Living drugs', *Science as Culture* 18:2, 123–31.

Gaudillière, J.-P. (2005), 'Better prepared than synthesized: Adolf Butenandt, Schering Ag and the transformation of sex steroids into drugs (1930–1946), *Studies in History and Philosophy of Biological and Biomedical Sciences* 36:4, 612–44.

———— (2008), 'How pharmaceuticals became patentable: the production and appropriation of drugs in the twentieth century', *History and Technology* 24: 2, 99–106.

Gaudillière, J.-P. and Hess, V. (eds) (2012), *Ways of Regulating Drugs in the 19th and 20th Centuries* (Basingstoke: Palgrave Macmillan).

Gaudillière, J.-P. and Thoms, U. (eds.) (2013), *Pharmaceutical firms and the construction of drug markets: from branding to scientific marketing*, special issue of *History and Technology* 29 (2), DOI 10.1080/07341512.2013.828867.

Gijswijt-Hofstra, M., Van Heteren, G. M. and Tansey, E. M. (eds) (2002), *Biographies of Remedies: Drugs, Medicines and Contraceptives in Dutch and Anglo-American Healing Cultures* (Amsterdam: Rodopi).

Goodman, J. and Walsh, V. (2001), *The Story of Taxol: Nature and Politics in the Pursuit of an Anti-cancer Drug* (Cambridge: Cambridge University Press).

Gordon, L. (2002), *The Moral Property of Women: A History of Birth Control Politics in America* (Urbana: University of Illinois Press).

Gradmann, C. (2013), 'Sensitive Matters: The World Health Organisation and Antibiotic Resistance Testing, 1945–1975', *Social History of Medicine* 26, 555–74.

Green, J. A. (2007), *Prescribing by Numbers: Drugs and the Definition of Disease* (Baltimore: Johns Hopkins University Press).

Green, J. and Watkins E. S. (eds.) (2012), *Prescribed: Writing, Filling, Using and Abusing the Prescription in Modern America* (Baltimore: Johns Hopkins University Press).

Haraway, D. J. (1995), *Ciencia, cyborgs y mujeres. La reinvención de la naturaleza* (Madrid: Cátedra-Feminismos).

Harding, S. (1998), 'Gender, development and post-Enlightenment Philosophies of Science', *Hypatia* 13:3, 146–67.

Hobby, G. (1985), *Penicillin. Meeting the Challenge* (New Haven/London: Yale University Press).

Jordanova, L. (1993a), 'Gender and the historiography of science', *British Journal for the History of Science* 26, 469–83.

——— (1993b), *Sexual Visions: Images of Gender in Science and Medicine between the Eighteenth and Twentieth Centuries* (pp. 134–59) (Madison: University of Wisconsin Press).

Junod, S. W. and Marks, L. (2002), 'Women's Trials: The Approval of the First Oral Contraceptive Pill in the United States and Great Britain', *Journal of the History of Medicine* 57, 117–60.

Kissling, E. A. (2013), 'Pills, Periods, and Postfeminism. The new politics of marketing birth control', *Feminist Media Studies* 13:3, 490–504.

Kline, W. (2010), 'Bodies of evidence. Activists, patients, and the FDA regulation of Depo-Provera', *Journal of Women's History* 22:3, 64–87.

Leong, E. (2008), 'Making medicines in the early modern household', *Bulletin of the History of Medicine* 82:1, 145–68.

Lesch, J. E. (2007), *The First Miracle Drugs: How the Sulfa Drugs Transformed Medicine* (Oxford: Oxford University Press).

Levy, S. B. (1992), *The Antibiotic Paradox. How Miracle Drugs are Destroying the Miracle* (New York/London: Plenum Press).

Lie, A. K. (2014), 'Producing Standards, Producing the Nordic Region: Antibiotic Susceptibility Testing, from 1950–1970', *Science in Context* 27 (2) (in press).

Liu, T. (1991), 'Teaching the differences among women from a historical perspective: rethinking race and gender as social categories', *Women's Studies International Forum* 14:4, 265–76.

Lock, M. and Kaufert, P. (2001), 'Menopause, local biologies, and cultures of aging', *American Journal of Human Biology* 13:4, 494–504.

Löwy, I. (2005), 'Le féminisme a-t-il changé la recherche biomédicale?' *Travail, genre et sociétés* 2:14, 89–108.

——— (2006), *L'emprise du genre. Masculinité, féminité, inégalité* (Paris: La Dispute).

Löwy, I. and Rouch, H. (2003), 'Genese et développement du genre: les sciences et les origines de la distinction entre sexe et genre', *Cahiers du Genre* 34, 5–16.

Mamo, L. and Fosket J. R. (2009), 'Scripting the body: Pharmaceuticals and the (re)making of menstruation', *Signs* 34:4, 925–49.

Marks, H. (1997), *The Progress of Experiment: Science and Therapeutic Reform in the United States, 1900–1990* (Cambridge: Cambridge University Press).

Marks, L. V. (2001), *Sexual Chemistry: A History of the Contraceptive Pill*, New Haven/London: Yale University Press).

McCall, L. (2005), 'The complexity of intersectionality', *Signs: Journal of Women in Culture and Society* 30:3, 1771–800.

Metzl, J. (2003), *Prozac on the Couch: Prescribing Gender in the Era of Wonder Drugs* (Durham: Duke University Press).

Mol, A. (2002), *The Body Multiple: Ontology in Medical Practice* (Durham: Duke University Press).

More, E., Fee, E. and Perry, M. (eds) (2009), *Women Physicians and the Cultures of Medicine* (Baltimore: Johns Hopkins University Press).

Morgen, S. (2002), *Into Our Own Hands: The Women's Health Movement in the United States, 1969–1990* (New Brunswick: Rutgers University Press).

Nelson, R. R. (1986), 'Institutions supporting technical advance in industry', *The American Economic Review* 76:2, 186–9.

Oldenziel, R. and Zachmann, K. (2009), 'Kitchens as technology and politics: An introduction' in Oldenziel, R. and Zachmann, K. (eds) *Cold War Kitchen: Americanisation, Technology and European Users* (Cambridge, MA: MIT Press) pp. 1–29.

Ortiz-Gómez, T. (2006), *Medicina, historia y género. 130 años de investigación feminista* (Oviedo: KRK).

Oudshoorn, N. (1994), *Beyond the Natural Body: An Archaeology of Sex Hormones* (London/New York: Routledge).

——— (2003), *The Male Pill. A Biography of a Technology in the Making* (Durham/London: Duke University Press).

Parr, J. (2002), 'Editor's Introduction: Modern Kitchen, Good Home, Strong Nation', *Technology and Culture* 43:4, 657–67.

Petryna, A. (2009), *When Experiments Travel: Clinical Trials and the Global Search for Human Subjects* (Princeton: Princeton University Press).

Pieters, T. (2005), *Interferon: The Science and Selling of a Miracle Drug* (New York: Routledge).

Pieters, T. and Snelders, S. (2007), 'From King Kong pills to mother's little helpers – career cycles of two families of psychotropic drugs: the barbiturates and benzodiazepines', *Canadian Bulletin of Medical History/Bulletin canadien d'histoire de la medicine* 24:1, 93–112.

——— (eds) (2011), 'Standardizing psychotropic drugs and drugpractices in the twentieth century: Paradox of order and disorder', *Studies in the History and Philosophy of the Biological and Biomedical Sciences* 42:4, 412–14.

Podolsky, S. H. (2010), 'Antibiotics and the social history of the controlled clinical trial, 1950–1970', *Journal for the History of Medicine and Allied Sciences* 65(3), 327–67.

Preciado, B. (2008), *Testo yonqui* (Madrid: Espasa Calpe).

Quirke, V. (2008), *Collaboration in the Pharmaceutical Industry: Changing Relationships in Britain and France, 1935–1965* (Abingdon/New York: Routledge).

Quirke, V. and Slinn, J. (eds) (2010), *Perspectives on Twentieth-century Pharmaceuticals* (Oxford: Peter Lang).

Ramírez de Arellano, A. B. and Seipp, C. (1983), *Colonialism, Catholicism, and Contraception: A History of Birth Control in Puerto Rico* (Chapel Hill: University of North Carolina Press).

Rankin, A. (2007), 'Becoming an Expert Practitioner: court experimentalism and the medical skills of Anna of Saxony (1532-1585)', *Isis* 98:1, 23–53.

Rasmussen, N. (2008), *On Speed: The Many Lives of Amphetamine* (New York/London: New York University Press).

Rayner, J. A., Pyett, P. and Astbury, J. (2010), 'The medicalisation of 'tall' girls: A discourse analysis of medical literature on the use of synthetic oestrogen to reduce female height', *Social Science and Medicine* 71:6, 1076–83.

Riot-Sarcey, M. and Salines, E. (1999), 'The difficulties of gender in France: reflections on a concept', *Gender and History* 11:3, 489–98.

Riska, E. (2001), 'Towards Gender Balance: But will Women Physicians have an Impact on Medicine?' *Social Science and Medicine* 52:2, 179–87.

Roberts, C. (2007), *Messengers of Sex: Hormones, Biomedicine and Feminism* (Cambridge: Cambridge University Press).

Rodríguez-Ocaña, E. (2001), 'The Politics of Public Health in State-Managed Schemes of Healthcare in Spain (1940–1990)', in Löwy, I. and Krige, J. (eds) *Images of Disease: Science, Public Policy and Health in Post-war Europe* (Luxembourg: Office for Official Publications of the European Communities) pp. 187–210.

Rodríguez-Ocaña, E., Ignaciuk, A. and Ortiz-Gómez, T. (2012), 'Ovulostáticos y anticonceptivos. El conocimiento médico sobre 'la píldora' en España durante el franquismo y la transición democrática (1940–1979)', *Dynamis* 32:2, 467–94.

Romero de Pablos, A. (2011), 'Regulation and the circulation of knowledge: Penicillin patents in Spain', *Dynamis*, *31*: 2, 363–83.

Rosenberg, C. E. (1977), 'The Therapeutic Revolution: Medicine, Meaning and Social Change in Nineteenthcentury America', *Perspectives in Biology and Medicine* 20:4, 485–506.

——— (2002), 'The Tyranny of Diagnosis: Specific Entities and Individual Experience', *Milbank Quarterly* 80:2, 237–60.

Rosenbaum, J. A. H. (2004), 'Whose Bodies? Whose Selves? A history of American women's health activism, 1968–present', Doctoral Thesis (Ann Arbor: Brown University).

Sanabria, E. (2010), 'From Sub- to Super-Citizenship: Sex Hormones and the Body Politic in Brazil', *Ethnos* 75:4, 377–401.

——— (2013), 'Hormones et reconfiguration des identités sexuelles au Brésil', *Clio. Histoire, Femmes, Sociétés* 37, 83–102.

Santesmases, M. J. (2000), *Mujeres científicas en España: profesionalización y modernización social* (Madrid: Instituto de la Mujer).

——— (2011), 'Screening antibiotics: industrial research in CEPA and Merck in the 1950s', *Dynamis* 31, 407–27.

Santesmases, M. J., and Gradmann, C. (eds) (2011), *Circulation of Antibiotics: Historical Reconstructions, Dynamis* 31:1, 293–426.

Schiebinger, L. (1989), 'More than skin deep: The scientific search for sexual differences', in *The Mind has no Sex? Women in the Origins of Modern Science* (Cambridge, MA: Harvard University Press).

——— (2010), *Gender, Science and Technology. Expert Group Meeting Background Paper* (United Nations). Available at: http://www.un.org/womenwatch/daw/egm/gst_2010/Schiebinger-BP.1-EGM-ST.pdf [accessed: 8 March 2013].

Scott, J. W. (1986), 'Gender: A useful category of historical analysis', *The American Historical Review* 91:5, 1053–75.

Seaman, B. and Eldridge, L. (eds) (2012) *Voices of the Women's Health Movement, Vol. 2* (New York: Seven Stories Press).

Sengoopta, C. (2006), *The Most Secret Quintessence of Life: Sex, Glands, and Hormones, 1850–1950* (Chicago: University of Chicago Press).

Silies, E. (2010), *Liebe, Lust und Last: Die Pille als weibliche Generationserfährung in der Bundesrepublik 1960–1980* (Göttingen: Wallstein Verlag).

Simon, J. and Gradmann, C. (eds) (2010), *Evaluating and Standardizing Therapeutic Agents, 1890–1950* (New York: Palgrave Macmillan).

Skocpol, T., Evans, P. and Rueschemeyer, D. (1985), *Bringing the State Back In* (New York: Cambridge University Press).

Soto Laveaga, G. (2009), *Jungle Laboratories: Mexican Peasants, National Projects, and the Making of the Pill* (Durham NC: Duke University Press).

Swann, J. P. (1988), *Academic Scientists and the Pharmaceutical Industry: Cooperative Research in Twentieth Century America* (Baltimore: Johns Hopkins University Press).

Timmermans, S. and Berg, M. (2003), *The Gold Standard: The Challenge of Evidence-based Medicine and Standardization in Health Care* (Philadelphia: Temple University Press).

Tone, A. (2001), *Devices and Desires: A History of Contraceptives in America* (New York: Hill and Wang).

Tone, A. and Watkins, E. S. (eds) (2007), *Medicating Modern America: Prescription Drugs in History* (New York: New York University Press).

van der Geest, S., Whyte, S. R., and Hardon, A. (1996), 'The Anthropology of Pharmaceuticals: A biographical approach', *Annual Review of Anthropology* 25:1, 153–78.

von Oertzen, C., Rentetzi, M. and Watkins, E. S. (2013), 'Finding Science in Surprising Places: Gender and the geography of scientific knowledge', *Centaurus* 55:2, 73–80.

von Schwerin, A., Stoff, H. and Wahrig, B. (eds) (2013), *Biologics. A History of Agents Made From Living Organisms in the 20th Century* (London: Pickering & Chatto).

Wahrig, B. (2013), 'Gender Bias in Biomedicine, more than a buzzword', paper presented at the *Final Conference, Research Networking Program Standard Drugs and Drug Standards*, Berlin, 20 February 2013.

Watkins, E. S. (1998), *On The Pill: A Social History of Oral Contraceptives, 1950–1970* (Baltimore: Johns Hopkins University Press).

Whittle, K. L. and Inhorn, M. C. (2001), 'Rethinking Difference: A feminist reframing of gender/race/class for the improvement of women's health research', *International Journal of Health Services* 31:1, 147–65.

Williams, S. J., Gabe, J. and Davis, P. (2008), 'The Sociology of Pharmaceuticals: Progress and Prospects', *Sociology of Health and Illness*, 30:6, 813–24.

PART I
Gender and Women in Pharmaceutical Research, Consumption and Industry

Oestrogens and Butter Yellow: Gendered Policies of Contamination in Germany, 1930–1970

Heiko Stoff

Since the 1930s, biochemists and pharmacologists have defined cancer as a disease which can be experimentally produced through the use of radium, x-rays, ultraviolet light, and coal tar and its derivatives, notably azo dyes and aromatic hydrocarbons. A minor modification of the molecular structure of these compounds could influence their activity enormously. In the 1940s, two distinct substances, oestrogens as a biologically active drug and butter yellow as a food colourant, came under scientific scrutiny due to their presumed carcinogenic nature. While in Germany oestrogens, some of the most profitable biologics and of major importance for the new physiology of the gendered human body, were acquitted of the charge of having a cancer-causing steroidal structure, butter yellow, representative of the ills of industrial food production, was identified as a carcinogenic molecule. The history of oncologic theories of carcinogenic substances in the early twentieth century alone would be a worthwhile undertaking, but the history of oestrogens and butter yellow sheds new light on the holistic bias of the German women's movement. The German women's movement was, from the 1920s to well into the 1960s, in many regards a consumer movement concerned with defending the individual, the family and the collective body from contamination. The main question this essay seeks to answer is why German housewife organisations played such a crucial role in the prohibition of butter yellow in the 1940s but, at the same time, remained silent about oestrogens. Indeed, it was another thirty years before feminists engaged with the dangers of supposedly cancer-causing steroids in regard to hormonal therapy and the contraceptive pill. The history of chemically and biologically active agents cannot be written without consideration of the processes of their socialisation: discourses and narratives, modes of production, standardisation and regulation of procedures, problematisations and activations (Stoff 2013; Stoff 2012a, 7–24). In an important twist, the history of the German women's movement in the twentieth century must also take these precarious substances into account.

In the following pages I will not only retell the history of oestrogens and butter yellow during crucial stages in the 1930s/1940s and 1950s/1960s, but will also highlight the different reactions of women's organisations towards suspicious molecules. While this corresponded with a new theory of carcinogenesis, one which highlighted the cancer-causing effects of certain chemicals, it also newly defined *healthy naturalness* and *dangerous artificiality*. In Germany, new biochemical knowledge strengthened a discourse on the poisoning of the people by modern civilisation, which from the 1930s to the 1950s, fuelled the continuing protest over the use of food colourants. Oestrogens could have been declared to be as precarious as azo dyes, but played a far too important role in the state's population policy, in the endocrine innovations within gynaecology, in the profit rates of pharmaceutical companies and in the careers of biochemists and pharmacologists, to be so easily condemned.

Oestrogens (1929–1940)

Ovarian extracts had been used for organotherapeutic supplementation and substitution since the 1890s, the female body having been defined as a precarious reproductive unit, always lacking something, always in danger of developing deficiencies. Organotherapy, with ovarian substances or by transplantation, was used for menstrual regulation and climacteric problems, but also produced new knowledge about a female reproductive system functioning through internal secretion, not nervous action. Both the new physiology and the new therapy relied on the concept of a notoriously deficient female body, one which could be regulated through the activation of efficient chemical messengers produced in the ovaries, 'speeding from cell to cell along the blood stream' (Starling 1905, 340; Sengoopta 2000, 441–55). In the 1910s, ovarian therapy was indicated for infantilism, sterility, asiderosis, anaemia, dysmenorrhea, amenorrhea, menorrhagia, genital neurasthenia, epilepsy and Graves' disease. The most critical deficiency symptom in turn of the century population policy was sterility. At this time, 1900, the field of gynaecology changed dramatically; endocrine events transformed not only the representation and materiality of the female body, but also practices within the doctor's surgery, in the clinic, the labour ward and postpartum rooms (Sengoopta 2006, 39–45; Gaudillière 2004a, 527). In the 1920s, it appeared that 'the ovary produces an internal secretion which governs the phenomena of estrus' (Doisy, Rolls, Allen and Johnston 1924, 711). The concepts of internal secretion and endocrine regulation generated a version of femininity as delicate, precarious and never resilient; but this new female body, in contrast to the nineteenth century's enigmatic nervousness, was amenable to direct therapy and prophylaxis. The assemblage of the pharmaceutical industry, gynaecology, biochemistry, and governmental population policy produced a female *reproductive body*, always endangered by sterility, the deficient functioning of which was characterised by menstrual and climacteric disorders. The bio-political agenda was informed by the idea of a female *deficient body* caringly arranged by male gynaecologists.

The quality of ovarian extracts, however, was rather dubious; indeed, little advance had been made in ovarian therapy since the 1890s. Still missing in the 1920s was knowledge surrounding the chemical and physical character of the biologically-active substance. In the year 1923 anatomist Edgar Allen and biochemist Edward A. Doisy at the Washington University Medical School in St Louis developed an assay enabling the isolation and industrial production of oestrogen-active substances. Injections of ovarian extracts into spayed animals produced 'typical estrual hyperemia, growth, and hypersecretion in the genital tract and growth in the mammary glands'. These changes included a characteristic cornification in the vaginal walls. This observation constituted a test easily monitored in a living animal. The active agent of these alterations in rats and mice, a follicle hormone, appeared to be an efficient substitute for the endocrine function of the ovaries of a non-pregnant animal, which was, according to Allen and Doisy, 'sufficient to explain the mechanism of estrual phenomena in the genital tract in the absence of pregnancy' (Allen and Doisy 1923, 821). The bio-assay not only facilitated the isolation of hormones but also their dosage and representation in mice or rat units (Oudshoorn 1994, 42–8). Animal experiments to assess the optimal dosages of a functioning female body led to the molecularisation of menstruation and menopause (Gaudillière 2006, 151).

The isolation of sex hormones in 1929, achieved almost simultaneously by two groups, one centred around Doisy, the other with the German biochemist Adolf Butenandt, relied on an enormous amount of raw material, such as follicles or placenta, which could only be organised with the help of clinics and the pharmaceutical industry. In 1928, Selmar Aschheim and Bernhard Zondek simplified this problem significantly, demonstrating that chemically-treated urine from pregnant women and animals passed the Allen-Doisy test, and two years later, Zondek identified mare urine as a rich source of follicular hormone (Zondek 1928; Oudshoorn 1994, 73–9; Ratmoko 2010, 90–97). Oestrogens could then be produced in large amounts by pharmaceutical companies such as Organon in the Netherlands (*Menformon*), Schering in Germany (*Progynon*), or Ciba in Switzerland (*Ovocyclin*) (Ratmoko 2010; Gaudillière 2004a; Oudshoorn 1994). Sex hormones were both druglike and communicative substances; they could be industrially produced while also defining and explaining the modern body (Hawhee 2009, 80). In the 1930s, oestrogens were efficient agents able to cause cornification of the epithelial cells in ovariectomised rats; in contrast to other substances passing the Allen-Doisy test, they had a steroidal chemical structure. Oestrogens were regulators of female functions, could be industrially produced and activated for both clinical and bio-political treatment of sterility and supposed menstrual or menopausal disorders. Oestrogens were conceptualised as highly effective molecular substances, thereby creating a new ontology of the female body and producing a tool for the regulation and optimisation of female functions or even 'femininity' itself. Since then femininity has mostly been seen as an alterable state of estrogenic activity (Ratmoko 2010; Roberts 2007; Sengoopta 2006; Stoff 2004a, 435–69; Oudshoorn 1994).

In the 1930s, although testosterone and progesterone could already be synthesised, biochemists had not yet achieved the synthesis of oestrogens. According to Butenandt, the reason for this lay in the lack of methods for a partial dehydrogenation of the steran skeleton (Butenandt 1942, 11–12). In the years 1937 and 1938, Hans Herloff Inhoffen and Walter Hohlweg, both chemists with Schering, synthesised ethinylestradiol from oestradiol. But this oestrogen-active substance had severe side effects, making it useless for marketing and clinical activation. It took another 10 years until a lower-dosed ethinylestradiol could be sold as a drug for menopausal symptoms (Hohlweg and Inhoffen 1939, 78). The only alternative to oestrogens isolated from pregnant mare urine was the stilbene derivative diethylstilbestrol (DES), which Charles Dodds produced as an oestrogen-active compound in 1938. According to Viennese chemist Fritz von Wessely, DES resembled natural oestrogens in quality, but was even more effective when administered in equivalent quantities. Dodd's research had been funded by the British Medical Research Council; since it had not been patented, IG Farben was able to produce a rather cheap DES-remedy under the name *Cyren* in the summer of 1938. *Cyren* and *Progynon* were competing in a lucrative market for biologically-active substances in the late 1930s; the production of sex hormones was behind the prosperity of pharmaceutical companies like Schering, Organon or Ciba (Dodds, Goldberg, Lawson and Robinson 1938; Wessely 1940, 198–201; Gaudillière 2008). But a dark cloud overshadowed this commercial, therapeutic and epistemological success story of the cooperation of pharmaceutical industry, the medical clinic and biochemistry. The effectiveness of oestrogens to induce growth in an organism made them also suspect of generating toxic or even carcinogenic effects. While this concerned nearly all biologically-active substances, oestrogens posed a particular threat.

In 1915, the Japanese pathologists Katsusaburo Yamagiwa and Koichi Ichikawa induced skin cancer in rabbits by painting their ears with coal tar. A group working with Ernest L. Kennaway and James W. Cook blamed benzpyrene, a pure chemical compound present in coal tar, for the cancer-causing effects. Therefore, aromatic hydrocarbons in general were regarded as potentially carcinogenic substances in the 1920s. One of these aromatic hydrocarbons, methylcholanthrene, was related to steroids. It was even possible, as the leading chemists Heinrich Otto Wieland and Adolf Windaus demonstrated, independently of each other, to convert cholesterol and bile acid into methylcholanthrene. This finding raised the possibility that under certain circumstances steroids could also become carcinogenic. Because oestrogens were characterised by a partially aromatised hydrocarbon framework, these useful reproductive agents were suddenly the critical and non-therapeutic focus of cancer research (Butenandt 1940, 348; Deichmann 2001, 344). The assumption, that oestrogens were evidently dangerous because of their chemical structure, was a serious threat to biochemists, gynaecologists and pharmaceutical companies. In the late 1930s, these bio-political agents, tools for the optimisation of female reproductive functions, became precarious substances. The very moment they were standardised through bio-assay and chemical procedures, they were also established as autonomous agents of an individual structure, which acquired the ability to induce growth independent of the experimenter's will (Wahrig, Stoff, Schwerin and Balz 2008, 5, 10).

Adolf Butenandt, Germany's leading biochemist during the 1930s and director of the Kaiser-Wilhelm-Institute for Biochemistry in Berlin-Dahlem, who in close cooperation with Schering had isolated oestrone in 1929, was indeed shocked that Kennaway and Cook's thesis had gained the status of facticity in some scientific writings. At stake was an achievement of major importance for Butenandt's own career, gynaecological practice, the bio-political interests of the national socialist state, and finally and most of all, for Schering. In the summer of 1937, Butenandt, spurred to action by Schering, financed by the German Research Foundation and in cooperation with the gynaecologist Carl Kaufmann from the Charité in Berlin, organised a working group to address this suspicion. The story of this research project, which combined the interests of laboratory science, clinic and industry, has been written at length by the French historian of science Jean-Paul Gaudillière (Gaudillière 2006 and 2004b). Expectations were that oestrogens would be given the benefit of the doubt, but Butenandt, even though his success as a biochemist was based on cooperation with the pharmaceutical industry, saw himself as a respectable and autonomous scientist, who would never have produced unjustly favourable results. What Kaufmann and Butenandt did, was concentrate their research not on the chemical structure of oestrogens, but on the disposition of laboratory animals. Kaufmann, who in the 1930s had tested Schering's hormone products for optimal dosages and broader indications (he was an expert on the treatment of amenorrhoea, the lack of menstrual periods), administered oestrogens to three thousand mice. He concluded that even continuous administration would not increase the rate of tumours. Butenandt again referred back to experimental work carried out by Antoine Lacassagne, who in 1936 had injected male mice with follicle hormones, thereby inducing breast cancer. Sex steroids, Butenandt stated, affect genetic conditions which only exist in such mice breeds already demonstrating a high susceptibility to breast tumours (Butenandt 1940, 349). Oestrogens are therefore only the catalyst, not the cause of cancer; in the case of oestrogens the genetic precondition or intrinsic factor is the essential condition for cancer-causing hormonal effects. When Butenandt presented the results of the working group in June 1940, he summarised that oestrogens and DES could indeed induce breast cancer in genetically preconditioned mice, but that this had nothing to do with the specific chemical structure alone. Even if this report cleared oestrogens, Schering were not very pleased, as the statement gave *Cyren* the same innocent status as *Progynon*. Soon after this, however, both companies agreed that IG Farben would stop comparing its cheaper product to *Progynon*, while Schering would be quiet about the toxicity of *Cyren*. What remained from Butenandt and Kaufmann's animal experiments was the statement that oestrogen-active substances themselves – as steroids or as stilbene-derivatives – were not carcinogenic substances (Butenandt 1940, 349; Gaudillière 2008, 117).

Despite the fact that Kennaway and Cook's findings, as well as the results of Butenandt and Kaufmann's biological trials, were published in leading professional journals, there was no public debate. The actors involved in this story were merely male scientists like Butenandt, Kennaway and Cook, clinicians like Kaufmann and pharmaceutical companies like Schering and IG Farben. In the late 1930s, there was an ongoing discussion on the subject in professional journals, but as yet, no public debate (Druckrey 1940). The only physician to take up the accusation against oestrogens was Paul Gerhardt Seeger, who aroused the interest of Adolf Hitler himself, by claiming a cancer-causing stereoisomeric reversal of follicle hormones was provoked by the *wrong* femininity, pathology and mongrelisation (Seeger 1940; Proctor 1999, 317). But where were the persons concerned, where were the women? Why was there no outrage over this suspicion? While there were restrictions on dissent in Nazi Germany, as I will show in the next section, this was not the case for a campaign on butter yellow, another supposedly cancer-causing substance, which was mobilised by German housewives' organisations at the same time. Whereas oestrogens were bio-political agents controlled by male experts, the case of butter yellow was about food and therefore concerned female consumer interests. Even though there was a short period of medical consumerism in the 1920s in relation to oestrogens, women were patients dependent on expert opinions and bearing bio-political responsibility. The fast reaction of Germany's leading biochemist, Butenandt, had smothered any doubt over hormonal therapy in the cradle. But the silence of women and women's organisations can also be explained by the simple fact that the reproductive and bio-political issue was itself part of feminist discourse in the first decades of the twentieth century. While oestrogens, in a rather disburdening way, defined biological femininity, hormonal therapy held the promise of relieving women's physical and social pains. There was simply no interest in criticising this biomedical practice because sex hormones defined women as both sexual and reproductive beings, thereby connecting physiology with the prospect of liberation in a 'motherhood-eugenics consensus' (Grossmann 1995, 15). In the case of butter yellow, not only the same biochemical experts but also the women's organisations, reacted strongly against the azo dye, on the one hand because it was a neglectable substance and on the other because it concerned the holistic bias of life-reformist discourse.

Butter Yellow (1937–1941)

Critiques of modern food production had been common in all western nations since the last third of the nineteenth century. But while this criticism was largely focused on food fraud, in Germany, the highly influential interplay of diet reform and a new dietetics emphasised the need for a healthy diet based on nutritional value. This political discourse turned life reform into science and nutrition research into life reform (Melzer 2003, 101–42; Merta 2003, 119–28). A nutrition-political and civilisation-critical discourse distinguishing between natural purity and artificial contamination merged toxicology, pharmacology and cancer research. In 1931, Curt Lenzner published a book entitled *Gift in der Nahrung*, which can be literally translated as 'Poisoned Food'. According to Lenzner, diseases of civilisation, notably cancer, were based on plasmatic damnifications caused by a lack of vital substances and an overflow of chemicals hostile to life. The latter he identified with food additives such as bleaching agents, colourants and preservatives (Lenzner 1933, XI, 191, 193). One year later, Erwin Liek, the notorious enemy of the social and health security system of the Weimar Republic, proclaimed a connection between civilisation and cancer, actualised in chemicalised and technicalised food (Liek 1932; Kater 1990). Diet-reform advocates like Werner Kollath, the German guru of wholefood nutrition, denounced industrially-produced food as denaturalised and a danger to the fitness and vitality of the people. If denaturalisation caused cancer, the sole hope for the German people lay in a natural diet (Proctor 1999, 120–72; Fritzen 2006, 201–4; Heyll 2006, 201–28). This strong positioning of purity and a natural lifestyle gained even more strength with the empowerment of the National Socialists; the narrative of a holistic body threatened by foreign matter fitted well into Nazi ideology of a 'Volksgemeinschaft' endangered by elements foreign to the German race (Harrington 1999, 185–8). While there were inner contradictions and an open dispute between propagandists of pure food and advocates of strategically important 'ideal preservatives' during the war, Kollath's distinction between near-natural and non-natural, therefore 'dead', food was widely accepted (Kollath 1942, 14; Stoff 2013; Stoff 2012a, 253–79; Sperling 2011).

In this historical setting the case of butter yellow, an azo compound used to give butter an attractive yellow colour, caused tremendous public interest. Butter yellow had been synthesised by Peter Griess at the Royal College of Chemistry in London in the 1860s and had been used as a colourant in Germany since the 1870s. In the early 1930s, Tomizo Yoshida published experimental findings, suggesting that rats fed with scarlet red (o-Aminoazotoluol) developed bladder cancer and hepatic tumours. O-Aminoazotoluol was closely related to p-Dimethylaminoazobenzol, the chemical compound better known as butter yellow. Between 1932 and 1937, Japanese pathologist Riojun Kinosita proved that several azo dyes were carcinogenic. The German pharmacologist Hermann Druckrey confirmed these results (Kinosita 1940, 287–92; Brock, Druckrey and Hamperl 1940). In 1943, Richard Kuhn and Helmut Beinert stated that butter yellow was the most important representative amongst carcinogenic azo dyes. And one year later, Eugene L. Opie summarised that '(a)dministration of butter yellow produces multiple foci of focal hyperplasia, cystic ducts, and cholangiofibrosis, and corresponding with these lesions, which are precursors of tumour growth, multiple tumours are formed' (Kuhn and Beinert 1943, 904; Opie 1944, 244). As early as June 1939, the International Congress for Cancer Research had recommended the banning of butter yellow for colouring food. A few months later, Hans Reiter, president of the German Reich Health Office, had suggested a new German Colour Law. Robert Proctor, in his book on the history of cancer research in Nazi Germany, has outlined the complicated situation Reiter was in, as a sudden removal of colours during the war might have been interpreted as the application of inferior foodstuffs. On the other hand, however, there were already rumours circulating that coloured food was poisoning consumers. It was at this point that the women's organisations of Nazi Germany intervened, applying pressure to Reiter, and finally succeeded. As Proctor tells this story, in 1941 a member of Göttingen's 'NS-Frauenwerk' asked her superiors why cancer-causing substances were still allowed in butter and margarine. The regional women's leader informed Reiter that 'while women were certainly willing to sacrifice for the war, accepting the presence of cancer-causing agents in food was something else'. And indeed Reiter, who appreciated the housewives' organisation as allies in his efforts for wartime food security, rather successfully negotiated with the different groups producing and marketing coal tar dyes to reduce their use. Finally, even the almighty IG Farben ceased production of butter yellow (Proctor 1999, 165–70).

To sum this story up, it was a coalition of scientists, politicians and women's organisations who succeeded in bringing about the prohibition of butter yellow. Women's organisations, as has been shown in several studies, were deeply involved in Nazi Germany's health and nutrition policies; they were the core of the rising consumer movement and experts in their own right, as consumers and in their role as 'guardians of nature'. Housewives, far from being marginalised, were able to determine health policy decisions (Davis 1996). Papers on the pharmacology of cancer in the 1940s referred to two classes of carcinogenic compounds: azo dyes and aromatic hydrocarbons (Butenandt 1940). But until the late 1960s only the case of butter yellow generated legislative and scientific political action.

Butter Yellow (1948–1958)

In the 1950s and 1960s these two stories of silent and worried, of strengthened and endangered, of dependent and autonomous, of apolitical and political women convened. And it was again these two differing substances, a sex hormone and a food colourant, which catalysed the establishment of German feminism as a consumer movement. In the year 1948, Butenandt, the defender of oestrogens, did not hesitate before frightening the public by proclaiming that butter yellow, a proven carcinogenic substance, was still in use (Hartmann 1949, 247–8). Although this accusation was immediately denied by nutrition experts and representatives of the pharmaceutical industry, a debate was begun, which shaped food additive policies in Germany throughout the 1950s. Magazines and newspapers took up the story and just a few years after the end of the Nazi reign, dramatically asked if the Germans were now poisoned (Anonymous 1954). This narrative expressed itself in a new oncological theory introduced by the well-respected physician Karl-Heinrich Bauer, which downplayed the role of genetics while emphasising the significance of exogenous agents, such as rays or chemical compounds. Bauer based his assumption on the case of azo dyes, thereby reiterating the idea of a strong connection between civilisation and an apparent rise in cancer (Bauer 1950). According to Bauer's 'pharmacology of cancer causing substances' the rise in cancer was the result of a progressing chemicalisation and technicalisation of the environment and the development of external toxins, or 'Noxen' as Bauer called them (Bauer 1950, 33–4). These mere speculations gained scientific facticity through the collaboration of Druckrey, again, with the mathematician Karl Küpfmüller in 1948. Druckrey, a convinced Nazi who had to be whitewashed by Butenandt, himself a profiteer of Nazi science policy, after 1945, conducted animal tests with butter yellow; these experiments demonstrated that the production of tumours required a certain total dose, regardless of how this was distributed over 35 to 365 days. The latency period, Druckrey stated, was inversely related to the daily dose. If experiments were extended over the life span of the animals, a smaller dose was necessary to produce an effect: with increasing age, there was an increasing disposition to tumour development. Druckrey concluded that the carcinogenic effect of butter yellow was therefore, even at the smallest doses, irreversible from the beginning of the experiment during the entire life span of the animals, and was additive with further exposure without any modification, until, after a critical total dose has been exceeded, tumours would develop. Because of this latency period – the dose-effect and dose-time relation – it was practically impossible to decide whether a certain substance was carcinogenic or not. From this time on, it was chemical substances in everyday use that demonstrated the most risk (Druckrey and Küpfmüller 1948; Wunderlich 2005; Stoff 2012b).

Bauer, Druckrey and Butenandt were comrades in arms in the ongoing war against cancer. The field for this battle was the senate commission for food colourants of the German Research Foundation, in which, under the guidance of Butenandt and Druckrey, representatives of the pharmaceutical and foodstuff-producing industry, together with politicians, negotiated the use of food additives (Stoff 2009). During the early 1950s, German scientists even tried to establish this new theory of carcinogenesis as a European norm and install a preventive risk policy for food additives in the institutions EUROTOX and the Joint FAO/WHO Expert Committee on Food Additives (JECFA). In the late 1950s, however, the influence of Druckrey and Butenandt faded; the radical and life-reformist informed concept of risk prevention was replaced by a mere risk management, expressed in the concept of 'acceptable daily intake' (Jas 2013; Stoff 2012b).

While the commission worked behind closed doors, a public discourse about the 'toxic condition' of modern life and the negative role of the pharmaceutical and chemical industry gained strength. The catchphrase of a 'toxic total situation' ('toxische Gesamtsituation') coined by Fritz Eichholtz, director of the Pharmacological Institute at the University of Heidelberg, inspired a far-reaching debate on the boundaries of risk assessment and the dangers of chemical substances (Eichholtz 1956). At the same time, organised as well as independently acting women intervened, writing hundreds of letters to the ministries in charge. A certain Anneliese Conrad from Schöppenstedt in Lower Saxony, for example, demanded the Ministry of Food immediately ban food colouring. Cancer, she wrote, had so dramatically increased that it was the dictate of the moment to search for the reason for this German disease ('deutsche Volkskrankheit').[1] Marie Seeger, who identified herself as a housewife from Augsburg on a postcard she sent to the health committee in Bonn, pleaded with the committee to bring uncoloured and raw foodstuff to the consumer. It was an unscrupulous act without comparison to supply the population with poisoned food even in the smallest doses, she wrote. In the future, food should be identified as pure or impure. Whoever wanted coloured food should be able to obtain it, but she and her family did not want any of it.[2] There was also an open critique in which consumers were not represented, however, by the commissions for food additives established by the German Research Foundation during the 1950s. In Germany at this time no official consumers' association existed. It was up to the housewives' and women's organisations to resume their battle against poisoned food and the poisoning of the people. In February 1950, the German Women's Association ('Deutscher Frauenring') demanded measures be taken against the colouring of food. In a concerted action, Catholic and Protestant women's and housewives' organisations demanded that the ministries of health and of the interior prohibit food colouring with azo dyes. The Women's Information Service ('Informationsdienst für Frauenfragen'), which united 80 women's organisations and groups, applied to all relevant political representatives, requesting the passage of a new food law based on a white list of experimentally proven dangerous substances.[3] On 24 February 1956, members of parliament, Hedwig Jochmus (CDU), Käte Strobel (SPD), Marie-Elisabeth Lüders (FDP) and 43 other female delegates of the German Bundestag, presented an application that the Bundestag should request the Federal Government to produce a draft of a new food law. This proceeding was well prepared by Jochmus, Strobel and Werner Gabel, undersecretary in the Ministry of the Interior. The issue produced much laughter from male members of parliament, but the 'united front of female delegates' ('Einheitsfront der weiblichen Abgeordneten') provoked a strong response from the public and the media.[4] Indeed, the women's organisations succeeded in releasing a new and much stricter food law. An as yet unwritten history of German consumer organisations would have to address the role of women in the debate on 'poisoned food', while also explaining the masculinisation of the consumer movement in the 1960s. The politics of precarious substances, which

---

1   Conrad, A. (1952), Letter to Federal Department for Nutrition, 2 December, B 116/420. Koblenz: Bundesarchiv.

2   Seeger, M. (1958), Letter to Health Committee, Bonn, 24 April, B 142/1530. Koblenz: Bundesarchiv.

3   Deutscher Frauenring, Committee for National and Domestic Economy (1950), Letter to Federal Ministry of the Interior, Health Department, 14 February, B 116/419. Koblenz: Bundesarchiv.

4   German Bundestag (1956), 149th Meeting, Bonn, 8 June, B 142/15282, p. 7901. Koblenz: Bundesarchiv.

united women across party lines, emerged as a major topic in the feminist agenda during the second half of the twentieth century.

Oestrogens (1950–1970)

In the 1950s, Western European cancer research was concentrated on azo dyes. In the case of West Germany this meant an absolution for oestrogens. In 1940, when supporting the results of Butenandt and Kaufmann's experiments, Druckrey had officially proclaimed that follicle hormones were not 'real carcinogenic substances' like derivatives of benzanthracene (Druckrey 1940). This contrasted sharply with the debate in England happening at the same time. In 1950, Alexander Lipschütz, a veteran of hormone research, published a monograph under the title *Steroid Hormones and Tumors*. He emphasised the connection between organs controlled by hormones, such as the breast, uterus and prostate, which could be governed by hormonal therapy, and a vulnerability to tumours. Eric Stephen Horning from the London Royal Cancer Hospital took up this idea. Together with Hadley Kirkman from the Stanford University School of Medicine, he was able to experimentally produce renal tumour in hamsters through the use of oestrogens (Lipschütz 1950; Horning 1951; Kirkman 1957). During the 1940s and 1950s, there was a widespread belief, at least in the USA, that the intake of oestrogen-active substances such as DES could prevent miscarriages, therefore this was a highly controversial finding (Langston 2010, 48–60). Kirkman produced a long list of questions relating to the relationship between hormones and cancer:

> Which hormones are tumorigenic, which carcinogenic? Do these hormones act directly or indirectly in producing neoplastic change? Do carcinogenic or tumorigenic hormones act only on normal physiological target tissues? Do the neoplastic changes occur in normal or in injured cells? Most hormonally induced tumors are dependent, but upon serial transfer some of them become autonomous. What is the nature of this transition from dependency to autonomy, and does the transition occur abruptly as a single step or is it a gradual process involving several or many steps? (Kirkman 1957, 757)

In West Germany the outcomes of these new experiments were mostly rejected. A remarkable exception was Walter Büngeler, director of the institute for pathology at the University of Munich, who attempted to re-examine Kirkman's and Horning's findings, but encountered harsh reactions from his colleagues. In 1959, Herwig Hamperl even tried to prevent the funding of Büngeler's research by the German Research Foundation.[5]

---

5 Büngeler, W. (1959), Application. Experimentelle Untersuchungen über die Bedeutung hormoneller Faktoren bei der Geschwulstentstehung (Leberveränderungen), 2nd September, Bü 1/17. Bonn: Archive of the German Research Foundation (DFG).

In the mid 1960s, however, the debate surrounding potentially carcinogenic hormones also flared up in West Germany. It was the translation of the bestseller *Feminine Forever*, written by the gynaecologist Robert A. Wilson, which raised tempers in the German public and amongst German physicians. Wilson recommended hormonal replacement therapy with oestrogens for the treatment of menopausal symptoms (Roberts 2007, 120–28; Houck 2003; Watkins 2001; Wilson 1966). The main discussion point was whether menopause was a natural condition to which women should adapt, or a deficiency symptom to be taken care of by gynaecologists. 'Wilson wants to abolish menopause with oestrogens', read one of the many headlines in the German press. Menopause, lectured the gynaecologist, Josef Zander, when interrogated by Germany's leading news magazine, *Der Spiegel*, is a deficiency disease based on a lack of oestrogens. The only question for Zander was whether acute or prophylactic measures should be taken. He opted for long-term treatment with oestrogens because, according to him, these highly potent substances had exceptional medicinal benefits (Müller and Petermann 1966, 149). The gynaecologist, Gerhard F. Winter, distanced himself from those he called conservative physicians, who regarded menopause as a simple physiological state and therefore not requiring any kind of therapy. Instead, he associated himself with a group of modern American physicians, 'who demand hormonal substitution in every situation and maintain this substitution until old age' (Winter 1967). But Wilson's book also caused a heated debate on the dangers of hormone replacement therapy. *Der Spiegel* even referred to a 'hormone-war' ('Hormon-Krieg'). In the weekly *Die Zeit*, Georg Schreiber listed a whole compendium of dangerous side effects associated with hormone replacement therapy (Schreiber 1966). The drug commission of the German Medical Association also published a joint statement (Anonymous 1966). Even though some physicians warned that, quite apart from heavy side effects, such a use of oestrogens could induce uterine and breast cancer, barely any experts mentioned the experiments conducted in the 1930s. The gynaecologists, Gisela Dallenbach-Hellweg and Frederick D. Dallenbach, were the exception, reminding their colleagues that 60 years earlier, oestrogens had already been accused of causing tumours in mice (Dallenbach-Hellweg and Dallenbach 1971). By contrast, Butenandt's verdict that a genetic proclivity was necessary for hormonally induced breast cancer was alive and well in the 1960s. Zander was, after all, a disciple of Butenandt.

Due to the authoritative statements made by German gynaecologists, the 1966 hormone-war had been long forgotten when, during the Whitsun holidays in 1969, another gigantic headline in the tabloid *Bild* frightened the West-German public: 'Shock for women! Lump in the breast due to birth control pill!' ('Schock für Frauen! Knoten in der Brust durch Anti-Baby-Pillen') (Köhler 1969). Animal testing had shown that a new oral contraceptive called *Neonovum* could induce breast cancer. Until this unexpected scandal the dangers of the contraceptive pill had mostly been discussed in relation to thrombosis (Marks 2001, 138–57). But there had already been warning voices in the early 1960s. In 1964, Hamburg gynaecologist Oskar Guhr had reported that the pill might induce uterine cancer.

Given his statement had been based on only 80 cases, Gregory Pincus examined a thousand women who took the pill and, according to his enthusiastic statement, appeared to be completely healthy. The journalist, Thomas von Randow, reminded *Die Zeit* readers of the sad case of Thalidomide some years previously: 'Even the fact that the pill is taken by millions of women cannot comfort us until Guhr's outrageous suspicion is refuted' (Randow 1964). Generally throughout the 1960s, the contraceptive pill had appeared to be much more of an ethical than a health problem (Ignaciuk, Ortiz-Gómez and Rodríguez-Ocaña, this volume; Thoms, this volume). But in 1969, an immediate and intensive debate began on the methods of steroid toxicology and the interpretation of experiments. This focused on the selection of laboratory animals, as research on Neonovum had been based on experiments with Beagles prone to breast cancer (Anonymous 1970, 198). In accordance with the Druckrey-Küpfmüller equation, the latency period between exposure and clinical manifestation called for long-term studies with a huge amount of investigations. But even such long-term studies were barely convincing. In 1973 the statistician, Karl Überla, realised that an increase in the risk of breast carcinoma following oestrogen treatment could not be claimed with sufficient certainty. With resignation, however, he added that this did not sufficiently invalidate the suspicion (Plotz et al. 1973, 371). The controversy on carcinogenic substances was not settled by knowledge, facts, or nature itself (Latour 1987, 96–100).

The story of the contraceptive pill, which has been written in great detail, is complicated because there were – in dramatic contrast to the 1940s debate on oestrogens – so many actors: self-proclaimed progressive scientists such as Carl Djerassi; neo-malthusianists and population politicians; conservative, pro-natalist and bio-political physicians; a new media hunting for headlines and fanning the fear of breast cancer; the famous papal encyclical; and last but not least, a far from homogenous women's movement (Marks 2001; Silies 2010). It was probably astonishing for actors like Djerassi that the women's movement, which had been associated with sexual reform and sexual emancipation since the 1920s, turned into a consumer movement during the 1960s, valuing bodily integrity higher than sexual fulfilment (Duden 2008, 595–6; Marks 2001). On one hand, sexual reform was consumerist itself, sexuality being a 'consumer choice' (Birken 1988). On the other, the German consumer movement was deeply influenced by the life-reform discourse of a holistic body endangered by poisons, as expressed in the fight against butter yellow and for a new food law in the 1950s. The 1970s West German debate on potentially cancer-causing oestrogens followed this argument against poisoned food and was led by the trope of a toxic total situation, which led the German environmental movement.

In the late 1970s, the modern utopia of liberated sexuality was questioned in various ways. This new feminist topic, claiming that the alleged sex wave only benefited men, while women had to bear the risk of a chemicalised body, echoed Michel Foucault's famous dictum that 'the irony of this deployment (of sexuality, H.S.) is in having us believe that our "liberation" is in the balance' (Foucault 1976, 159). For those advocating sexual consumerism, suspicion of cancer was the argument of a conservative-feminist conspiracy. In 1973, two projects studied the role of the 'subjective side-effects' of oral contraceptives, as social psychological factors and religious moral values (Frick, Kessler and Pferdmenges 1973; Blättler, Blättler and Hauser 1973). These factors seemed to explain the critical position towards the contraceptive pill so many women adopted in the early 1970s. For supporters and beneficiaries of sexual liberation, like *Der Spiegel*, the papal encyclical of 1968 was the same type of propaganda against the contraceptive pill as exaggerated medical objections (Anonymous 1968, 85). Contemporary journalists, like social scientists, were unable to trace the new feminist position towards oestrogens back to the case of butter yellow, the identity of women's and consumer movements, and the trope of poisoning.

Thirty years after the silent acceptance of expert opinion on oestrogens, these precarious substances became a political issue. In 1970, female members of parliament, Hedda Heuser (FDP) and Käte Strobel (SPD), who had already played a major role in the amendment of German food law, again organised a non-party inquiry regarding the dangers of the contraceptive pill. Feminists, overcoming the former, hierarchical separation of experts and patients, not only utilised the expertise of those scientists who proved the dangers of oestrogen-active substances, they also referred to the experiences of women, their unease and discontent with the pill. As part of a consumer movement, the feminist critique of the pill was raised against elitist negotiations of risks, which neglected or redefined women's interests. The controversy surrounding the pill, as Barbara Duden has summarised, accelerated the transformation of women from immature patients to self-determined consumers. The gendered promise of autonomy, youth, beauty and health merged with an optimised life designed by experts, self-care and steroids (Duden 2008; Stoff 2004b, 238). While today the quarrel about oestrogens as potentially cancer-causing substances remains unresolved, the female body is both a contested side of consumerism, activated for consumption and defended in the name of consumer rights, and a residuum of purity and holism. In Germany, the narrative of the poisoning of the female body started around 1940 with butter yellow, influenced the German consumer movement in the 1950s, and finally affected the feminist movement in the 1970s.

The German women's movement as a consumer movement inherited the life-reform discourse and critique of civilisation from the 1940s. It gained its political strength through the battle against butter yellow and its short lived victory in the instalment of a new food law in 1958 (which in the following years was diluted by much laxer resolutions). Feminists in the 1970s took up the holistic discourse and rhetoric of the women's movement while also questioning sexual liberalism and male expert definitions of the female body. The history of the German feminist movement does not have to be rewritten, but following the actions of and quarrels about molecules can help reveal motives and discourses which would otherwise remain invisible.

References

Allen, E. and Doisy, E. A. (1923), 'An Ovarian Hormone. Preliminary Report on its Localization, Extraction and Partial Purification, and Action in Test Animals', *Journal of the American Medical Association* 81, 819–21.

Anonymous (1954), 'Werden wir vergiftet? Gebleichte, gefärbte, konservierte, 'geschönte' Lebensmittel' *Die Zeit*, 17 June. Available at: http://www.zeit. de/1954/24/werden-wir-vergiftet [accessed 23 March 2012].

———— (1966), 'Was Brunst erzeugt' *Der Spiegel* 20:11, 137–9.

———— (1968), 'Last und Lust', *Der Spiegel* 22:32, 82–90.

———— (1970), 'Bilanz: Nach wie vor zu Gunsten der Pille', *Der Spiegel* 24:12, 197–202.

Bauer, K.-H. (1950), 'Über Chemie und Krebs – dargestellt am Anilinkrebs', *Langenbecks Archiv für Klinische Chirurgie* 264, 21–44.

Birken, L. (1988), *Consuming Desire: Sexual Science and the Emergence of a Culture of Abundance, 1871–1914* (Ithaca and London: Cornell University Press).

Blättler, I., Blättler, W. and Hauser, G.A. (1973), 'Einfluß der Massenmedien auf Nebenwirkungen der Ovulationshemmer', *Archiv für Gynäkologie* 214, 254–5.

Brock, N., Druckrey, H. and Hamperl, H. (1940), 'Die Erzeugung von Leberkrebs durch den Farbstoff 4-Dimethylamino-azobenzol', *Zeitschrift für Krebsforschung* 50, 431–56.

Butenandt, A. (1940), 'Neuere Beiträge der biologischen Chemie zum Krebsproblem', *Angewandte Chemie* 53, 345–52.

———— (1942), 'Entwicklungslinien in der künstlichen Darstellung natürlicher Steroidhormone', *Die Naturwissenschaften* 30, 4–17.

Dallenbach-Hellweg, G. and Dallenbach, F.D. (1971), 'Besteht ein morphologisch faßbarer Zusammenhang zwischen Oestrogen und Carcinogenese?', *Archiv für Gynäkologie* 211, 198–200.

Davis, B. (1996), 'Food scarcity and the empowerment of the female consumer in World War I Berlin' in de Grazia, V. (ed.) *The Sex of Things: Gender and Consumption in Historical Perspective* (Berkeley: University of California Press) pp. 287–310.

Deichmann, U. (2001), *Flüchten, Mitmachen, Vergessen. Chemiker und Biochemiker in der NS-Zeit* (Weinheim: Wiley-VCH).

Dodds, E. C., Goldberg, L., Lawson, W. and Robinson, R. (1938), 'Estrogenic Activity of Certain Synthetic Compounds', *Nature* 141, 247–8.

Doisy, E. A., Rolls, J. 0., Allen, E. and Johnston, C. G. (1924), 'The extraction and some properties of an ovarian hormone', *Journal of Bioligical Chemistry* 61, 711–27.

Druckrey, H. (1940), 'Über oestrogene und cancerogene Wirkung', *Zeitschrift für Krebsforschung* 50, 27–9.

Druckrey, H. and Küpfmüller, K. (1948), 'Quantitative Analyse der Krebsentstehung', *Zeitschrift für Naturforschung* 3b, 254–66.

Duden, B. (2008), 'Frauen-,Körper: Erfahrung und Diskurs (1970–2004)' in Becker, R. and Kortendiek, B. (eds) *Handbuch Frauen- und Geschlechterforschung: Theorie, Methoden, Empirie. 2., erweiterte und aktualisierte Auflage* (Wiesbaden: VS-Verlag) pp. 593–607.

Eichholtz, F. (1956), *Die toxische Gesamtsituation auf dem Gebiet der menschlichen Ernährung: Umrisse einer unbekannten Wissenschaft* (Berlin, Göttingen and Heidelberg: Springer).

Foucault, M. (1976), *The History of Sexuality. Vol. 1: The Will to Knowledge* (London: Penguin).

Frick, V., Kessler, S. and Pferdmenges, J. (1973), 'Psychologische Aspekte der Nebenwirkungen oraler Kontraceptiva', *Archiv für Gynäkologie* 214, 252–3.

Fritzen, F. (2006), *Gesünder leben: Die Lebensreformbewegung im 20. Jahrhundert* (Stuttgart: Steiner).

Gaudillière, J.-P. (2004a), 'Genesis and Development of a Biomedical Object: Styles of Thought, Styles of Work and the History of the Sex Steroids', *Studies in History and Philosophy of Biological and Biomedical Sciences* 35, 525–43.

——— (2004b), 'Biochemie und Industrie. Der "Arbeitskreis Butenandt–Schering" während der Zeit des Nationalsozialismus' in Schieder, W. and Trunk, A. (eds) *Adolf Butenandt und die Kaiser–Wilhelm–Gesellschaft. Wissennschaft, Industrie und Politik im Dritten Reich* (Göttingen: Wallstein) pp. 198–246.

——— (2006), 'Hormones at Risk. Cancer and the Medical Uses of Industrially-Produced Sex Steroids in Germany, 1930–1960' in Schlich, T. and Tröhler, U. (eds) *The Risks of Medical Innovation. Risk Perception and Assessment in Historical Context* (London and New York: Routledge) pp. 148–69.

——— (2008), 'Professional or Industrial Order? Patents, Biological Drugs, and Pharmaceutical Capitalism in Early Twentieth Century Germany', *History and Technology* 24, 107–33.

Grossmann, A. (1995), *Reforming Sex: The German Movement for Birth Control and Abortion Reform, 1920–1950* (New York and Oxford: Oxford University Press).

Harrington, A. (1999), *Reenchanted Science: Holism in German Culture from Wilhelm II to Hitler* (Princeton: Princeton University Press).

Hartmann, F. (1949), '55. Tagung der Deutschen Gesellschaft für innere Medizin', *Die Naturwissenschaften* 36, 245–9.

Hawhee, D. (2009), *Moving Bodies: Kenneth Burke at the Edges of Language* (Columbia: University of South Carolina Press).

Heyll, U. (2006), *Wasser, Fasten, Luft und Licht: Die Geschichte der Naturheilkunde in Deutschland* (Frankfurt/Main: Campus).

Hohlweg, W. and Inhoffen, H. H. (1939), 'Pregneninolon. Ein neues per os wirksames Corpus luteum-Hormonpräparat', *Die Naturwissenschaften* 18, 77–9.

Horning, E. S. (1951), 'Hormones and Carcinogenesis', *British Medical Journal* 2, 834–5.

Houck, J. A. (2003), 'What Do These Women Want?: Feminist Responses to *Feminine Forever,* 1963–1980', *Bulletin of the History of Medicine* 77, 103–32.

Jas, N. (2013), 'Adapting to "Reality": The Emergence of an International Expertise on Food Additives and Contaminants in the 1950s and early 1960s' in Boudia, S. and Jas, N. (eds.) *Toxicants, Health and Regulation since 1945* (London: Pickering & Chatto) 2013, 47-69.

Kater, M. H. (1990), 'Die Medizin im nationalsozialistischen Deutschland und Erwin Liek', *Geschichte und Gesellschaft* 16, 440–63.

Kinosita, R. (1940), 'Studies on the cancerogenic azo and related compounds', *Yale Journal of Biology and Medicine* 12, 287–300.

Kirkman, H. (1957), 'Steroid Tumorigenesis', *Cancer* 10, 757–64.

Köhler, O. (1969), 'Pfingst-Verkehrs-Stille', *Der Spiegel* 23:23, 179.

Kollath, W. (1942), 'Natürliche Nahrung, wissenschaftliche Ernährungslehre und ihre Synthese' *Die Ernährung* 7, 7–14.

Kuhn, R. and Beinert, H. (1943), 'Über das aus krebserregenden Azofarbstoffen entstehende Fermentgift', *Berichte der deutschen chemischen Gesellschaft* 76, 904–9.

Langston, N. (2010), *Toxic Bodies: Hormone Disruptors and the Legacy of DES* (Yale: Yale University Press).

Latour, B. (1987), *Science in Action. How to follow scientists and engineers through society* (Cambridge, MA: Harvard University Press).

Lenzner, C. (1933), *Gift in der Nahrung. Zweite umgearbeitete und erweiterte Auflage* (Leipzig: Verlag der Dykschen Buchhandlung).

Liek, E. (1932), *Krebsverbreitung, Krebsbekämpfung, Krebsverhütung* (München: Lehmanns).

Lipschütz, A. (1950), *Steroid Hormones and Tumors. Tumirogenic and antitumirogenic actions of steroid hormones and the steroid homeostasis: experimental aspects* (Baltimore: Williams & Wilkins).

Marks, L. V. (2001), *Sexual Chemistry. A History of the Contraceptive Pill* (New Haven and London: Yale University Press).

Melzer, J. M. (2003), *Vollwerternährung. Diätetik, Naturheilkunde, Nationalsozialismus, sozialer Anspruch* (Stuttgart: Steiner).

Merta, S. (2003), *Wege und Irrwege zum modernen Schlankheitskult. Diätkost und Körperkultur als Suche nach neuen Lebensstilformen 1880–1930* (Stuttgart: Steiner).

Müller, R. S. and Petermann, J. (1966), 'Östrogen für alle Frauen?', *Der Spiegel* 20:11, 140–49.

Opie, E. L. (1944), 'The Pathogenesis of Tumors of the Liver Produced by Butter Yellow', *The Journal of Experimental Medicine* 80, 231–46.

Oudshoorn, N. (1994), *Beyond the Natural Body. An Archaeology of Sex Hormones* (London and New York: Routledge).

Plotz, E. J. et al. (1973), 'Nebenwirkungen oraler Kontrazeptiva: eine Kritik der Prüfungsmethoden', *Archiv für Gynäkologie* 214, 367–73.

Proctor, R. N. (1999), *The Nazi War on Cancer* (Princeton: Princeton University Press).

Randow, T. V. (1964), 'Statt Baby Angst vor Krebs? Fatales Sensationsgeschrei um einen umstrittenen Befund', *Die Zeit* 30 October. Available at: http://www.zeit.de/1964/44/Statt-Baby-Angst-vor-Krebs [accessed 21 February 2012.]

Ratmoko, C. (2010), *Damit die Chemie stimmt. Die Anfänge der industriellen Herstellung von weiblichen und männlichen Sexualhormonen 1914–1938* (Zürich: Chronos).

Roberts, C. (2007), *Messengers of Sex: Hormones, Biomedicine and Feminism* (Cambridge: Cambridge University Press).

Schreiber, G. (1966), 'Doktor Wilsons Allheilmittel. Ärzte verschreiben, was die Illustrierte den Frauen suggeriert', *Die Zeit* 11 February. Available at: http://www.zeit.de/1966/07/Doktor–Wilsons–Allheilmittel [accessed 21 February 2012].

Seeger, P.G. (1940), 'Über die Beziehung des Follikelhormons zur Ätiologie maligner Tumoren und seine Bedeutung für die Krebsgenese', *Klinische Wochenschrift* 19, 107–12.

Sengoopta, C. (2000), 'The Modern Ovary. Constructions, Meanings, Uses', *History of Science* 38, 425–88.

———— (2006), *The Most Secret Quintessence of Life. Sex, Glands, and Hormones, 1850–1950* (Chicago and London: Chicago University Press).

Silies, E.-M. (2010), *Liebe, Lust und Last. Die Pille als weibliche Generationserfahrung in der Bundesrepublik 1960–1980* (Göttingen: Wallstein).

Sperling, F. (2011), *"Kampf dem Verderb mit allen Mitteln?" Der Umgang mit ernährungsbezogenen Gesundheitsrisiken im Dritten Reich am Beispiel der chemischen Lebensmittelkonservierung* (Stuttgart: Deutscher-Apotheker-Verlag).

Starling, E. H. (1905), 'The Croonian Lectures on the Chemical Correlations of the Body', *Lancet* 2, 339–41.

Stoff, H. (2004a), *Ewige Jugend. Konzepte der Verjüngung vom späten 19. Jahrhundert bis ins Dritte Reich* (Köln and Weimar: Böhlau).

———— (2004b), 'Janine. Tagebuch einer Verjüngten. Weibliche Konsumkörper zu Beginn des 20. Jahrhunderts' in Bruns, C. and Walter, T. (eds) *Von Lust und Schmerz. Eine Historische Anthropologie der Sexualität* (Köln and Weimar: Böhlau) pp. 217–38.

———— (2009), 'Hexa-Sabbat. Fremdstoffe und Vitalstoffe, Experten und der kritische Verbraucher in der BRD der 1950er und 1960er Jahre' *N.T.M.* 17, 55–83.

———— (2012a), *Wirkstoffe. Eine Wissenschaftsgeschichte der Hormone, Vitamine und Enzyme, 1920–1970* (Stuttgart: Steiner).

———— (2012b), 'Summationsgifte. Zum Evidenzproblem einer Pharmakologie krebserregender Substanzen in den 1950er Jahren' in Moser, G., Kuhn, J. and Stöckel S. (eds) *Die statistische Transformation der Erfahrung. Beiträge zur Geschichte des Evidenzdenkens in der Medizin* (Freiburg: Centaurus) pp. 33–62.

——— (2013), 'Vital Regulators of Efficiency. The German Concept of "Wirkstoffe", 1900-1950' in Schwerin, A., Stoff, H. and Wahrig B. (eds.) *Biologics. A History of Agents Made From Living Organisms in the 20th Century* (London: Pickering & Chatto) 89–104.

Wahrig, B., Stoff, H., Schwerin, A. v. and Balz, V. (2008), 'Precarious Matters. An Introduction' in Balz, V., Schwerin, A. v., Stoff, H. and Wahrig, B. (eds) *Precarious Matters /Prekäre Stoffe. The History of Dangerous and Endangered Substances in the Nineteenth and Twentieth Centuries* (Berlin: MPIWG) pp. 5–14.

Watkins, E. S. (2001), 'Dispensing with Aging: Changing Rationales for Long-term Hormone Replacement Therapy, 1960–2000', *Pharmacy in History* 43, 23–37.

Wessely, F. v. (1940), 'Über synthetische Östrogene', *Angewandte Chemie* 53, 197–202.

Wilson, R. A. (1966), *Feminine Forever* (New York: Evans & Co).

Winter, G. F. (1967), 'Natürliche konjugierte Östrogene im Klimakterium', *Zentralblatt für Gynäkologie* 89, 296–300.

Wunderlich, V. (2005), 'Zur Entstehungsgeschichte der Druckrey–Küpfmüller–Schriften (1948–1949): Dosis und Wirkung bei krebserzeugenden Stoffen', *Medizinhistorisches Journal* 40, 369–97.

Zondek, B. (1928), 'Darstellung des weiblichen Sexualhormons aus dem Harn, insbesondere dem Harn von Schwangeren', *Klinische Wochenschrift* 7, 485–6.

Chapter 2

Rising from Failure: Testing Drugs and Changing Conceptions for Female Sexual Dysfunction[1]

Marta I. González García

The approval by the US Food and Drug Administration of sildenafil citrate (Viagra) as an oral therapy for the treatment of erectile dysfunction (ED) in 1998, and its striking success, triggered renewed interest in both male and female sexual dysfunction. In particular, and under the common assumption since Masters and Johnson's well known model of the Human Sexual Response Cycle that female and male sexualities are essentially the same, researchers have tried to establish the effects of Viagra (and other drugs) on sexual response in women. Assessing the efficacy of sex drugs in women, however, has been far more challenging than was expected. As a consequence of the methodological and conceptual difficulties encountered in this research program, intended to find a magic pill that would solve women's sexual problems, researchers have therefore turned their attention towards the specificities of female sexuality. While male sexual problems are assumed to be both simple and simply diagnosed and repaired, female sexuality appears to be more complex, and intermixed with social and psychological factors. Nevertheless, this assumed complexity does not rule out research on drug therapies for female sexual problems, nor does it overcome commonplace, entrenched ideas on the nature of women and men, their bodies and their minds.

Recent research on female sexual dysfunction has addressed relevant questions in the fields of science studies and recent feminist analyses of corporality. On the one hand, it represents one of the most notorious examples of the 'extension of medical jurisdiction over health itself' (Clarke et al. 2003, 162; Fishman 2004) that characterises the biomedicalisation process. In this respect, interest in redefining female sexual dysfunction has been criticised as a case of 'disease mongering' (Moynihan 2003; Tiefer 2006), a strategy of pharmaceutical companies to 'sell sickness' in order to promote drug sales (Payer 1992). While the literature on disease mongering uncovers and denounces the often suspect practices of the pharmaceutical industry, designed to broaden their markets, it leaves central questions relating to how bodies act and are enacted in the origins of new diseases

---

1   This contribution has been possible thanks to financial support provided by the Spanish National R&D&I Plan (MICINN-12-FFI2011-24582).

unanswered (Law and Mol 2008). Thus, I will present the coproduction of diseases, drugs and patients that occur in the process of the search for a female Viagra as an appropriate locus for exploring these issues. I will employ various approaches from within science studies that have described scientific practice as the interplay between heterogeneous elements, both human and non-human, that are at the same time producers and produced (see, for instance, Pickering 1995; Pickering and Guzik 2008; Malafouris and Knappet 2008). The 'dance of agency' in the search for the pink Viagra also raises gender issues at the core of contemporary feminist debates on the body, with conceptions about sameness or difference between women and men at stake. Therefore, to address these issues, and to complement attempts by Celia Roberts (2007), Barbara Marshall (2009) and Anne Fausto-Sterling (2000) to recover the materiality of the body in feminist analyses, women's bodies will appear here, not as passive recipients of drug companies' attempts to sell more drugs, but as active agents in the production of sexes and genders.

Based on scientific literature, FDA reports, documents and transcriptions of the Advisory Committee for Reproductive Health Drugs meetings, and current discussions concerning revisions proposed by the DSM-5 Sexual and Gender Identity Disorders Work Group, this contribution will focus on drug companies' attempts to find a product for women that would mirror the success of Viagra for men. In this search for a pharmacological fix to women's sexual problems, both the definition of female sexual dysfunction (FSD) and the success criteria of the proposed drugs are continuously being modified, in order to address the difficulties and failures encountered in the processes of drug testing: difficulties that arise from the resistance of women's bodies to the 'Viagra model'. In each successive attempt and failure, diagnosis categories and success criteria are being shaped and reshaped in an attempt to match the drug's effects.

Changes in the identification of the organic root of women's sexual problems, from a vascular problem to a hormonal one, and from hormones to neurotransmitters, following the promises of different drugs, point to the persistence of a pharmaceutical logic and its influence on the conceptualisation of disorders.[2] As a result, certain commonplace beliefs are revisited: sex is in the mind, and female sexuality is more emotional, while male sexuality is more genital-based. These revised stereotypes are reinforced in the complex interactions of bodies and drugs, women, researchers, clinicians and pharmaceutical companies.

---

2 Barbara Marshall (2009) has described the working of what she calls the 'pharmaceutical imagination' in the narratives of sexual problems in the post-Viagra era. The 'pharmaceutical imagination' assumes an organic basis for every sexual dysfunction and anticipates pharmaceutical solutions for them. However, sexual dysfunctions are not preexisting entities; they are produced as 'therapeutic targets' in the same processes as their medical treatments.

Rising from Failure I: We Have the Drug ... What's the Problem?

Immediately following the approval of Viagra, female sexual dysfunction began to receive increasing attention through epidemiological, clinical and basic research studies. It is not surprising that researchers and companies attempted to take advantage of Viagra's success and increase the number of potential users even more. After all, if the sexual response of women and men is basically the same, why wouldn't women benefit from the treatment of their sexual problems with Viagra?

FSD classification systems are typically based upon the Human Sexual Response Cycle model proposed by Masters and Johnson (1966). Their 'cycle' presents the development of the sexual act in four universal and non-sex specific steps: arousal, plateau, orgasm and resolution. Helen Kaplan (1977) later introduced 'desire' as the first step of the process.[3] Minor differences were conceded. Women might move through the steps more slowly or present variations in their orgasmic response (orgasm might be multiple or not present at all), but the overall message was clear: women and men are essentially the same in terms of their sexual functioning. The division of sexual activity into autonomous stages enabled the identification of dysfunctions within each step and facilitated the search for specific therapeutic solutions, even though, in practice, different disorders frequently coexist.

Studies into the prevalence of sexual dysfunctions, however, have revealed a sex disparity. According to a study by Laumann et al. published in 1999 in the *Journal of the American Medical Association* and widely cited in both academic literature and the popular media, 43 per cent of American women experience some kind of sexual problem, while the prevalence among American men is 31 per cent. This does indeed represent a large market for the expansion of any therapy intended to treat female sexual dysfunction and was systematically referred to as a reason to promote research on FSD and its treatment (see, for instance, Basson et al. 2000, Basson et al. 2004).

Without losing any time, an international multidisciplinary consensus development conference, sponsored by pharmaceutical companies, to redefine FSD and adapt it to the new times was convened in Boston in 1998.[4] The four

---

3 Actually, Lief (1977) and Kaplan (1977) simultaneously introduced 'desire' as the first step of the cycle.

4 Consensus conferences are organised around controversial topics in medicine. They bring together different kinds of experts in a particular field to assess and discuss the available information and reach an agreement on scientific evidence and best practices. In the US, The National Institutes of Health Consensus Development Program has been organising conferences since 1977 without accepting funding from non-government entities in order to avoid any potential influence. However, drug companies also sponsor meetings aimed at producing expert consensus and guidelines for clinical practice (Healey 2006). The 1998 conference on FSD was funded by eight drug companies, and 18 of the 19 authors of the consensus statement disclosed financial relationships with 22 different companies (Irvine 2005, 245).

major categories of dysfunction described in the DSM-IV-TR (Diagnostic and Statistical Manual of Mental Disorders) and the ICD-10 (the World Health Organization International Classification of Diseases) – disorders of desire, of arousal, of orgasm, and pain disorders – were maintained, although minor changes were made to their definitions (American Psychiatric Association 2000; World Health Organization 1992). Masters and Johnson's model thus continued to provide a good basis for diagnosis.

As Viagra had been shown to work wonders on problems of male sexual arousal, assessed directly through penile erection, work on FSD began to focus on performance outcome measures such as genital vasocongestion and vaginal lubrication. However, researchers were puzzled by the difficulty of measuring arousal in women. Not only is the female sexual response hard to quantify objectively, it is also difficult to perceive by women themselves: several studies found an important discordance between arousal measured by technical devices and women's subjective experience of arousal (Shields and Hrometz 2006). Despite these problems, in order to achieve the same therapeutic success as in the treatment of ED, sexual arousal disorder in women had to be defined in the same terms: those of measurable vasculogenic activity. Thus, 'vaginal engorgement and clitoral erectile insufficient syndromes' made their appearance as the female equivalent of 'erectile dysfunction' for men, and the target of clinical trials with Viagra for women (Goldstein and Berman 1998). In this case, as Barbara Marshall has suggested, the already existing cure appeared to define the disorder (Marshall 2002, 142). Sildenafil produced a confusing ambivalence: it improved physiological measures of genital engorgement, but had no significant effect on the psychological perception of arousal. It was therefore difficult to assess the drug's success. As the initial clinical trials of vasoactive drugs for the treatment of FSD had been disappointing, Pfizer did not even submit Viagra for approval by the FDA for its use by women.

This failure coincided with the revision of the diagnostic categories based on Masters and Johnson's model and the reassessment of the question regarding the sameness and difference of female and male sexualities. Masters and Johnson's egalitarian model, as reflected in the DSM-IV-TR and the ICD-10 classificatory systems, was now in crisis. Although the Boston consensus conference, organised by the American Foundation for Urological Disease (AFUD) in order to redefine FSD promptly after the approval of Viagra in 1998, maintained, in general terms, a classification system with a classical structure based on the steps of Masters and Johnson's cycle (Basson et al. 2000), the Second International Consultation on Sexual Medicine held in Paris in 2003 introduced noticeable modifications addressing the mismatches found in clinical trials of Viagra for women (Basson et al. 2004).[5] The arousal disorder in women, well defined in men as 'erectile dysfunction', was now divided into a 'subjective sexual arousal disorder' and

---

5   See, in general, Hatzimouratidis and Hatzichristou (2007), and Meston and Bradford (2007). A Third International Consultation was held in Paris in 2009.

a 'genital sexual arousal disorder', adding the possibility of the diagnosis of a combined genital and subjective arousal disorder.

The 'pharmaceutical imagination' promotes the search for the right drug for each disease (Marshall 2009). In this case, however, the challenge was to find the right disease for the existing drug. There was a pharmacological solution, Viagra, for which a physiological basis of women's sexual problems was needed. However, confronted with the resistance of women's bodies to the simplicity of Viagra's effects, efforts were instead focused on redefining classification systems and the search for a successful match between a magic drug and its corresponding disease in other, more promising steps of the sexual response cycle.

Rising from Failure II: From Arousal to Desire

The failure to expand the market of Viagra prompted exploration of other areas of FSD more amenable to medical treatment. After all, the difference in the prevalence of sexual dysfunction between men and women was not only quantitative: women appeared to complain more often of sexual problems, and studies have also identified sex differences in the most common kinds of dysfunction (Laumann et al. 1999). While men tend to suffer with problems of arousal or orgasm, the most common sexual dysfunction for women lies in the first step of the cycle: lack of desire. The focus of research therefore shifted to hypoactive sexual desire disorder (HSSD).

This focus on women's desire was associated with the testing of hormonal therapies. Recent discussions on the proposal of a new disorder, 'female androgen insufficiency', reveal the attempt to couple problems of desire with a hormonal deficit. The new promise of a 'female Viagra', however, resulted in additional problems related to the definition of dysfunctions and the success criteria for drug tests.

The 'female androgen insufficiency' syndrome first appeared in 2002, a result of the interdisciplinary consensus conference held in Princeton in 2001, designed to assess 'the evidence for and against androgen insufficiency as a cause of sexual and other health-related problems in women and of making recommendations regarding definition, diagnosis, and assessment of androgen deficiency states in women' (Bachmann et al. 2002). The Princeton Consensus statement defined the syndrome as 'a pattern of clinical symptoms in the presence of decreased bioavailable T and normal estrogen status'. Among these symptoms, and featuring as one of the most notorious, was 'impaired sexual function', characterised by low libido, decreased sexual receptivity and pleasure (Bachmann et al. 2002).

Along with the category of 'female androgen insufficiency', participants proposed recommendations for laboratory tests, a diagnosis algorithm, and some directions for future research. They acknowledged the scarce attention devoted to the role of androgens in women, and the difficulties of their measurement: there are no reliable laboratory tests for androgen levels in women, which are lower than male levels. Moreover, it is not clear what the appropriate measure would be for a 'normal' level: whether it should be total testosterone, free testosterone, or bioavailable testosterone, and so on. Due to the scant amount of epidemiological and clinical data, the low reliability of available tests, and the absence of data on normal levels of androgens in women, experts proposed a 'pragmatic' definition of the syndrome, mostly based on unspecific clinical symptoms, such as fatigue, dysphoric mood, reduced libido, bone loss or poor memory. As these symptoms are common to other diseases and are affected by a good number of variables, the diagnosis also requires taking into account estrogen and testosterone levels.[6]

The new syndrome was presented with caveats, as proponents were aware of the myriad problems it posed. Apart from those factors already mentioned, androgen levels may vary in relation to age, race or reproductive cycle phase. The unspecificity of the symptoms makes differential diagnosis with other disorders such as stress, thyroid or metabolic diseases or, simply, difficulties in the relationship, complex. To make things worse, androgen therapy has potential risks that are not well known. The consensus statement thus created a new disorder, though with a good number of reservations, and the consequent recommendation of more research in order to clarify these doubts.

The emergence of the 'female androgen insufficiency syndrome' generated considerable debate in professional circles. Its main weakness is that no evidence of a relationship between testosterone levels and sexual desire in women exists; testosterone levels do not correlate with measures of sexual functioning or desire. In this scenario, although the controversy embraced all the aforementioned uncertainties in the definition of the syndrome, the most controversial issues were those related to androgen treatment. The new syndrome only appeared to make sense if androgen therapy was accepted. The North American Menopause Society (NAMS) (Shifren et al. 2005) and the Endocrine Society (Wierman et al. 2007) in particular, engaged in a harsh dispute over the syndrome and testosterone therapy. The NAMS, while acknowledging the problems of definition and diagnosis, defended the validity of the new syndrome, arguing that testosterone did in fact relieve symptoms. The Endocrine Society, however, did not recommend the diagnosis, due to the potential risks of long-term treatment.

In this debate, what was initially presented as a controversy surrounding a new diagnosis category turned into a controversy regarding hormonal therapies for the treatment of female sexual dysfunction. Once again, the 'pharmaceutical imagination' underlies the search for the right disease-drug dyad. However, as it is not possible to diagnose androgen insufficiency in women on the basis of hormonal levels, would the fact that testosterone therapy improves women's desire constitute a reason to support the new syndrome? Insofar as testosterone therapy

---

6 Estrogen levels must be normal and free T concentration should be at or below the lowest 25th percentile of the normal range for premenopausal women (Bachmann et al. 2002).

works, it would do so not as a replacement, but as a pharmacological therapy. But, does it really work?

In 2004, two years after the first appearance of the female androgen insufficiency syndrome, Procter & Gamble presented a new product to the FDA for approval: a testosterone patch under the commercial name of Intrinsa. Intrinsa was developed for a specific subset of women: those who become menopausal through the surgical removal of their ovaries and who were also on estrogen therapy, although it was immediately made clear in the marketing campaign that the intended number of users was much larger (Tsao 2004).

Intrinsa underwent FDA evaluation with clinical trials demonstrating that women who before treatment had, on average, a baseline of three satisfying sexual encounters in a four-week period, had five such episodes in a four-week period after using Intrinsa patches for six months.[7] Women who used placebo patches had, on average, four episodes in a four week period at the end of the study. The FDA Advisory Committee concluded that, although statistically meaningful, the improvements registered in patients using the testosterone patches were not clinically meaningful. Moreover, the Committee also pointed out that any possible risks, such as breast cancer or cardiovascular problems (Schover 2008), resulting from the long-term combined use of testosterone and estrogen could not be revealed by surveys conducted in the short term. The cautious resolution of the FDA contrasts with the approval of Intrinsa by the European Medicines Agency in 2006.[8]

There are no simple answers to the question 'Does Intrinsa work?' It is not even possible to assert that it has succeeded in Europe and failed in the United States. Enthusiasm is lacking in the European context and there are a growing number of critical voices opposing its prescription (Iheanacho 2009). We find a very different

---

7 'Satisfactory sexual events' were taken as the primary 'efficacy endpoint' of the clinical trials following the guidelines issued by the FDA in 2000 for the development of drugs for the treatment of female sexual dysfunction. To assess the efficacy of treatments for problems of desire in terms of 'satisfactory sexual events' is problematic. According to the FDA guideline, a 'satisfactory sexual event' may include: satisfactory sexual intercourse, sexual intercourse resulting in orgasm, oral sex resulting in orgasm, and partner initiated or self-masturbation resulting in orgasm (FDA 2000). These criteria have been criticised because of the emphasis on numbers, the high subjectivity of the concept of 'satisfaction' and the influence of context in the frequency of sexual events (Althof et al. 2005).

8 The rejection of Instrinsa by the FDA occurred immediately after the results of the Women's Health Initiative on hormonal therapy for menopausal women were released. The Women's Health Initiative was established in 1991 by the US National Institutes of Health to address the most common causes of death, disability and impaired quality of life in postmenopausal women. Results on replacement hormonal therapy, published in 2002 (Writing Group 2002), shed serious doubts on a treatment that had become commonplace in the 1990s. Although risks were identified in relation to estrogen and progestin therapies, these findings may have had an influence on the FDA's decision. Occurring during the same years, the Vioxx scandal may also have influenced this rejection.

picture on the other side of the Atlantic. After the rejection of Intrinsa, publications discussing and opposing the FDA decision flourished. There was an urgent need, it was argued, for an approved drug to treat female sexual dysfunction. After all, women were already using testosterone to solve their sexual problems: different testosterone products, approved for androgen deficiency in men or used in transsexual treatments, were being prescribed to women (Seibel 2005).

Despite the complications and complexities, hormonal therapy still remains a strong candidate to treat female sexual dysfunction. New drugs are being tested, such as Libigel (a gel formulation of testosterone), which has not yet been submitted for approval to the FDA by BioSante. However, other paths are also being explored, in which women's desire has returned from the bodily flow of hormones to the mind.

Rising from Failure III: Flibanserin ... Sex is in the Brain

With hormonal therapies under discussion and clinical practice that often resorts to drugs approved for other disorders, new research on the pharmacological cure for female sexual dysfunction and, specifically, for problems of desire has focused on central action drugs (Brown, Blagg and Reynolds 2007). Some data, such as the relevance of the placebo effect found in all the clinical trials, together with the fact that subjective arousal in women may be differentiated from genital arousal, have prompted this strategy (Brown, Blagg and Reynolds 2007; Nappi et al. 2010). For women, sex may be in the brain. This new turn, however, has encountered its own difficulties, and in June 2010, the Advisory Committee for Reproductive Health Drugs of the FDA voted against the approval of Flibanserin for the treatment of hypoactive sexual desire disorder in women.

As in the case of Viagra, a failed heart drug, serendipity had turned Flibanserin, a poor antidepressant, into the next candidate to be women's Viagra. Boehringer Ingelheim, the German manufacturer company, originally studied Flibanserin for the treatment of depression in both women and men. The drug failed to demonstrate efficacy for depression, but in phase II trials little sexual dysfunction was noted. For that reason, subsequent studies included the Arizona Sexual Experiences Scale (ASEX) for comparison of Flibanserin with an approved antidepressant and a placebo in improving the sex drive of subjects. The company hence decided on a change in identity for Flibanserin, from antidepressant to the new promise for solving women's sexual problems.

Desire disorders in women, it was now argued, were caused by neurotransmitter abnormalities in the brain (FDA 2010a). Flibanserin increases the levels of dopamine and noradrenalin while controlling those of serotonin, which is believed to act as a sexual satiety signal. However, the drug's actual mechanism of action in the treatment of hypoactive sexual desire disorder (HSDD), according to the documentation provided for the meeting of the Reproductive Health Drugs Advisory Committee of the FDA, was 'unknown' (FDA 2010b).

In this case, 'hypoactive sexual desire disorder' was maintained as defined in the DSM-IV-TR, as 'the persistent or recurrent deficiency or absence of sexual thoughts, fantasies, and/or desire for sexual activity, which causes marked distress or interpersonal difficulty'. HSDD is a kind of disorder that does not point to a single cause in the sense that 'female androgen insufficiency syndrome' did. It was therefore possible to translate female sexual problems from hormones (where Intrinsa could not have the expected success) to the brain, with the promise of a new medical treatment whose mechanism of action was not well known. Flibanserin made its way into the headlines and reignited the debate on female sexual dysfunction.

The evidence supporting the efficacy of Flibanserin treatment for problems of desire in women presented by Boehringer Ingelheim was based on clinical trials with premenopausal women, both in North America and Europe, designed to test the efficacy and long-term safety of the therapy. Flibanserin was submitted to the FDA for approval with the claim that clinical trials demonstrated an increase in sexually satisfying events, an increase in desire and a decrease in distress related to problems of desire. However, the Committee voted ten to one that the drug was not significantly better than a placebo in the treatment of HSDD. They also voted unanimously that the benefits did not outweigh potential adverse effects (FDA 2010c).

Once again, the rise and fall of Flibanserin illustrates the problematic definition of desire disorders in women and the consequent difficulties in assessing the efficacy of any proposed treatment. The combination of these obstacles with concerns surrounding side effects led to its rejection. As in the case of the Intrinsa trials, the rise in the number of 'satisfactory sexual events' was taken as the primary 'efficacy endpoint', following the guideline issued by the FDA in 2000. Apart from the intrinsic difficulties of defining a 'satisfactory sexual event', it is not clear that changes in their number have a direct relation to changes in desire. Thus, the quantitative indicator has to be complemented with measurements of sexual desire and distress as co-primary and secondary endpoints. In the case of Flibanserin, an electronic diary (eDiary), in which women registered sexual activity and their perception of sexual desire on a daily basis, was agreed on by the company and the FDA as an instrument of measurement.

Conclusions from the three main trials presented by the applicant were once more open to interpretation. While Flibanserin was associated with statistically significant improvements in the number of satisfactory sexual events, it did not significantly improve desire compared to a placebo, as shown by eDiary entries. The company, arguing that women did not adequately comply with the daily requirement of the eDiary, then attempted to introduce a different measurement of desire, the Female Sexual Function Index (FSFI), a validated scale administered at clinic visits, thus assuring 100 per cent compliance. As the use of the FSFI was not agreed on beforehand with the FDA, the Commission decided the applicant had failed to demonstrate the drug's efficacy.

Concern about safety also contributed heavily to the rejection of Flibanserin. More Flibanserin-treated subjects discontinued the trials prematurely than those on placebo due to adverse events, with dizziness, nausea, insomnia, anxiety, fatigue and somnolence being the most common side effects. An increased frequency of depression, syncope and accidental injury was also recorded. Moreover, Flibanserin interacted with a high number of drugs, making it a bad candidate for use in the general population. Together with the ambiguous evidence regarding its efficacy, the safety assessment inclined the Commission towards rejection.

The FDA applied rigorous standards of safety both in the case of Intrinsa and Flibanserin, prompted by underlying doubts regarding the diagnosis of HSSD, its causes, and the adequacy of medical treatment. These doubts were also raised in the meeting of the Advisory Committee, where sociologist Thea Cacchioni and sexologist Leonor Tiefer argued against the diagnosis and its pharmacological fix. The question posed by Tiefer reflects this approach: 'But how did this application for a brain-changing drug that was going to be prescribed for women to take daily to treat something vague, variable and unmeasurable called hypoactive sexual desire disorder, even get this far?' (FDA 2010b). For Tiefer, and the 'New View Campaign of Women's Sexual Problems' she leads (Tiefer 2001), Flibanserin represented a 'spurious, profit-driven effort to treat an ill-defined nonmedical disorder with a new, poorly understood medication'. Other voices, namely those of women who spoke at the hearing in the name of a silent majority of sufferers, defending the reality of the disorder and the need for a medical cure, did not succeed in their goal.

However, the Committee did adopt a cautionary stance, recognising HSDD as a real condition and encouraging the search for treatment. Thus, the rejection of Flibanserin did not seem to be such a hard blow to the wide array of actors committed to female sexual dysfunction and its medical solution. As a result, however, answers to questions such as what is desire, when is it 'normal', how can it be measured, what are the causes of its decrease, and how should it be treated, have become ever more elusive following each new pharmaceutical promise of a pink Viagra.

Side Effects of the Endless Search for the Female Viagra

The female sexual dysfunction market still represents a challenge to pharmaceutical companies: there is no clear definition of disorders, or of success criteria or endpoints for clinical trials. Moreover, the placebo effect makes it difficult to prove the efficacy of treatments statistically, and regulatory bodies such as the FDA carefully monitor safety issues related to women's health, rigorously applying the precautionary principle.

However, the unending search for the pink Viagra has left its mark on the definition of female sexual problems. Actually, it would be more accurate to say that the main consequence of the endless search for a fine tuning between drugs and disorders has not been a magic pharmacological fix, but rather the redefinition of models of sexual response and diagnostic categories of sexual dysfunction in women.

Each successive failure, from Viagra to Flibanserin, has highlighted the problems inherent in the definition of disorders, and in establishing criteria for the success of clinical trials. What was simple in the case of men poses continuous problems when applied to women. Women's sexual problems appear to be more elusive and difficult to understand and treat than men's. The list of sexual disorders for women, developed on the basis of the Masters and Johnson sexual response cycle in meetings and consensus conferences sponsored by the pharmaceutical industry (problems with desire, arousal and orgasm, and pain), does not work well. There are no unambiguous biological measures to slot women into one category or another, and women's descriptions of arousal and desire often overlap. Many women report several complaints. Moreover, although the drugs tested so far have some identifiable effects (Viagra affects genital measures of blood flow, Intrinsa and Flibanserin raise the frequency of 'satisfactory sexual events'), it is difficult to discriminate their effect from that of the placebo and they do not improve sexual distress and desire in a consistent, clear-cut manner.

These difficulties have led scientists to revise the universal model of human sexual response. After decades of approaching sexual behaviour in terms of sameness, new models are now being proposed for female sexual response. At the same time, the classification of female sex disorders is being accordingly modified.

Rosemary Basson (2002)[9] has revised Masters and Johnson's model under the assumption that women are definitely different. Basson's alternative model of the female sexual response cycle – intimacy-based, as she names it – is circular rather than lineal and begins with evidence that 'desire', the first stage in Masters and Johnson's cycle, means very different things to women and men. The presence of sexual thoughts, fantasies and an innate urge to experience sexual tension and release, alone or with a partner, have been considered the markers of desire. However, according to Basson, this is how it works for men. Women, only sometimes, mainly at the beginning of a relationship, engage in sex to satisfy a truly 'sexual' need. In general, they have other reasons for being sexually active or receptive: to feel emotionally close to their partner, to show love and affection, to share physical pleasure, to increase a sense of attractiveness or commitment, or simply to relax. A woman frequently begins a sexual experience 'sexually neutral' and, for 'intimacy-based' reasons, deliberately finds or receives sexual stimuli that could potentially move her to a state of sexual arousal. In this model, it is arousal that triggers desire and the need to seek release of sexual tension (orgasm is no longer the endpoint of the sexual cycle). As the reasons are intimacy-based, so are the goals.

---

9   Rosemary Basson is a Canadian-based researcher funded by Pfizer, Lily, Procter & Gamble and other pharmaceutical companies in the search for a medical fix of women's sexual problems.

Basson's model accounts for the difficulties experienced by women in distinguishing between desire and arousal, and the common lack of both. At the same time, it supports the review of female sexual disorders classification proposed by the Sexual and Gender Identity Disorders Work Group of the APA (American Psychiatric Association) for the DSM-V, released in 2013.

The diagnostic and practical consequences of revising the meaning of women's desire was addressed in proposals at the Second International Consultation on Sexual Medicine held in Paris in 2003. A suggestion was made that the narrowly defined 'hypoactive sexual desire disorder' of the DSM-IV-TR be replaced by 'Women's Sexual Interest/Desire Disorder'. Although the distressing absence of sexual thoughts and fantasies remains a criteria of the new diagnostic category, the main markers were the lack of motivations (in the sense of reasons or incentives) to become sexually aroused and the lack of responsive desire. Thus, it is assumed that women need 'reasons' to engage in sex, and female desire is now understood as a reaction to external stimuli (Basson et al. 2004).

The APA Workgroup took one step further towards a broader definition by getting rid of the problematic desire and subsuming interest and arousal under the same diagnostic category: 'Female sexual interest/arousal disorder.'[10] The label 'hypoactive desire' was definitively rejected in order to avoid the connotation of a deficit of testosterone or a deficiency of activity. Desire has now completely disappeared, acknowledging the difficulties of its definition and normalising the lack of sexual fantasies and biological urges in women. 'Desire' is replaced by 'interest', and the common empirical finding of an overlap between interest and arousal in women justifies their combination under the same heading. In the case of male disorders, however, the traditional labels of 'hypoactive sexual desire disorder' and 'erectile disorder' remain the same. The rationale for this new disorder also aims to recognise the multifactorial nature of sexual dysfunctions, with the introduction of a number of 'specifiers' relating to partner, relationship, cultural, medical or individual vulnerability factors.

Criticism of Masters and Johnson's model of the sexual response cycle, however, does not mean that alternative models, such as Basson's (2002), are more empirically adequate to account for female sexuality. From the scarce empirical studies available, only one conclusion is possible: there is no 'universal' model of female sexual response (Sand and Fisher 2007; Brotto 2010).

Although Basson's model takes emotional factors into account in female sexual response, it was not welcomed by feminist sex therapists. Sexologist Leonor Tiefer (2001) and her 'The New View Campaign' group have criticised the classificatory systems based on Masters and Johnson's model. Even in the context of Basson's circular and 'intimacy based' version, sex problems such as lack of desire are still defined as medical problems. Tiefer proposes a radically different way of categorising sexual dysfunctions that addresses causes rather than the distance from an idealised universal model of sexual behaviour. She distinguishes

---

10   More information can be found at http://www.dsm5.org/.

four categories of sexual problems: (1) problems resulting from socio-cultural, political or economic factors; (2) problems relating to partner or relationship; (3) problems resulting from psychological factors; and (4) problems resulting from medical factors (Tiefer 2010).

The proposal of The New View group takes the multidimensional nature of sexual problems seriously. However, even though Tiefer's system has many advantages over both Masters and Johnson's and Basson's models, and there is some empirical evidence suggesting drug therapy may not be the best way to treat most women's sex problems,[11] the DSM-V Workgroup did not consider such a radical transformation in the classification of dysfunctions. The reform of the DSM confronted the challenge of reflecting the results of a decade of efforts in the search for the female Viagra, within a professional context committed to the continuity of traditional categories.

The rupture with Masters and Johnson prompted a debate about the differences between female and male sexuality and the convenience of a parallel revision of male disorders. Actually, the changes suggested for female dysfunctions reflect the intense research that has taken place in recent years in failed attempts to find the female Viagra. Paradoxically, Viagra's success in the treatment of erectile dysfunction did not foster a comparable amount of research into male sexuality. Hence, there is no reason to reject the category of 'erectile disorder' as a kind of problem clearly separated from those of desire: Viagra is not open to appeal. However, some work, although limited, is already being done on the diversity of desire and the overlap between desire and arousal in men. The question of the sameness or difference of men and women's sexuality has only partial, contextual answers.

Discussion

When Viagra hit the market, pharmacological logic began to look for similar disease-drug dyads for the treatment of female sexual dysfunction. However, the idea of a simple medical remedy for a single disorder encountered the resistance of women's bodies again and again. Viagra failed because of difficulties in achieving a clear operational definition of female arousal; difficulties that seemed to imply that genital and subjective arousal were different entities in women. Viagra's failure changed the focus of research to desire problems and testosterone therapy, but hormones turned out not to be the appropriate messengers of sex (Roberts 2007) researchers and companies were seeking. The problems encountered with the

---

11   Nicholls (2008, cited by Brotto 2010) provides an empirical test in which Tiefer's classification system is confronted with women's accounts of their sexual problems. 98 per cent of the sexual difficulties described by women could be classified according to the New View scheme, most of them (65 per cent) in the category of problems relating to partner or relationship, and only 7 per cent in the category of medical problems.

'female androgen insufficiency syndrome' clearly illustrate the shortcomings of the pharmaceutical imagination. Sex may be, after all, in women's brain, although the Flibanserin trials yet again revealed the problems involved in defining desire and measuring the success of the drugs being tested. Consequently, each new attempt and failure to find the female Viagra has had profound consequences on the conceptualisation of female sexual response and female sexual dysfunction.

Models and classificatory systems are modified in efforts to accommodate the resistance of women's bodies to medicalisation, in a complex play whose actors are researchers, physicians, drug companies, hormones, neurotransmitters, gels, patches and pills, regulatory bodies, professional societies, feminists and, of course, women themselves. However, the fine tuning among these heterogeneous elements,[12] the successful coupling of a drug and a disease, has remained elusive.

New models and classificatory systems have resulted in a growing distance between an unquestionable male sexuality and a mysterious female sexuality that hinders every attempt to enroll it in pharmaceutical logic. As the distance grows, stereotypes about an essentially emotional female sexuality and a basically genital male sexuality become naturalised.

The new requirement of different models of sexual response for men and for women and, consequently, of different ways of classifying their dysfunctions, far from revealing the true nature of sex differences, is merely a consequence of the processes of trying to extend the market of sex drugs to women. The classification of dysfunctions becomes dichotomised as a result of an approach that divides humans into two separate categories and does not allow for any difference apart from that which sorts women from men. Diversity is therefore limited to only two modes of sexual behaviour. While Viagra turned male sexual response into a homogenous black box, female sexual response resists black-boxing attempts, demonstrating the contextual nature of sex and desire. However, the problems encountered in the search for the female Viagra were not enough to overcome the basic model of desire-arousal-orgasm in the revisions proposed by the medical community for the classification of female sexual dysfunctions. Rather, efforts are devoted to avoiding the dissolution of the female sexual response cycle by proposing complex subdivisions that attempt to account for the difficulties encountered without giving up the old schemes.

The question regarding differences between male and female sexual response does not have a single answer. The feminist insight that sex is not a natural, but rather a social and cultural act (Tiefer 1995) seems to be confirmed with each new female Viagra that has been endorsed and failed. There is no biologically-determined sexual response. At the same time, however, women's bodies are the locus of resistance and the promoters of changes in models and disorders. It is women's biology that has led to industry-funded researchers now considering how to include the 'other factors' (emotional, social, economic, cultural, and partner-related) in their models and classificatory systems of disorders.

---

12   The dialectic of 'accommodation and resistance' (Pickering 1995).

In consensus conferences and working groups, models and disorders are produced discursively: experts define sexual response cycles, the taxonomy of sexual problems, the endpoints of clinical trials, the boundary between what is normal and what is pathological, between desire and arousal, androgen sufficiency and insufficiency, between men and women, their sameness and difference. Women's bodies are also constituted and redefined through these discursive practices, and through cultural practices that impose demanding criteria on sexual performance in the post-Viagra era. However, discursive practices are not the only relevant ones. In laboratories, clinics, in each sexual act, the discursive production of bodies meets their materiality, and struggles to articulate the rebel corporality of women with the limitations imposed by a pharmacological framework.

Women's bodies and their physiological reactions are active agents in the constitution of the 'sexual response', in addition to being located in complex biosocial systems. The material body resisting biomedicalisation is a cultural and situated body. Failures in the search for a pharmacological fix for female sexual dysfunction have already resulted in researchers paying increasing attention to the agency of women and their situated bodies: acknowledging that models of sexual response lack an appropriate empirical basis, and promoting research that attends to women's voices on their own experiences of sex and desire (see for example Brotto et al. 2009). However, would a framework guided by the 'pharmacological imagination' be able to listen to and integrate these voices?

References

Althof, S. E. et al. (2005), 'Current perspectives on the clinical assessment and diagnosis of female sexual dysfunction and clinical studies of potential therapies: a statement of concern', *Journal of Sexual Medicine* Supplement 3, 146–53.

American Psychiatric Association (2000), *DSM-IV-TR: Diagnostic and Statistical Manual for Mental Disorders*, 4th Edition (Arlington: APA).

Bachmann, G. et al. (2002), 'Female androgen insufficiency: the Princeton consensus statement on definition, classification, and assessment', *Fertility and Sterility* 77:4, 660–65.

Basson, R. (2002), 'Rethinking low sexual desire in women', *BJOG: An International Journal of Obstetrics and Gynaecology* 109, 357–63.

Basson, R. et al. (2004), 'Revised definitions of women's sexual dysfunction', *Journal of Sexual Medicine* 1:1, 40–48.

Basson, R. et al. (2000), 'Report of the international consensus development conference on female sexual dysfunction: definitions and classifications', *The Journal of Urology* 163, 888–93.

Braunstein, G. D. (2007), 'The Endocrine Society Clinical Practice Guideline and The North American Menopause Society Position Statement on androgen therapy in women: another one of Yogi's forks', *Journal of Clinical Endocrinology and Metabolism* 92:11, 4091–3.

Brotto, L. A. (2010), 'The DSM diagnostic criteria for hypoactive sexual desire disorder in women', *Archives of Sexual Behavior* 39:2, 221–39.

Brotto, L. A. et al. (2009), 'Narratives of desire in mid-age women with and without arousal difficulties', *Journal of Sex Research* 46:5, 387–98.

Brown, A. D., Blagg, J. and Reynolds, D. S. (2007), 'Designing drugs for the treatment of female sexual dysfunction', *Drugs Discovery Today* 12, 17–18, 757–66.

Clarke, A. et al. (2003), 'Biomedicalization: technoscientific transformations of health, illness, and U.S. biomedicine', *American Sociological Review* 68:2, 161–94.

Fausto-Sterling, A. (2000), *Sexing the Body. Gender politics and the construction of sexuality* (New York: Basic Books).

FDA (2000), *2000 Draft Guidance for Industry Female Sexual Dysfunction: Clinical Development of Drug Products for Treatment*. Available at http://www.fda.gov/ScienceResearch/SpecialTopics/WomensHealthResearch/ucm133202.htm [accessed 1 November 2011].

———— (2010a), Background document for meeting of the Advisory Committee for Reproductive Health Drugs (June 18, 2010). NDA 22-526. Flibanserin (Proposed trade name: Girosa). Boehringer Ingelheim. http://www.fda.gov/downloads/AdvisoryCommittees/CommitteesMeetingMaterials/Drugs/ReproductiveHealthDrugsAdvisoryCommittee/UCM215437.pdf, accessed 7 November 2011.

———— (2010b), Transcript for the June 18, 2010 Meeting of the Advisory Committee for Reproductive Health Drugs. Available at http://www.fda.gov/downloads/AdvisoryCommittees/CommitteesMeetingMaterials/Drugs/ReproductiveHealthDrugsAdvisoryCommittee/UCM248753.pdf [accessed 7 November 2011].

———— (2010c), Minutes for the June 18, 2010 Meeting of the Advisory Committee for Reproductive Health Drugs. Available at http://www.fda.gov/AdvisoryCommittees/CommitteesMeetingMaterials/Drugs/ReproductiveHealthDrugsAdvisoryCommittee/ucm210869.htm [accessed 7 November 2011].

Fishman, J. R. (2004), 'Manufacturing desire: the commodification of female sexual dysfunction', *Social Studies of Science* 34:2, 187–218.

Goldstein, I. and Berman, J. R. (1998), 'Vasculogenic female sexual dysfunction: vaginal engorgement and clitoral erectile insufficiency syndromes', *International Journal of Impotence Research* 10: Suppl. 2, S84–90.

Hatzimouratidis, K. and Hatzichristou, D. (2007), 'Sexual dysfunctions: classifications and definitions', *Journal of Sexual Medicine* 4:1, 241–50.

Healey, D. (2006), 'Manufacturing consensus', *Culture, Medicine and Psychiatry* 30, 135–56.

Iheanacho, I. (2009), 'Testosterone patches for female sexual dysfunction', *Drug and Therapeutics Bulletin* 47, 30–34.

Irvine, J. (2005), *Disorders of Desire: Sexuality and Gender in Modern American Sexology*, 2nd Edition (Philadelphia: Temple University Press).

Jutel, A. (2010), 'Framing disease: the example of female hypoactive sexual desire disorder', *Social Science and Medicine* 70:7, 1084–90.

Kaplan, H. S. (1977), 'Hypoactive sexual desire', *Journal of Sex and Marital Therapy* 3, 3–9.

———— (1979), *Disorders of Sexual Desire* (New York: Brunner/Mazel).

Laumann, E. O. et al. (1999), 'Sexual dysfunction in the United States: prevalence and predictors', *Journal of the American Medical Association* 281, 537–44.

Law, J. and Mol, A. (2008), 'The actor-enacted: Cumbrian sheep in 2001' in Malafouris, L. and Knapett, C. (eds) pp. 55–77.

Lief, H. I. (1977), 'Inhibited sexual desire', *Medical Aspects of Human Sexuality* 7, 94–5.

Malafouris, L. and Knappett, C. (eds) (2008), *Material Agency: Towards a Non-Anthropocentric Approach* (New York: Springer).

Marshall, B. L. (2002), '"Hard Science": gendered constructions of sexual dysfunction in the "Viagra age"', *Sexualities* 5:2, 131–58.

———— (2009), 'Sexual Medicine, Sexual Bodies and the "Pharmaceutical Imagination"', *Science as Culture* 18:2, 133–49.

Masters, E. H. and Johnson, V. (1966), *Human Sexual Response* (Boston: Little Brown & Co).

Meston, C. M. and Bradford, A. (2007), 'Sexual dysfunctions in women', *Annual Review of Clinical Psychology* 3, 233–56.

Moss, P. and Teghtosoonian, K. (eds) (2008), *Contesting Illness. Processes and Practice* (Toronto: University of Toronto Press).

Moynihan, R. (2003), 'The making of a disease: female sexual dysfunction', *British Medical Journal* 326, 45–7.

Nappi, R. E. et al. (2010), 'Management of hypoactive sexual desire disorder in women: current and emerging therapies', *International Journal of Women's Health* 2, 167–75.

Nicholls, L. (2008), 'Putting the New View classification scheme to an empirical test', *Feminism and Psychology* 18, 515–26.

Payer, L. (1992), *Disease-Mongers: How Doctors, Drug Companies, and Insurers Are Making You Feel Sick* (New York: John Wiley).

Pickering, A. (1995), *The Mangle of Practice* (Chicago: Chicago University Press).

Pickering, A. and Guzik, K. (eds) (2008), *The Mangle in Practice. Science, Society and Becoming* (Durham: Duke University Press).

Potts, A. (2008), 'The Female Sexual Dysfunction Debate: Different "Problems", New Drugs – More Pressures?', in Moss and Teghtosoonian (eds).

Roberts, C. (2007), *Messengers of Sex: Hormones, Biomedicine and Feminism* (Cambridge: Cambridge University Press).

Sand, M. and Fisher, W. A. (2007), 'Women's endorsement of models of female sexual response: The nurses' sexuality study', *Journal of Sexual Medicine* 4, 708–19.

Schover, L. R. (2008), 'Androgen therapy for loss of desire in women: is the benefit worth the breast cancer risk?', *Fertility and Sterility* 90, 129–40.

Seibel, M. M. (2005), 'Men, Women, and testosterone: Why did the FDA fail Intrinsa?', *Sexuality, Reproduction and Menopause* 3:1, 1–2.

Shields, K. M. and Hrometz, S. L. (2006), 'Use of sildenafil for female sexual dysfunction', *Annals of Pharmacotherapy* 40:5, 931–4.

Shifren, J. L. et al. (2005), 'The role of testosterone therapy in postmenopausal women: position statement of the North American Menopause Society', *Menopause* 12, 497–13.

Snabes, M. C. and Simes, S. M. (2010), 'Approved hormonal treatments for HSDD: an unmet medical need', *Journal of Sexual Medicine* 6:7, 1846–9.

Tiefer, L. (1995), *Sex is not a Natural Act and Other Essays* (Boulder: Westview).

——— (2001), 'A new view of women's sexual problems: Why new? Why now?', *Journal of Sex Research* 38: 1–23.

——— (2006), 'Female sexual dysfunction: a case study of disease mongering and activist resistance', *PLoS Medicine* 3:4, e178.

——— (2010), 'Beyond the medical model of women's sexual problems: A campaign to resist the promotion of "female sexual dysfunction"', *Sexual and Relationship Therapy* 25:2, 197–205.

Traish, A. M. et al. (2007), 'Are the Endocrine Society's Clinical Practice Guidelines on androgen therapy in women misguided? A commentary', *International Society for Sexual Medicine* 4, 1223–35.

Tsao, A. (2004), 'Can Intrinsa be Viagra for Women?' *Businessweek,* (published online 28 October 2004) http://www.businessweek.com/bwdaily/dnflash/oct2004/nf20041028_8091_db016.htm [accessed 23 March 2012].

Wierman, M. E. et al. (2006), 'Androgen therapy in women: An Endocrine Society Clinical Practice Guideline', *Journal of Clinical Endocrinology and Metabolism* 91, 3697–710.

World Health Organization (1992), *International Statistical Classification of Diseases and Related Health Problems* (Geneva: WHO).

Writing Group for the Women's Health Initiative Investigators (2002), 'Risk and benefits of estrogen plus progestin in healthy postmenopausal women. Principal results from the Women's Health Initiative Randomized Controlled Trial', *Journal of the American Medical Association* 288, 321–33.

Chapter 3

Gender in Research and Industry: Women in Antibiotic Factories in 1950s Spain

María Jesús Santesmases

At 6:30 am on 23 December 1954, Sagrario Mochales, a young woman with a university degree in natural sciences, took the underground to Atocha station in Madrid. There she got on a truck – like the military ones covered in canvas that used to carry soldiers – to go to the factory of the Spanish penicillin-manufacturing firm, CEPA (Compañía Española de Penicilinas y Antibióticos), for her first day of work. Every day, CEPA workers took this transportation, provided by the factory, to go from Atocha to the facilities at Méndez Alvaro, in an industrial neighbourhood in southeast Madrid. After boarding with the help of a small ladder they remained standing for the journey.

Having been selected the previous day by the director of CEPA's department of quality control to work in a newly created research department, Mochales would be screening for new antibiotics alongside a physician and a chemist, both male. The three of them were beginning their training as interns in the CEPA laboratories immediately before Christmas 1954. When two women in the quality control department left to begin their married lives, Mochales and the technical director, Carmela Viejo, were the only women at the factory with university degrees from the early 1950s until 1966, when another female graduate, Isabel Martín, joined the CEPA research program.[1]

Other women did work at the factory. Their portraits can be found in news reports and advertising published by CEPA and Antibiotics SA from the mid 1950s onwards, when these two penicillin-manufacturers began to bottle the new antibiotic for sale within Spain. CEPA and Antibiotics SA were the only industrial firms approved by the Franco government to meet the national need for penicillin, at a time when its antibacterial activity was globally renowned. Up until then, penicillin had been scarce in Spain, distributed by a Commission from the Department of Health or sold 'de estraperlo', on the Spanish black market (Santesmases 2010; Santesmases 2014 in press).

1   I am grateful to Sagrario Mochales for the information provided in two interviews, in 2002 and recently in 2012, about her career in CEPA and Merck and to Isabel Martín, interviewed in 2013. Unless otherwise noted, the translations of Mochales's texts included in this chapter are Lori Gerson's.

In August 1950, penicillin advertisements began to be published in Spanish daily newspapers. They depicted factory woman seated at devices for the weighing, bottling and labelling of penicillin. Female workers appeared in a lot of advertising and were also included in news reports about this new national industry. The recurrent representations of women at work in the penicillin factories suggest they were deliberately selected, so as to promote Spain's antibiotic production industry and apparently to emphasise women's participation as industrial workers.

This chapter will give women agency in the history of Spanish antibiotics production and research. When highlighting women, an apparent social order is seen in which gender is articulating a hierarchy in the workplace. In these images, women remain seated at benches on which new, innovative devices are positioned, while men are standing up, monitoring the large fermentation devices. Women in white coats and men in blue overalls can be read as a history of antibiotics that from the beginning segregated the sexes, and the promotional strategies of which chose women to represent the technical innovation and cleanliness of an industrial process that offered a new – purifying – medicine: penicillin. A woman working in the research laboratory also wore a white coat, but this had a different meaning; that of 'research', while in the factory line of the bottling plant it denoted 'working girl'.

Having briefly introduced the early history of penicillin production in Spain, in the second part of this chapter I draw on newspaper images to explore the social life of gender, articulated in an antibiotics manufacturing plant by a dichotomised hierarchy. In the third part I reconstruct the trajectory of Sagrario Mochales, a researcher at the research laboratory of one of the companies. Mochales's recollections of her career enable analysis of the circulation of gender within the antibiotics factory to go further, as a part of everyday factory life. Gender as an analytical category places women at the centre of this study of industrial manufacturing, as agents in drug history and production in both the production line and the research laboratory, so as to reconstruct the history of early antibiotics production in Spain with women as the focal point.

Women's contributions to the history of antibiotics are, as yet, not included in any account. Men remain the main characters in archival material and in reconstructions, as men were the directors, inspirers, and recognised agents in the history of these antimicrobial drugs (see, for example, Hobby 1985; Lesch 2007; Bud 2008; Santesmases and Gradmann 2011), and it is usually taken for granted that any women represented were subordinates (for a challenge to this portrayal, see Oldenziel 1999). Therefore, this contribution is, in part, a reflexive analysis intended to include women in the historical narrative, and to understand the extent to which their historical experience has been concealed by historians' insufficient consideration of women's contributions. This lack of scrutiny has largely gone unchallenged: only within the history of *the pill* has the agency of women been examined in any depth (see Ignaciuk, Ortiz and Rodríguez Ocaña, this volume; Thoms, this volume, and references in both).

One reason for this combined analysis, of women in the manufacturing process and of a woman in the research department, is spatial: the research laboratory studied here belonged to one of the firms manufacturing penicillin in Spain, and its facilities were located within a factory building. As I have argued elsewhere, this singularity illustrates a particular case of research produced within a factory, as if knowledge – in this case microbiological knowledge – was an industrial object, produced by an industrial culture that also occupied the laboratory space (Santesmases 2011).

My main reason for studying gender in a research laboratory and a manufacturing space in the same chapter is to demonstrate that by using gender as an analytical category, these two gendered spaces of production reveal the similarities between the production of scientific and medical knowledge, and the production of industrial objects. Objects and knowledge are alike, in that both are commodities that contemporary societies manufacture. In both, gender remains encoded, with men controlling the management of the work place and the access to and the distribution of recognition. In both, women's activity has contributed to changing cultural and social norms, to the modification of symbolic values attached to particular skills in the workplace and in society at large (see, among many others, Rossiter 1995; Schiebinger 1989; Rose 1994; Álvarez Ricart 1988; Ortiz 2006; Magallón 1998; Santesmases 2000; on women in factories, see Downs 1995; on women, men and machines, see Oldenziel 1999).

Penicillin Manufacture in Spain

During the 1950s, Spain began to recover from the devastating effects of the civil war (1936–1939) and from the hardships of the 1940s. Hunger and poverty combined with corruption and the black market of basic products – bread and drugs among them – during the national isolation in the early decades of Franco's dictatorship (del Cura and Huertas 2007; Catalán 1995; Cazorla 2009). The economic and political misery of the1940s included the violent repression of those considered disloyal to the dictatorship, and harsh living and working conditions for the working class (Mir et al. 1997; Saz and Roda 1999; Cenarro 2008 and 2009).

This isolation was twofold, composed of the policy of the Franco autarchy for promoting national production, and the policy of the allies toward the dictatorship, which prevented Spanish membership in those international organisations that emerged following WWII (Portero 1989; Guirao 1998). At times this double scenario conflicted; at others the two aspects reinforced each other. This duality of practices, the politics of the dictatorship and of the allies towards it, was the basis of Spain's recovery from the civil war and the misery of the 1940s, as well as one of the bases for the longevity of Franco's dictatorship.

On 1 September 1948, the Spanish government took up the challenge of a growing demand for penicillin. On that day, the Ministry of Industry approved a decree entitled 'Penicillin: its manufacture is of national interest', which was published in October, launching an open public competition for the establishment of two factories (*Boletín Oficial del Estado* 1948). By considering penicillin production to be of national interest, the authorities assumed control over its manufacture and included penicillin among the government's industrial priorities. In August 1949, the government approved two firms to produce penicillin: Compañía Española de Penicilinas y Antibióticos (hereafter CEPA, as the directors and workers referred to the company) was authorised to build a penicillin factory in Madrid, and the Industria Española de Antibióticos SA (hereafter Antibióticos SA) to build a penicillin production plant in León. Antibióticos SA was created by a group of Spanish pharmaceutical laboratories in collaboration with US pharmaceutical firm Schenley. CEPA was a combination of firms dedicated to the production of chemicals, an industrial bank – Banco Urquijo – and US pharmaceutical manufacturer, Merck (Santesmases 1999).

Contracts signed with foreign firms were submitted to government industrial authorities for their approval (Santesmases 2010). Both firms were private, even though the State legally controlled their financial and foreign relation activities (Puig 2004). Agreements with foreign companies suggest that nationalism and state-controlled industry coexisted with the importation of both the drug and its production process. From then on, purchasing patents came to be a regular feature of Spanish industrial life (Cebrián 2004; Romero de Pablos 2011).

The official NoDo newsreel of Fleming's visit in 1948, in which penicillin was publicly praised, became propaganda at a time when the news regarding its curative effects was well-known and widespread. A transformation of penicillin was taking place, from the scarce hero it had been in the 1940s, to the cultural icon associated with industrial innovation and prosperity that it became in 1950 (on the construction of penicillin as an icon in Britain, see Bud 2008).

Women Factory Workers and Social Order

'Spain is going to have enough penicillin to cover its needs', proclaimed the double page of propaganda published in September 1950 (*Abc* Sevilla, 10-9-1950, pp. 4–5; same text in *La Vanguardia* 29-8-1950, p. 5). In the summer of that year, CEPA and Antibióticos SA started bottling penicillin imported in bulk from the US, and began their campaigns to advertise their industrial endeavour as manufacturers of one of the most popular wonder drugs of the time. A long text and two large photographs depicting women's participation in penicillin production were part of the same pages of advertising (see Figures 3.1 and 3.2). The pictures included in CEPA advertisements are very similar to those included in news reports, suggesting the firm had done some marketing to boost coverage. Images from both sources are used in this chapter for reconstructing the representation of gender in a Spanish antibiotic factory.

The images of penicillin factories were presented to the public at the end of the poor and miserable decade following the Spanish Civil War as a visual rhetoric of

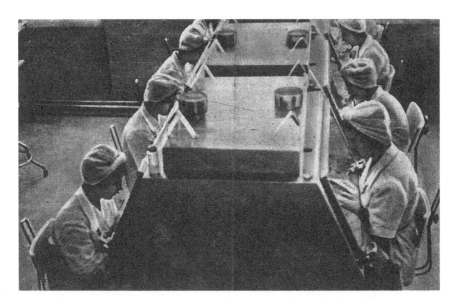

Figure 3.1   Lines of women weighing penicillin, CEPA bottling plant, Madrid
Source: *Abc* Sevilla 10-9-1950, p. 4

national achievement. In these photographs, antibiotic production is shown through the women sitting in a factory line and their participation in innovative technical practices. Lines of women in the bottling plant of a penicillin factory are seen; women seated at tables, white-coated, their hair covered with white caps as if they were nurses, factory nurses taking care of a new wonder product – penicillin – that required safe conditions for its bottling. They wear uniforms; they are standardised and thus, as standards, remain a collective of dissolved individualities, as in many production-line assemblies. It is from this collective that they offer an identity, one based on their role as women industrial workers (on women workers, see Kaplan 2008; Borderías 1993).

These women are not looking at the camera; instead, they are in a working stance, their heads bent forward, carefully examining the contents of the glass cases: that is, according to the wording alongside, pure, sterile penicillin powder. All are bent at the same angle, a uniformity that exhibits safety and order. A perfect similarity between the women in the photograph makes them not only equal but also anonymous, indistinguishable from one another.

These images became evidence for a historical narrative (Burke 2001; Park 2011; Daston and Lunbeck 2011). Thinking visually and analysing visual representations aims to unveil the rhetoric of images, their cultural meaning (Jordanova 1989 and 1992). As visual records of factory production – the early industrial task that was weighing, bottling and labelling of penicillin that was received in bulk directly from US factories – women's presence in the factory

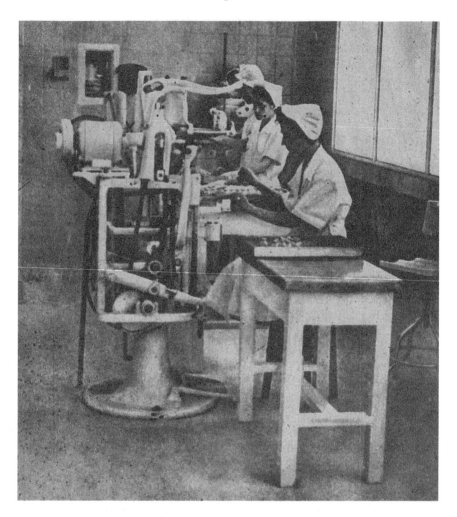

Figure 3.2   Women labelling penicillin flasks, CEPA bottling plant, Madrid
Source: *Abc* Sevilla 10-9-1950, p. 5

space encoded professional technicians who were women (Gewurtz 2006 has been
an inspiration for my analysis). Women workers are shown as segregated, and this
segregation makes them stand out as the preferred *manpower* for some gendered
workplaces in an apparently stable social order (see Borderías 1993, 10, for an
analysis of women working at a telephone company).

A woman's hands were also shown (*La Vanguardia* 29-8-1950, p. 5). Two hands
wearing gloves 'as if surgeons', demonstrate the central role of the precision scale,
one of the technical devices also praised, and the leading role of which reinforces
the precision of the women's work. According to the text of the advert, a sterile

environment was of major importance in the penicillin purification and bottling process: women took compulsory showers and adhered to other strict hygienic measures, suggesting the purified environment that efficient bottling of penicillin required and which these women provided (*La Vanguardia* 29-8-1950, p. 5).

'To be really efficient, penicillin needs two conditions: absolute purity and exact quantities.' This can be read in the account of women's tasks in the factory (*Abc* Madrid 10-9-1950). Praising women was praising cleanliness and safe handling; that is, praising penicillin itself. The representation selected to advertise the drug was composed of women dressed in white, in front of stainless steel boxes and purified flasks. The impact was doubly symbolic: of the drug and its wondrous effects, and of the women's work while handling it safely in this innovative, technical environment.

The narrative of these images associates women with the new, innovative devices and exhibits the set – women and devices – as safety innovation in the manufacturing of a product whose function was to therapeutically provide cleanliness and purity. The cleanliness and purity of women's images represent this promotion of the new drug in these poor times. The women's uniforms were washed and ironed every day, and the environment kept clean by automatically closing double doors; workshops were located in small rooms for the same objective of cleanliness. Hermetically sealed, stainless steel cases were provided with two ultraviolet light lamps to kill any germs, with the air circulating inside passing through many filters. The two gloves already mentioned were used to handle the products inside the glass cases (Figure 3.3) (*Abc* Sevilla, 10-9-1950, p. 5).

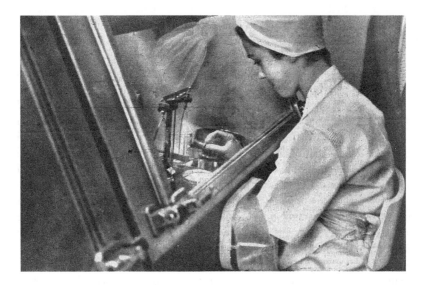

Figure 3.3   Woman weighing penicillin, CEPA bottling plant, Madrid
Source: *Abc* Madrid 16-8-1950, p. 4

Our eyes are trained in the contemporary rules of industry, photography and advertising, and by a gendered culture which has formed our way of seeing (Alpers 1983; Kemp 2006). The photographs presented here attest to the origins and trajectories of a social life segregated by sex that naturalised and normalised differences fuelled by industrial life experience. This sexual division is part of contemporary culture and its narrative, thus illustrating the strength of a system of symbols and cultural values bisected by a sexual classification that became a cultural dichotomy.

The audience these images addressed – those who read newspapers – was composed of people who needed to feel safe consuming a previously scarce healing product. Following a decade of poverty and a scarcity of medications, modernisation and prosperity were depicted in the photographs of the penicillin factory. It was a direct promotion of penicillin: assuring the public that penicillin would no longer be scarce –'a major problem has been solved' declares the text of the report (*La Vanguardia* 29-9-1950, p. 5).

Men were also portrayed in these images, in tie and on foot. Their male clothing and their standing position at the factory's door encoded the power of a male hierarchy that selected the representation of men as authority and women working in the factory line as user participants in technical innovation. Visual narratives of gender change over time, and men would recover their main role as technicians, when a year later they were depicted in blue overalls standing at the foot of the fermentation tanks, handling the stopcocks and main taps of the circulating liquids and gases (*Abc* Madrid 18-7-1951; *Abc* Madrid 30-6-1957). Men were in charge of the section composed of big devices: steam boilers, air filters, devices for water depyrogenation (removal of pyrogens or substances that can produce fever, mostly bacteria) and deionisation, steam pressure reducers, and detergent tanks (Figure 3.4). 'Each device is a pattern of perfection and modernity', proclaimed the news report (*Abc* Sevilla, 10-9-1950, p. 5). The shape of the new buildings was also emphasised, part of the expanding industry antibiotics manufacturing was becoming: property as power.

Women could be taken for granted as subordinate factory workers involved in bottling and labelling at the time, but a major question remains to be posed, regarding the gendered 'logic' of this distribution of tasks which was also a distribution of space. Such a distribution evokes older associations of women with caring tasks and duties: caring for children, the sick and the aged, as well as providing food and daily remedies beyond their families and households. It is through the perspective of this feminist approach to the history of care, that those women in white shown in the factory lines as images to publicise industrial development, can be seen, viewed, observed and retrieved (Ortiz 1993; on retrieving women and their workplaces, see Cabré 2008; on the kitchen as women's workplace and technology, see Oldenziel and Zachmann 2009).

This at least partial feminisation of particular types of industrial work, such as the handling of sensitive, delicate products on a production line, was promoted – more than simply permitted – during the Franco dictatorship. At the end of the first

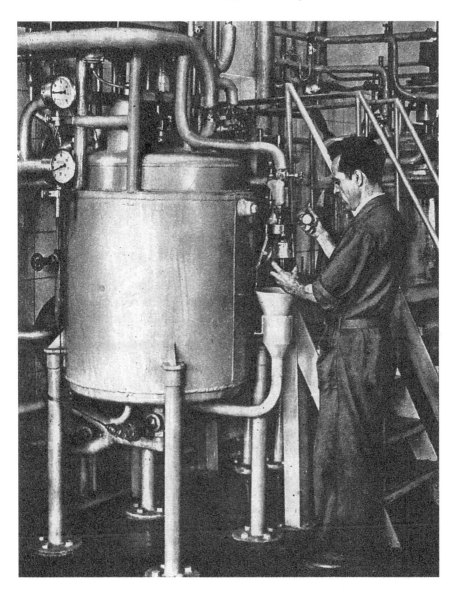

Figure 3.4   A man at the tank, CEPA bottling plant, Madrid
Source: *Abc* Madrid 18-7-1951, p. 23

miserable decade of Franco's rule in the 1940s, a high number of young, single women were able to fit both the requirements defined by the (male) managers of a factory line and the norms of the dictatorship, which kept married women in the home. Once they entered the factory, many single women got married and had children while at the same time keeping their jobs (see below, the testimony of Sagrario Mochales).

This social order, both in the factory and the laboratory, was in harmony with a Western society that had sent women back to their homes following WWII (Rossiter 1995; Vicedo 2009). In the case of Spain, discrimination was reinforced by the laws of the Franco dictatorship and its representation of maleness in the form of the army's hierarchical order: that of Franco as the generalissimo of the Spanish army, navy and air force, who governed the country through its recovery from the miseries of the civil war and the post war years of the 1940s, until 1975 (Gallego Méndez 1983).

The poverty among Western societies, together with trends toward industrial recovery and development, brought women to work in the factories. The contemporary construction of femaleness was appropriate for factory work: seen as conscientious, women workers handled pure products and small, new factory devices with care. Women were included among the factory workers in the two penicillin production plants from the late 1940s on. In caring for penicillin production, women took part as careful technicians (on women's carefulness, Menéndez and Medina 2003; Medina and Menéndez 2005; Ortiz 1993; and on women, feminism and medicine, Ortiz 2006). They were thus regarded as reliable contributors to the manufacturing line and, in so doing, became part of the active population available for hire by a growing national industry (Borderías, Sarasúa and Pérez Fuentes 2010; Sarasúa and Gálvez 2003; Segura 2004).

Between 1940 and 1950, there were a high number of single women in Spain between the ages of 21 and 40 – 45 per cent of all Spanish women – while fertility rates decreased throughout the decade. As the number of single women decreased, the number of women in the workplace increased. This suggests that single women, once they entered the labour market, were very likely to stay there after marriage and childbirth (Cabré 2007; Delgado 1993; Garrido 1993; Santesmases 2000). Women entered the labour market while young and single, when the norms of the dictatorship regarded married women unsuitable for work; they should be fully dedicated to their work at home (Sarasúa and Gálvez 2003; see also Sarasúa and Molinero 2008). Among the single were those 'working girls' who sat at the bottling table in penicillin production plants, which by the end of 1950 had bottled more than a million doses of the drug (*Abc* Madrid 31-12-1950).

The image of the technical director of CEPA, Carmela Viejo, is also presented here. It illustrates that women participated at various levels within the hierarchical management of the manufacturing plant. The image of Carmela Viejo that has been preserved shows her white-coated, guiding the factory managers through the workshops and aisles. Having graduated with a degree in pharmacy, she was regarded as a highly competent director, skilled and smart, who achieved everything she set her mind to. She was also an attractive person (Mochales 2012). We see her with the directors of the company, Justo Martínez Mata, Antonio Robert and Antonio Gallego, visiting the basements of the bottling plant – the plumbing of the sterile facilities surrounding them. Although dressed in white, she was part of the same job category as Martínez Mata. As Mochales remembers, Carmela Viejo always wore a white coat. She wore it as medical doctors did, as did technicians – the term used to refer to those university graduate workers in the factory research laboratory. White conveyed educational level and scientific recognition.

A Woman in the Industrial Research Laboratory

As part of the industrial policy of the Franco dictatorship during the 1940s, a tax was levied on the incomes of every industrial firm. In the case of the iron, steel and concrete industries this was between 0.5 and 1 per cent of sales. While for other industries the contribution was portrayed as a donation, it was in fact a hidden tax. The resulting funds were supposedly dedicated to applied research, with some invested in useless projects, and others in promoting research in such areas as organic chemistry. These taxes became part of the funding for applied research at the Consejo Superior de Investigaciones Científicas, the research institution created by Franco immediately following the Civil War (López García 1994 and 1996). Instead of donating a percentage of its income, CEPA was authorised to create a research centre in 1950 at the University of Madrid, School of Medicine. Named the Instituto de Farmacología Española (IFE), it was initially dedicated to physiology, the discipline in which the director of CEPA, Antonio Gallego, was a professor. Gallego's research interests were broader, however, and prompted a negotiation with Merck, after the building of the penicillin factory, and the establishing of a new program in search of antibiotics which ran from 1954 (Santesmases 1999 and 2001, ch. 4).

Between the autarchy norm and the promotion of international scientific collaboration circulating in Europe in the early 1950s, the research department was created at the CEPA penicillin factory on Méndez Álvaro road in 1954. Based on an agreement with Merck (Rahway), the research agenda for what was called the 'screening program' was the search for new antibiotics. The Spanish group was to identify antibacterial activity in samples collected from soil – the style of work established by Selman Waksman's research group at Rutgers University, which had led to the identification and isolation of streptomycin – by using a set of microbiological techniques for culturing microbes and testing the activity of cultures against a previously established list of bacteria. It was a small group whose scientific identity remained attached to the factory and its industrial interests (Santesmases 2011).

The CEPA research laboratory shared its director with the department of quality control: Justo Martínez Mata MD remained in charge for over two decades. The head of the research laboratories was Sebastián Hernández

MD. Coming from quality control, Hernández went to the Merck facilities in Rahway to be trained in how to set up a screening department and the techniques to be used. Following his return, the three interns were selected and started work. As university graduates, they remained in a category apart from the factory workers. Some of the factory 'girls' did move to the new laboratories as assistants – 'they were smart girls, already trained in factory work', Sagrario Mochales (2012) remembers. Mochales started as an intern at the research department in 1954 and soon gained a young female assistant. The number of assistants the group employed increased over the next few years as the work became more intensive. At the time of Mochales's selection, a discussion had taken place among CEPA directors about whether a woman should be part of the research group, but Antonio Gallego, the scientific director of the factory, had finally acquiesced. Two women chemists were also selected to work at the Quality Control Department and a woman pharmacist, Carmela Viejo, was hired as the factory technical director.

Managerial capitalism was compatible with the family firm that to a certain extent CEPA was at that time. Personal relationships were instrumental and remained a source of interns – Mochales was the niece of a clinical expert in infectious diseases, Francisco Baquero, who had a good professional and personal relationship with CEPA. Mochales grew up in Madrid, attended one of the very few private schools that did not belong to a religious order, and entered the University of Madrid in the late 1940s. She belonged to a well-educated middle-class family. Her father, a cashier at the industrial Urquijo bank that created CEPA, was able to overcome the difficulties of the Spanish Civil War and keep his job.

Methods for the collaborative research program of CEPA with Merck in the screening for new antibiotics remained artisanal, as microbiology was in general. Every extract was treated separately, with portions placed in Petri dishes and the antimicrobial agent revealed by the clear zones that appeared surrounding the colonies. Through this collaboration with CEPA, Merck shifted its major screening programme to Spain and initiated new research at Rahway, on such problems as dental caries (Woodruff 1981, 23). The screening programme became part of the biographies of CEPA and Merck, firms whose main task was to manufacture antibiotics, and whose research was conceived as support for this manufacturing (Gadebusch, Stapley and Zimmerman 1992). After being created to produce penicillin in Spain, CEPA became an industrial firm that also carried out research, with a small department established inside the bottling plant.

Merck provided laboratory equipment, reagents and methods for isolating and testing the soil extracts the CEPA research program received from Merck sales agents all over the world. 'We imported instruments and exported results' (Mochales 2012). Spanish researchers were cheaper than US ones according to Mochales, which suggests she regarded US Merck training skills and technical equipment for research as superior to her own capabilities as a scientist and researcher.

When reconstructing her work at the research group, Mochales perceives her identity as a scientific one. She was very young at the beginning, and single – a requirement at the time for a woman to be hired:

> I was the youngest of the group and all of them soon became my friends, friends who, of the ones who remain, are still my friends. What happened? Simply, at that time no one questioned male superiority ... It seemed to be a better tactic not to give importance to the 'principles' of the society I lived in. I defended myself by showing, step by step, my convictions because I thought they were right. (Mochales 2002)

The space she found to construct her professional identity was that of discussions conducted in the group meetings she joined in Madrid, and in Rahway, during her annual visits to report on the Madrid results and receive training in new methods and objectives. In the early years, she joined the chief of the laboratory, Sebastián Hernández, on these trips to the US. Later, however, she was on her own for these annual three-week visits. In her account she emphasises how her work style differed:

> In all the most important meetings, either here [in Madrid] or in the US, in which I remained the sole woman until the very end, I was famous because I overwhelmed them with papers in which our work was summarised in detail. Papers in which, fortunately, there were few objections. When there were, I humbly accepted the objections, sincerely gave my thanks and recognised publicly my mistake, which was very surprising to them. (Mochales 2002)

They said she was 'too direct':

> I took it as a compliment. I knew how to accept the so-called male dominion, but knowing, both them and myself, that this acquiesence was more theoretical than real. The result is that, at the end of my professional career, I had gained the respect of all my numerous bosses. (Mochales 2002)

The program was expected to be very productive and indeed it was. For a decade, however, despite the work being very intensive, not one antibiotic was discovered:

> What really made me happy was the laboratory work. My years as a technician, this was the category at the time, were the happiest of my life. Many trials dedicated to the discovery of new drugs depended on me. I used all the care possible so that the microorganisms we isolated would be in conditions we considered optimal because our big dilemma was that we worked with unknown microorganisms, they didn't talk to us, so trial and error was the usual tool. I used all my intuition and growing experience to select those small activities produced by the cultures in which my beloved microorganisms grew. (Mochales 2002)

Careful handling and patient observation of 'tiny' antibacterial activity appeared here as a value: in her reconstruction, she stands out by situating herself in the social order of the laboratory. She says she never rebelled. This was her strategy as a smart and skilled technician, at the beginning of the screening program, and later as a respected scientist. It was in her workplace at the laboratory that she became defined as different from the men as a professional norm.

In a sample taken from the soil in the Levante region in 1966, Sagrario Mochales detected a weak antibacterial activity with the SPHERO screen (Silver 2012). This method, designed by Merck microbiologist, Eugene Dulaney, involves detection of the physical effects produced by cell wall antimicrobials. As the microbe's cell wall is digested, membrane tension causes the cell to acquire a characteristic spherical shape, known as a spheroplast. The soil sample was taken in April 1966, and Mochales detected its activity in May. A month later the activity was confirmed, and a sample lyophilised (dried for transportation as a solid powder) once its purity had been tested in the CEPA laboratories. The extract identified by Mochales immediately became part of the research agenda of the screening group – consisting of the two women, Mochales and Isabel Martín, and Tomás Cubillo and Sebastián Hernández – and became an intensively researched object. It turned out to be active *in vitro* against a set of bacteria, both Gram-negative and Gram-positive, by inhibiting cell-wall synthesis, according to the test she herself performed. When tested in mice, even without being purified, the first extracts displayed high activity against many experimental infections. This meant that the substance was more active *in vivo* than *in vitro*, a fact that attracted a great deal of attention to the product: a product the existence of which was based on the ability of Mochales to detect minute activity within a Petri dish (Hendlin et al. 1969). This high activity prompted the group to carry out further research on the extracts in order to identify the substance responsible. The extracts were partly purified – the concentration in the sample increased – and sent to the Merck laboratories at Rahway, where the substance was isolated as a calcium salt, and turned out to be an unusual chemical compound – a phosphonic acid (Martínez Mata 1974).

Microbiology has been an instrumental discipline in the funding and manufacturing of antibiotics. As an artisanal craft, it required the careful handling and observation of minute activity that would reveal prospective new antibiotics in a culturing media in which activity emerged as visual evidence, sometimes so tiny that both sensitivity and training were needed, as was careful handling of the culture. This suggests a gendered way of developing microbiological skills at the screening laboratory, which resonates with the meticulousness of the women workers at the bottling facilities of the factory, suggesting a gendered construction of both manufacturing and research skills. Research results were sometimes encouraging, as antibacterial activity could be identified in many of the culture mediums handled. However, some had already been identified or were not considered suitable. 'But success was also with us, with five products discovered' (Mochales 2002). The samples that displayed antibacterial activity created an atmosphere of excitement that led, at least four times, to new products entering the market following extensive trials. For Mochales, this feeling of success appears to have pushed aside any sense of segregation or lack of recognition.

Fosfomycin came to be known as the first Spanish antibiotic, identified and cultured in the CEPA research laboratory (Heindlin et al. 1969; Christinesen et al. 1969; Stapley et al. 1969). Isolated and chemically characterised in Merck research laboratories, the patent application submitted in May 1968 was signed by Sagrario Mochales together with David Heindlin and Edward O. Stapley, both from Merck, and the director of the CEPA research department, Justo Martínez Mata. Mochales remembers that her name had not originally been included – neither women nor technicians usually signed – but Heindlin insisted, and her name can be found on both the application and the 1972 patent awarded by the US Patent Office (Heindlin, Stapley, Mochales and Martínez Mata 1972). By the time of the application, Sagrario Mochales was already married and pregnant, and as it was not considered suitable that a married woman keep a job outside the home, her job was at risk. According to her recollections, Mochales's signature on the patent application protected her. With the support from Carmela Viejo she was allowed to stay: eventually the CEPA director accepted her as a married woman, a researcher and a mother.

The new antibiotic, initially labelled Fosfomycin and later marketed as Fosfocina, entered the Spanish market in 1975. After a long process of chemical identification and development in a pilot plant at Rahway, the manufacturing process was set up at the CEPA facilities under the advice of Merck experts. Some came to Madrid to supervise the entire process of building the production line. Fosfomycin was a powerful symbol of CEPA research and its partnership with Merck; an emblem for the laboratory, the success of the whole program was concentrated in it and, as such, it was celebrated by the director of the department and the scientific director of CEPA when it came out on the market. No women were included in the promotional photographs for the new Spanish antibiotic.

Mochales's reconstruction displays the pride of a pioneer:

> [W]e enjoyed the best conditions to grow as modern scientists, as part of the most advanced world of research that then existed. For example, penicillin and streptomycin [manufacturing] had been developed by Merck Research Laboratories and the group of scientists dedicated [in Merck Research Laboratories] to the discovery of natural products was a leader in the field in the US. Some of them were our teachers, our sources of information on new techniques and new microbiological advances, about all that was part of the scientific avant-garde landscape. (Mochales 2002)

Mochales was the sole woman in the research group for over a decade, until in 1966 Isabel Martín began working in the group. During this period, up until the mid 1970s, the research department was composed of a small group of people

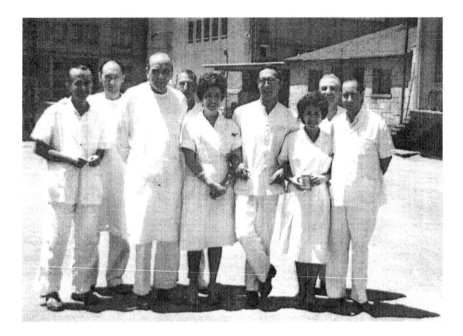

**Figure 3.5   Isabel Martín and Sagrario Mochales with their technician
colleagues at the research laboratory at CEPA**

Courtesy Sagrario Mochales

whose scientific identity remained attached to the factory and its industrial interests (Santesmases 2011).

Following the success of Fosfomycin, Sagrario Mochales and slightly later Isabel Martín participated in the screening that led to identify new antibiotics: Thienamycin, and Cephamycin were also detected at the CEPA research laboratory (Figure 3.5) (Mochales 1994). All were marketed, along with various chemical modifications thereof, such as Cefoxitin and Imipenem, during the research partnership between Merck and CEPA. These discoveries joined the 'evolving family of biological molecules' (Pieters 2005, 8):

> It's difficult for me to say, but it's true that it was me who first saw, selected
> as interesting and did studies to test the initial activities of the microbiological
> cultures that became, after long research by our American friends [at Merck],
> fosfomycin and thienamycin. (Mochales 2002)

These antibiotics are, Mochales says, 'not as old as I am but they are marketed products still in clinical use, even if they're no longer as innovative as they were at the beginning' (Mochales 2002). The research work shared with the factory both a culture of industrial production – the program examined almost 100,000 samples in the first three years (Hernández, Mochales, Martínez Mata and Gallego 1958) – and a space in the manufacturing plant. The culture of industrial production was at the intersection of the space shared by the research department and the factory line, where women represented careful, meticulous work.

This genderising was also displayed in the hierarchies of the factory and the laboratory:

> When I was appointed director [in the 1980s, after 30 years of work and many successful detections of antimicrobial activity] there was only one other woman in the whole research department which I belonged to, with around four hundred people or maybe more … All this changed at the end of the 1980s. Starting from the 1980s, the number of women researchers in our centre increased until it exceeded the number of men, which left a positive mark in the [research] program. (Mochales 2002)

Here, Mochales identifies both her achievements and the barriers to be crossed by her and other women – by the end of her professional life, a transformation had occurred: more women, more medicines, and everything going well for her in a highly divided social order of gendered authority. And she had been part of the transformation: she herself had changed, obtaining recognition in her appointment as director and gaining personal satisfaction:

> So I can say that, till the end, a part of my life, the most difficult, the furthest from my beloved laboratory benches, the most stressful without any doubt, I lived in a world of male executives, men from the US. And it worked out well for me. (Mochales 2002)

Was Penicillin Female? The Circulation of Gender as a Cultural Category in the Factory and the Laboratory

The aim of this chapter had been to retrieve women in the early history of antibiotics; to acknowledge the contribution women have made in this history in Spain, both in industrial manufacturing and research. It is concerned with the relationship of women and men in industrial history and the history of science, and the connections between past and present social practices regarding the differentiation of the two sexes (Scott 1986; Jordanova 1993; Löwy and Rouch 2003).

In conclusion, I would like to draw attention to images of women and their representation in the factory space, on the manufacturing line and in the research laboratory, and the circulation of gender in this space.

As part of the Western geography of the history of industry during the post-WWII era, the Spanish government was laying foundations for the economic expansion of the 1960s. In the antibiotic factory, at the bottling tables of sterilised workshops and the benches for carefully culturing microorganisms in the research laboratory, gender circulated; women and men themselves shouldered this category. Factory images are taken as representations of the industrial setting in which gender condensed as a category and unveiled itself as dynamic. Gender invaded the space of practices, and women have been made visible, both by the industrial environment of the time and by my own narrative.

Experiences as collective practices have been structured within political and geographical settings, where time and place have played a part. This gender circulation broke the norms regarding women's place in society; norms established by the Western biopolitics of the time, and reinforced by a political regime that denounced women working outside the home. Women, however, became an increasing part of *human resources* for working places outside the household. Their participation in the antibiotics factory and the research laboratory of the factory, as conscientious workers privileged by gender categorisation, illustrates their agency in producing changes in the factory, the research laboratory and society at large. Women participated in the industrial space being created.

What women's representation in these images reveals is the impact of women's presence on antibiotic production. What is found in these images is a recognised collective of women in white as a representation of prosperity. By recognition I mean they were represented in the images because women or, more likely, their workplaces in the bottling plant, were worth showing. Their worthiness meant that images of women became agents for the credibility of the factory, for what was manufactured there and for the tasks involved. This was part of the wonder of penicillin: the values attached to it when it circulated. Attached to penicillin, gender as a category was also moved, mobilised and carried by penicillin propaganda.

In the history of antibiotics, men have been the main characters. To counter this asymmetry, I introduce here the idea of women as otherness, with images considered as displays of social interaction. In this eye-witnessing exercise that I propose, visual images of women in an antibiotic factory are shown as representations of women's social condition, read by juxtaposing text and pictures and their historical and geopolitical location. Biological models – sexualised bodies – became embedded in lifestyle and social roles, and were agents in the construction of gender as a cultural category capable of being analysed (inspired by Jordanova 1992, 57).

The distribution of physical space at the factory and the different symbolic and physical spaces segregated the sexes. This separation in antibiotics manufacturing took the form of the social and cultural relationships that have been presented: in men wearing ties, in the dark suits of white collar workers and in blue overalls standing beside big fermentation tanks, while women dressed in white coats and white caps, like pure, clean nurses in the purified atmosphere of the bottling workshop, worked with smaller devices. Through examination of the spaces they occupied within the factory, a social order emerges: collectives of women and men, and the distribution of recognition, agency and authority of the two sexes.

Working women were selected as strategic representations of prosperity and the modernisation of early antibiotic production in Spain. These representations emphasise women's roles and their skills in the finishing processes assigned to them. Women provided credibility and demonstrated the innovative techniques of the factory's facilities while, as a group, they remained a set of shared yet dissolved identities. Research was also a space for professional recognition, where a young women, Sagrario Mochales, was initially accepted, but was not welcome as a mother. This was the same workplace in which she constructed her professional identity and gained scientific recognition, qualities she almost lost when becoming pregnant. However, along with the directors of the Spanish and US research laboratories she had signed a patent for a new antibiotic, and had been supported by the female technical director of the factory, Carmela Viejo. 'I loved my work', she stated modestly. From technician to director, Mochales spent her professional life searching for and finding new therapeutic agents.

In the finishing stages of production – the bottling, sealing and labelling – women were gentle representations of the clean, exquisite manners of modern innovations in penicillin manufacturing. Women were able to contribute to the manufacturing of a product that saved lives because they were clean and created cleanliness. Images of women at benches, operating automatic devices, brought attention to innovation and modern production: female values were shown to be associated with penicillin. It was as if penicillin condensed female symbolic values, as if it was also female. To some extent, gender circulated toward the meaning of penicillin itself. It was a caregiver, a saviour, a clean, pure final product from the manufacturing line that was able to cure; a task the delicacy of which could be associated with that of someone at the screening laboratory bench, searching a Petri dish for antimicrobial activity.

The carefulness of women handling the drug was symbolically attached to the way in which mothers care. Therefore the rhetoric of women remaining in the home would not have been contradictory to allowing women to work in the factory. Women were reliable agents of purity and cleanliness, and this permission reinforced the political discourse of women's limited rights precisely by letting them leave home to do what they, according to the norms of the time, really knew how to do: to provide care. And with their skill for purity and cleanliness, women fitted into the social order while they also broke it.

It has been the aim of this chapter to question the construction of women's identities and the systems of representation that have defined and stabilised the feminine and the masculine in antibiotics industrial production, in the contemporary system of production of goods and knowledge, and in the culture at large. In the late 1950s, Franco's government was attempting to increase national production, as were governments all over Europe. Changes were introduced when women took part, although male authority remained in both visual representations and managerial practices. The white colour offered both scientific authority at the research laboratory and technical sensitivity at the bottling workplace. Men in blue retained a physical power, as male workers who stood up in front of big apparatuses, and when in ties they showed managerial authority. The distribution of colours and workplaces turned out to be mutually reinforcing.

As Sagrario Mochales's own reconstruction suggests, some women remained in work during the post-war era despite the Western trend of sending women back to the home and the Franco dictatorship's policy against married women working. Political and economic circumstances played a part: women were hired and retained at work – an increase in female workers that coincided with the highest birth rate in twentieth-century Spain (Garrido 1993). A double presence and a double biography – a job and a family – should be considered part of women's strategies at that time. This took effect in the form of cultural changes regarding the social meaning of gender; that is – to limit the comments to the spaces studied here – regarding the role played by, and assigned to women in industry, research and society.

As workers, as social agents, women's individual and collective identities were permanently reconstructing order in a sex-segregated space of activity. The subjective identity has been explored in the case of Sagrario Mochales, who provides a part of this history, as do the images, a representation of the gendered hierarchies in manufacturing plants. Mochales mobilised resources to keep her workplace at the factory and remained in it. In this workplace, gender was constructed, as in the labour market, the research laboratory and the factory, all arenas where the differences between men and women were repeatedly reinforced – every day, by every skilful gesture that was part of workplace practice. By using gender as an analytical category to study the work at the research laboratory, together with that at the manufacturing plant, the similarities between the production of knowledge and of industrial drugs become visible, which demonstrates the overlapping capacity of women as agents in the contemporary history of both research and industry.

Acknowledgements

I would like to thank Cristina Borderías, Ilana Löwy, Teresa Ortiz and the participants in the workshop Gendered Drug Standards, held in Granada, November 2011, for their comments and suggestions about an earlier version of this chapter. My main debt is to Sagrario Mochales, who has repeatedly answered my questions, to Isabel Martín, and to Roberto Gallego, who gave me access to his father's papers and told me the CEPA story. Librarians at the Hemeroteca Municipal de Madrid and at the Biblioteca Regional de Madrid Joaquín Leguina deserve special thanks for providing access to originals and the best quality copies available for the figures. I am also grateful to Joanna Baines and Lori Gerson for insightful copyediting. The research for this essay was supported in part by funding provided by the Spanish ministry of Science and Innovation (FFI2009-07522) and the Spanish ministry of Economy and Competitiveness (FFI2012-34076).

References

Alpers, S. (1983), *The Art of Describing* (Chicago: University of Chicago Press).

Álvarez Ricart, C. (1988), *La mujer como profesional de la medicina en la España del siglo XIX* (Barcelona: Anthropos).

Boletín Oficial del Estado (1948), 6 October.

Borderías, C. (1993), *Entre líneas: trabajo e identidad femenina en la España contemporánea. La compañía telefónica, 1924–1980* (Barcelona: Icaria).

Borderías, C. and Renom, M. (eds) (2008), *Dones en movement(s)* (Barcelona: Icaria).

Borderías, C., Sarasúa C. and Pérez-Fuentes P. (2010), 'Gender inequalities in family consumption: Spain 1850–1930' in Addabbo, T., Arrizabalaga, M. P., Borderías, C. and Owens, A. (eds) *Gender Inequalities, Households and the Production of Well-being in Modern Europe* (Burlington, VT: Ashgate) pp. 179–95.

Bud, R. (2008), *Penicillin: Triumph and Tragedy* (Oxford: Oxford University Press).

Burke, P. (2001), *Eyewitnessing: The Use of Images as Historical Evidence* (London: Reaktion Books).

Cabré, A. (2007), 'Cuarto aproximaciones explicativas a las tendencias de nupcialidad y fecundidad' in Cabré, A. (ed.) *La constitución familiar en España* (Madrid: Fundación BBVA).

Cabré, M. (2008), 'Women or healers? Household practices and the categories of health care in late Medieval Iberia', *Bulletin of the History of Medicine* 82, 18–51.

Catalán, J. (1995), *La economía española y la segunda guerra mundial* (Barcelona: Ariel).

Cazorla, A. (2000), *Políticas de la Victoria: la consolidación del Nuevo Estado franquista (1938–1953)* (Madrid: Marcial Pons).

Cebrián, M. (2004), 'Technological imitation and economic growth during the Golden Age in Spain: 1959–1973', Doctoral Thesis (Florence: European University Institute).

Cenarro, Á. (2008), 'Memories of repression and resistance. Narratives of children institutionalized by Auxilio Social in postwar Spain', *History and Memory* 20:2, 39–59.

——— (2009), *Los niños del Auxilio Social* (Madrid: Espasa Calpe).

Christinesen, B. G., Leanza, W. J., Beattie, T. R., Patchett, A. A., Arison, B. H., Ormond, R. E., Kuehl, F. A., Albers-Schonberg, G. and Jardetzky O. (1969), 'Phosphonomycin: Structure and Synthesis', *Science* 160, 123–5.

Daston, L. and Lunbeck, E. (2011), 'Observation observed' in Daston, L. and Lunbeck, E. (eds) *Histories of Scientific Observation* (Chicago: University of Chicago Press) pp. 1–14.

del Cura, I. and Huertas, R. (2007), *Alimentación y enfermedad en tiempos de hambre: España, 1937–1947* (Madrid: Consejo Superior de Investigaciones Científicas).

Delgado, M. (1993), 'Cambios recientes en el proceso de formación de la familia', *Revista Española de Investigaciones Sociológicas* 64, 125–54.

Downs, L. L. (1995), *Manufacturing Inequality. Gender Division in the French and British Metalworking Industries, 1914–1939* (Ithaca and London: Cornell University Press).

Gadebusch, H. H., Stapley, E. O. and Zimmerman, S. B. (1992), 'The discovery of cell wall active antibacterial antibiotics', *Critical Reviews in Biotechnology* 12, 225–43.

Gallego Méndez, T. (1983), *Mujer. Falange y franquismo* (Madrid: Taurus).

Garrido, L. (1993), *Las dos biografías de la mujer en España* (Madrid: Instituto de la Mujer).

Gewurtz, M. S. (2006), 'Looking for Jean Daw: Narratives of women and missionary medicine in modern China' in Shteir, A.B. and Lightman, B. (eds).

Guirao, F. (1998), *Spain and the Reconstruction of Western Europe, 1945–57* (London: Macmillan).

Heindlin, D., Stapley, E. O., Mochales, S. and Martínez Mata, J. (1972), assignors to Merck & Co., Inc., Rahway, NJ. Antibacterial composition containing (-) (cis-1,2-epoxipropyl)phosphoric acid, United States Patent Office. Patented February 1, 1972.

Hendlin, D., Stapley, E. O., Jackson, M., Wallik, H., Miller, A. K., Wolf, F. J., Miller, T. W., Chaiet, L., Kahan, F. M., Foltz, E. L., Woodruff, H. B., Mata, J. M., Hernández, S. and Mochales, S. (1969), 'Phosphonomycin: A new Antibiotic produced by Strains of Streptomyces', *Science* 166, 122–3.

Hobby, G. (1985), *Penicillin. Meeting the Challenge* (New Haven and London: Yale University Press).

Jordanova, L. J. (1989), *Sexual Visions: Images of Gender in Science and Medicine between the Eighteenth and Twentieth Centuries* (New York and London: Harvester, Wheatsheaf).

——— (1992), 'Natural facts: a historical perspective on science and sexuality' in MacCormack, C.P. and Strathern, M. (eds) *Nature, culture and gender* (Cambridge: Cambridge University Press) pp. 42–69.

——— (1993), 'Gender and the historiography of science', *British Journal for the History of Science* 26, 469–83.

Kaplan, T. (2008), 'Social movements of women and the public good' in Borderías, C. and Renom, M. (eds), pp. 19–47.

Kemp, M. (2006), *Seen/Unseen: Art, Science and Intuition from Leonardo to the Hubble Telescope* (Oxford: Oxford University Press).

Lesch, J. E. (2007), *The First Miracle Drugs: How the Sulfa Drugs Transformed Medicine* (Oxford: Oxford University Press).

López García, S. (1994), *El saber tecnológico en la política industrial del primer franquismo*, Doctoral Thesis (Madrid: Universidad Complutense).

——— (1996), 'La investigación científica y técnica antes y después de la guerra civil' in Gómez Mendoza, A. (coord.), *Economía y sociedad en la España moderna y contemporánea* (Madrid: Síntesis).

Löwy, I. and Rouch, H. (2003), 'Genèse et development du genre: les sciences et les origines de la distinction entre sexe et genre', *Cahiers du Genre* 34, 5–16.

Magallón, C. (1998), *Pioneras españolas en las ciencias* (Madrid: CSIC).

Martínez Mata, J. (1974), 'La investigación de antibióticos en la industria farmacéutica española. Historia de un descubrimiento: la fosfomicina', *Química e Industria* 20:1, 51–9.

Medina-Doménech, R. M. and Menéndez-Navarro, A. (2005), 'Cinematic representations of medical technologies in the Spanish official newsreel, 1943–1975', *Public Understanding of Science* 14, 393–408.

Menéndez Navarro, A. and Medina Doménech, R. M. (2003), 'Ausencia y primor: mujer, tecnologías médicas e identidad nacional en el discurso visual del No-Do' in Amador, P. and Ruiz Franco, R. (eds) *Representación, construcción e interpretación de la imagen visual de las mujeres* (Madrid: Instituto de Cultura y Tecnología Miguel de Unamuno) pp. 395–403.

Mir, C., Corretgé, F., Farré, J. and Sagués, J. (1997), *Repressió econòmica i franquisme. L'actuació del Tribunal de Responsabilitats Politiques a la provincia de Lleida* (Barcelona: Publicacions de la Abadía de Montserrat).

Mochales, S. (1994), 'Forty years of screening programmes for antibiotics', *Microbiología SEM* 10, 331–42.

———— (2002), Untitled talk at the Residencia de Estudiantes, Madrid, 25 July.

———— (2012), Interview with the author, Madrid, 4 May 2012.

Oldenziel, R. (1999), *Making Technology Masculine: Men, Women and Modern Machines in America* (Amsterdam: Amsterdam University Press).

Oldenziel, R. and Zachmann, K. (2009), 'Kitchens as technology and politics: An introduction' in Oldenziel, R. and Zachmann, K. (eds) *Cold War Kitchen: Americanisation, Technology and European Users* (Cambridge, MA: MIT Press) pp. 1–29.

Ortiz, T. (1993), 'Luisa Rosado, una matrona en la España ilustrada', *Dynamis* 12, 323–46.

———— (2006), *Medicina, historia y género. 130 años de investigación feminista* (Oviedo: KRK).

Park, K. (2011), 'Observation in the margins, 500–1500' in Daston, L. and Lunbeck, E. (eds) *Histories of Scientific Observation* (Chicago: University of Chicago Press) pp. 15–44.

Portero, F. (1989), *Franco aislado. La cuestión española (1945–1950)* (Madrid: Aguilar).

Puig, N. (2004), 'Networks of innovation or networks of opportunity? The making of the Spanish antibiotics industry', *Ambix* LI, 167–85.

Quirke, V. and Slinn, J., (eds) (2011), *Perspectives on Twentieth Century Pharmaceuticals* (Oxford: Peter Lang).

Romero de Pablos, A. (2011), 'Regulation and the circulation of knowledge: penicillin patents in Spain', *Dynamis* 31, 87–108.

Rose, H. (1994), *Love, Power and Knowledge. Toward a Feminist Transformation of the Sciences* (Cambridge: Polity Press).

Rossiter, M. (1995), *Women Scientists in America: Before Affirmative Action 1940–1972* (Baltimore: Johns Hopkins University Press).

Santesmases, M. J. (1999), *Antibióticos en la autarquía. Banca privada, industria farmacéutica, investigación científica y cultura liberal en España, 1940–1960* (Madrid: Fundación Empresa Pública), documento de trabajo.

—— (2000), *Mujeres científicas en España: profesionalización y modernización social* (Madrid: Instituto de la Mujer).

—— (2001), *Entre Cajal y Ochoa: ciencias biomédicas en la España contemporánea* (Madrid: CSIC).

—— (2010), 'Distributing penicillin: The clinic, the hero and industrial production in Spain, 1943–1952' in Quirke, V. and Slinn, J. (eds) pp. 91–117.

—— (2011), 'Screening antibiotics: industrial research by CEPA and Merck in the 1950s', *Dynamis* 31, 131–51.

—— (in press), 'The Long Post-War and the Politics of Penicillin: Early Circulation and Smuaggling in Spain, 1944–1954', *Medicina nei Secoli*, forthcoming 2014.

Santesmases, M. J. and Gradmann, C. (eds) (2011), *Circulation of Antibiotics: Historical Reconstructions*, *Dynamis* 31:2, 17–152.

Sarasúa, C. and Gálvez, L. (eds) (2003), *¿Privilegios o eficiencia? Mujeres y hombres en los mercados de trabajo* (Alicante: Publicaciones de la Universidad de Alicante).

Sarasúa, C. and Molinero, C. (2008), 'Franquismo, trabajo y niveles de vida. Un estado de la cuestión desde una perspectiva de género' in Borderías, C. (ed.) *Historia de las Mujeres. Perspectivas actuales* (Barcelona: Icaria) pp. 309–54.

Saz, I. and Roda, A. G. (eds) (1999), *El franquismo en Valencia* (Valencia: Episteme).

Schiebinger, L. (1989), *The Mind has no Sex?* (Cambridge, MA: Harvard University Press).

Scott, J. (1986), 'Gender a useful category in historical analysis', *American Historical Revue* 91:5, 1053–75.

Segura, C. (2004), 'Mujeres, trabajo y familia en las sociedades industriales' in I. del Val y otras (coords.) *La historia de las mujeres: una revisión historiográfica* (Valladolid: Universidad de Valladolid-AEIHM).

Shteir, A. B. and Lightman, B. (2006), *Figuring it out. Science, Gender and Visual Culture* (Hanover, NH: Darmouth College Press).

Silver, L. L. (2012), 'Rational Approaches to Antibacterial Discovery: Pre-Genomic Directed and Phenotypic Screening' in Dougherty, T. J. and Pucci, M. J. (eds) *Antibiotic Discovery and Development* (New York: Springer) pp. 45–6.

Stapley, E. O., Hendlin, D., Mata, J. M., Jackson, M., Wallick, H., Hernández, S., Mochales, S., Currie, S. A. and Miller, R. M. (1969), 'Phosphomycin. I. Discovery and In Vitro biological characterisation', *Antimicrobial Agents and Chemotherapy* 9, 284–90.

Vicedo, M. (2009), 'The father of ethology and the foster mother of ducks: Konrad Lorenz as expert on motherhood', *Isis* 100, 263–91.

Woodruff, H. B. (1981), 'A soil microbiologist's odyssey', *Annual Review of Microbiology* 35, 1–28.

PART II
Contraceptives for Women:
Between Users and Prescribers

Chapter 4

Spermicides and their Female Users After World War II: North and South

Ilana Löwy

Spermicides: From Disreputable Preparations to 'Ethical Drugs'

Birth control is a very complicated issue: it has biological aspects and socio-cultural ramifications, and articulates anatomy and physiology, psychology and sexual desire, culture, religion, law, economy and politics. On the other hand, the fundamental problem of birth control can be presented as a simple one: how to prevent a fertilising encounter between a sperm and an egg. Before the advent of hormonal contraception, this could be done through the use of mechanical devices that prevented contact between sperm and egg, such as a diaphragm, cervical cap or condom; through the use of chemical substances which, when placed in the vagina, inactivated sperm cells; or through a combination of these two approaches. Contraceptive preparations dwelled for a long time on the boundary between official and quack medicine. They suffered from a double opprobrium: religious and cultural resistance to birth control, and the proximity between contraception and the prevention of sexually transmitted diseases. So-called 'female hygiene' products – frequently a code name for substances designed to prevent conception or produce abortion – were sold in pharmacies alongside condoms as protection against venereal infections, and were therefore associated with an amoral life. Links with sexually transmitted infections (STIs) facilitated the diffusion of contraceptives, but at the same time, strengthened their marginal status (Woycke 1988; McLaren 1990; Brodie 1994; Tone 2001).

In the 1920s and 1930s, efforts to limit conception focused on women-controlled contraceptives: that is, on strongly gendered technologies (Cowan 1989 and 2001). Advocates of birth control – at that time a heteroclite coalition of liberal physicians and scientists, feminists, and activists – had multiple goals: to help all women improve the quality of their sexual life and therefore strengthen their partnerships; enable birth spacing and improve maternal and child health; reduce suffering and misery among the poor; and limit the number of children born to lower class parents. A sincere wish to help women who suffered from the economic, social and emotional consequences of unplanned pregnancies was frequently intermingled with eugenic aspirations (Soloway 1995a and 1995b).

In the interwar era, scientists, physicians and activists who promoted birth control strived to dissociate contraception from its disreputable connections with illicit sex and prostitution, and transform it into a mainstream activity. This endeavour included a systematic effort to transform contraceptives– especially chemical contraceptives (or spermicides) used by women – into ethical drugs, sold in mainstream pharmacies and regulated in the same way as legitimate pharmaceutical preparations. They promoted scientific testing of spermicides in the laboratory, and their presentation as specific drugs, aimed solely at conception prevention. The new image of spermicides aspired to dissociate these preparations from dubious links with STIs. In the post war era, promoters of birth control in industrialised countries continued their efforts to improve contraceptive preparations. At that time, however, the status of 'chemical contraceptives' had undergone a radical shift. The fear of a 'population explosion' legitimated a large scale diffusion of contraceptives among the 'exploding populations' of the Global South, perceived as a threat to the economic and political stability of the Western world. The key issue was no longer respectability, but efficacy. The main promoters of chemical contraceptives were population experts, whose principal aspiration was to slow down population growth through the transformation of women from colonial and post-colonial countries ('targets') into 'faithful contraceptors' (Connelly 2008; for a feminist perspective see Hartmann 1987). The chemical preparations were often the same, but the expectations linked with these preparations were not.

Testing Spermicides in the Clinic: the US Experience

In the interwar era, birth control clinics in Europe and North America promoted the diaphragm-jelly method. This method combined the use of a diaphragm, a mechanical device that prevented the entry of sperm to the fallopian tubes, and a spermicidal jelly, a chemical preparation that killed spermatozoids (Himes 1949). The superiority of the 'diaphragm and jelly' method was deduced from theoretical considerations. Nevertheless, doctors observed that when used faithfully by motivated couples this approach worked reasonably well. In his review of a 1928 book on sexual behaviour in man, Bronislaw Malinowski, an enthusiastic supporter of birth control (he corresponded with many key activists in this area, including Margaret Sanger, Robert Lou Dickinson, Marie Stopes, Cecil Voge and Norman Hines), explained that in all human societies marriage was related to sex and sexual pleasure, but 'the true innovation of our time is the ubiquity of sex, the extraordinary freedom of movement of young and adults alike, the ease of prevention of conception'.[1] Thanks to the availability of contraception, Malinowski argued in the late 1920s, the sexual revolution had already taken place.

The diaphragm-jelly method, although viewed in the interwar era as the best method for preventing conception, had major drawbacks. The diaphragm had to

---

1   Malinowski, B. (n.d. c1928/1929), Review of Schmalhausen's book of 1928, Bronislaw Malinowski's papers, 29:16. London: London School of Economics' Archives.

initially be fitted by a health professional. Then women had to be taught how to use the method and follow instructions faithfully, a process many found messy and unpleasant. But perhaps the most severe limitation of this contraceptive method was that it was very difficult to use by women who lived in crowded conditions and had no access to a private bathroom. Hence the aspiration to develop simple spermicides: chemical preparations that when placed in the vagina before a sexual encounter would prevent conception. An ideal chemical contraceptive was expected to be safe, reliable, easy to apply, pleasant, and inexpensive. Such a preparation had a double goal: to ease the lives of all women, and promote the use of contraceptives among those poor women unable or unwilling to use existing birth control methods. In the interwar era, researchers attempted to develop better spermicides, or, alternatively, to encourage manufacturers of commercial spermicidal preparations to improve their products (Soloway 1995b; Löwy 2011). In the UK, efforts to produce an ideal spermicide led to the manufacture of Volpar (for VOLuntary PARenthood), a product hailed by the manufacturer as vastly superior to its competitors (Baker, Ranson and Tynen 1938). In the US, comparative tests of spermicides and the introduction of evaluation of these substances by the publication *Consumer Reports*, led to a greater homogenisation of physicochemical properties, chemical composition and shelf life of commercially sold spermicides.[2]

In the 1920s and 1930s the efficacy of spermicides was investigated nearly exclusively in a test tube (Voge 1933; Baker 1935; Brown, Levenstein and Becker 1943). New preparations, such as Volpar, were marketed after a very limited testing of their ability to prevent conception (Baker, Ranson and Tynen 1938). Scientists who studied contraception recognised, however, that an activity measured in the laboratory did not necessarily parallel activity in a woman's body (Millman 1952). They also understood that the real-life efficacy of a contraceptive preparation reflected not only its technical efficacy, but also its acceptability: that is, women's willingness to use the preparation in a consistent way. Hence the importance of spermicide field trials. A few small-scale trials of chemical contraceptives conducted in the 1940s confirmed that, when used regularly, chemical contraceptives did reduce fertility. These studies also indicated that the superiority of the diaphragm and jelly method over spermicide alone was exaggerated, because the theoretical advantages of a double protection were often nullified by the practical difficulty of applying the method correctly (Garvin 1944; Siebels 1944; Eastman 1949; Eastman and Siebels 1949). The latter conclusion needed, however, to be confirmed in large-scale field trials. Participants of such trials were generally recruited among clients of birth control clinics, thus among poorer and less educated women (middle class women often received contraceptive prescriptions from their physicians), often seen as inconsistent and unreliable. Lydia deVillbis, a physician who tested 'simple contraceptives'

2 Consumers Union of USA (1937), Analysis of contraceptives [Leaflet] Clarence J. Gamble papers, 1920–1966, HMS c23. Boston: Countway Medicine, Depository of Rare Books (subsequently, Gamble papers, 119: 3154).

among Black women in Florida, explained she had learned even a simple method would not be used on every occasion by the class of patients in her investigations (deVilbiss 1938, 19).

A study of the clinical efficacy of contraceptive suppositories, conducted by the pioneer of contraceptive studies, Clarence Gamble (1894–1966), illustrates this point. Heir to the Procter & Gamble fortune, Gamble studied medicine and initially attempted to become an academic medical researcher. He was not happy, however, with this career choice. Thanks to a chance encounter with the director of the National Committee for Maternal Health (NCMH), Robert Lou Dickinson, Gamble learned about the need to develop scientific research on contraception, and decided to dedicate all his efforts, and part of his personal fortune, to such research (Williams 1978; Reed 1978). In the interwar era, Gamble was mainly interested in the improvement and standardisation of commercial preparations of local contraceptives marketed in the US. He developed laboratory tests of the spermicidal activity of these preparations, and published annual comparisons of the test-tube activity of substances on the US market (Löwy 2011). Gamble studied contraceptive suppositories together with Christopher Tietze, the head statistician of NCMH, in a study funded by the Alabama State Board of Health and Alabama League of Planned Parenthood, recruiting women from impoverished rural areas in Alabama. Later, Gamble and Tietze asserted that the decision to conduct an investigation in this setting had been a mistake, as it was impossible to trust the information provided by the women. Participants provided inaccurate data about their sexual history, sexual life, and their use of contraceptives. Women who did not get pregnant claimed to use the contraceptive suppositories as instructed, but once a pregnancy had occurred, two out of three 'admitted' an irregular use. The trial was condemned to failure, Gamble and Tietze concluded, because the population they studied was 'backward, poorly educated, shiftless and irresponsible' (Tietze and Gamble 1948, 36).

The most ambitious effort to organise a large scale clinical trial of chemical contraceptives was made in the late 1950s and early 1960s by Mary Steichen Calderone, medical director of the Planned Parenthood Federation of America (PPFA) (Meldrum 1994 and 1996; Marks 2000). Calderone aspired to demonstrate that, if correctly instructed, women of all social strata could learn how to control their fertility. A secondary goal was to show that the diaphragm, increasingly seen at that time as poorly adapted for mass distribution due to its low acceptability, was not essential; that a 'chemical contraceptive' alone could provide reasonable protection from unwanted pregnancies. The Clinical Investigation Program (CIP), coordinated by Calderone, was conducted in numerous PPFA-affiliated clinics. Its aim, Calderone explained, was to rate methods, not products. The CIP, planned and supervised by Tietze and his wife, the statistician Sarah Levitt, put a strong emphasis on a correct methodology of experimentation in clinics, especially concerning randomisation, an element absent from earlier field trials of contraceptives. Another important innovation was direct collaboration with the pharmaceutical laboratories supplying the products under test. Despite the careful preparation of this clinical trial, birth control centres that participated in CIP systematically reported difficulties in ascertaining whether the women who participated were faithfully employing the prescribed method and providing accurate data about protected and unprotected sexual encounters.[3]

The CIP confirmed earlier indications that the use of chemical contraceptives alone, in field conditions, was only marginally less efficient than the use of a barrier method and spermicide. 'The best method for the patient', Calderone explained, 'is the one the patient will use consistently'.[4] Hence the importance of providing women with a choice of contraceptive methods, and offering those who were not pleased with the first method they had selected the possibility to switch to a different one. The goal of transforming lower class women in industrialised countries into 'faithful contraceptors', CIP organisers concluded, could not be achieved without taking into consideration their tendency to vote with their feet. This tendency also explains why the CIP did not end as planned. In the early 1960s, patients enrolled in CIP became increasingly tempted away by a new, simple, and highly efficient contraceptive: the pill.

Among the products tested in the CIP trial were Durafoam vaginal tablets, manufactured by Durex Products. The Durex company (for DUrability, Reliability and EXperience) had initially specialised in condoms, but in the 1930s branched out to the production of lubricants and female contraceptives. Durafoam tablets were included in the general CIP trial, but were also tested in a separate field trial in Cleveland, conducted by Dr Janet Dingle. Although this trial was officially founded by NCMH, the money came from a different source. For Tietze this was an episode that illustrated the continuing lack of respectability that contraceptives held: 'some people on the board of the foundation wanted to give money for contraceptive research but others were against it, so they gave the grant indirectly, to NCMH, something that today may be called "laundering of money"'. The Cleveland project was indeed funded in a very complex way. In 1958, Nathaniel Elias, the director and owner of Durex Products, secured a grant of $10,000 from the New York Foundation, to test Durafoam tablets and compare their efficacy to an older product, Durex vaginal jelly. The money was then channelled by the New York Foundation to NMHC, which provided a respectable front. Frederick Osborn, the director of the Population Council – a Rockefeller-founded organisation officially dedicated to the investigation of a broad range of population issues, but in practice

---

3   Mary Calderone to Mrs Fergunson, February 26, 1960; Mary Calderone, memorandum, 29 September, 1959. Harvard University, Schlesinger Library, (Cambridge, MA), Mary Steichen Calderone papers, 1904–1983, 179/ M-125 (subsequently, Calderone's papers), 5:69; CIP, reports from individual testing centers, 1958–1960. Calderone's papers, 5:70–76, and 6:77–84.

4   Mary Calderone to Dr Goodrich Schauffler, July 14, 1960. Calderone's papers, 9:155; Calderone to Tietze, December 29, 1960. Calderone's papers, 9:192.

focused on the development of methods which would slow population growth – informed Tietze about the existence of this grant.[5]

At that time, the Population Council was interested in foam tablets. Frank Notestain, the Population Council's second director, believed that the Durafoam clinical trial was of great importance, because 'the foam tablet seems to be the most hopeful for the immediate use in those areas where simplicity of procedure and low costs are essential', a statement which can be directly related to the neo- and post-colonialist attitudes of the 'population control' entrepreneurs at that time (Connelly 2008). On the other hand, the Council did not wish to be directly associated with the testing of contraceptives. Tietze passed the information about a grant for testing the Durafoam tablets to one of his CIP correspondents, Julia Brown. Brown successfully applied for the grant and, together with Janet Dingle, organised the testing of tablets in birth control clinics in Cleveland. She understood, however, that the money came from the Population Council, and mentioned the Council in an early communication of the trial's result. The Population Council's president, Frederick Osborn, was distressed by this misunderstanding, and insisted the Council was able to recruit important sums of money from different foundations because it maintained its position as a scientific group not engaged in the practical application of birth control.[6]

Nathaniel Elias remained in close contact with Julia Brown and Janet Dingle, the coordinators of the Cleveland Durafoam trial. In 1960, through Tietze's mediation, he negotiated the prolongation and extension of the Cleveland clinical trial. Dingle was pleased by this expansion and added: 'I'm sure that we can work out a mutually satisfactory financial arrangement.' However, the trial's results were not encouraging. Durafoam tablets were not very efficient, and, moreover, many women found them more unpleasant to use than other spermicidal preparations (Dingle and Tietze 1963). Women who participated in the CIP held a similar opinion. Calderone wrote to Elias in 1961: 'I'm under the impression that as much as I have pushed the use of Durafoam tablets, it is one of the less popular methods, and this is the reason why tests on it are so difficult to arrange.'[7]

One of Durafoam's main competitors was Emko, a vaginal foam developed by a self-taught entrepreneur, Joseph Sunnen. Emko was popular with the CIP participants as it was easy to apply (it was packaged in single dose plastic applicators,

---

5   Frederick Osborn to Christopher Tietze, 5 June 1958. Sleepy Hollow, NY: Rockefeller Archives Center, Population Council papers, records group IVB4.4a, National Committee on Maternal Health materials (subsequently, NCMH papers), 75:1405.

6   Frank Notestein to David Heyman. 18 March, 1960. NCMH papers, 75:1405; Christopher Tietze to Julia Brown, 9.6.1958. NCMH papers, 75:1405; Frederick Osborn to Julia Brown, 22 September 1958, NCMH papers, 75:1405; Frederick Osborn to Christopher Tietze, 30 September, 1958. NCMH papers, 75:1405.

7   Nathaniel Elias to Janet Dingle, 22 September 1958. NCMH papers, 75:1405; Janet Dingle to Nathaniel Elias, 5 February 1960. NCMH papers, 75:1405; Mary Calderone to Nathaniel (Nat) Elias, 31 July, 1961. NCMH papers, 81:1540.

at that time a major innovation), and, unlike other spermicide preparations, had a pleasant aroma. Moreover, Sunnen enthusiastically and aggressively promoted his invention (Meldrum 1996).[8] Sunnen hoped to distribute Emko throughout both the US and developing countries, and financed several field trials of the product in Puerto Rico (Briggs 2002, 123–8). He was one of several 'contraceptive entrepreneurs' who combined, in unknown proportions, a desire to help women, especially those from lower social strata and poorer countries, a hope of reducing the (perceived) risks of uncontrolled population growth, and aspirations to sell their products on new, expanding markets. Such entrepreneurs became central to efforts to curb population control in developing countries through the sale of spermicides. However, in these countries – and only there – other activists were promoting an alternative approach: homemade contraceptives.

Clarence Gamble's Quest for 'Simple Methods'

In the aftermath of WWII, major advances in health care, especially those that had greatly reduced child mortality (vaccines, antibiotics, and improved nutrition) were perceived as a mixed blessing and a potential threat to humanity's future. Influential books, such as Fairfield Osborn's 1948, *Our Plundered Planet*, and William Vogt's *Road to Survival* of the same year, linked uncontrolled population growth to the destruction of natural equilibrium, which would lead to famine, war, the collapse of Western social order (identified with civilisation) and, a major fear for many, the rise of Communism. In 1952, Abraham Stone, medical director of the Margaret Sanger Research Bureau and a leading advocate of birth control, quoting from a 1950 speech by Jaime Rorres Bodet, Director General of Unesco, bemoaned the fact that a control of death, achieved through the recent progress of medicine, was not accompanied by a control of life: the reduction of birth rates. The combination of a rapid increase in population with an absence of a parallel increase in food resources was a recipe for future disaster. If food production could not be brought into balance with increases in population, humanity would face an unprecedented catastrophe (Stone 1952). The growing fear of the 'population bomb', led in 1952 to the foundation of two influential organisations: the above mentioned Population Council, and the International Planned Parenthood Federation (IPPF).

The diaphragm-jelly method, already difficult to promote in industrialised countries, was seen as impossible to advance among women in non-Western ones. Only a tiny fraction of upper class women in these countries were viewed by these international organisations as having the financial means, living arrangements, and necessary 'intelligence' to use this contraceptive approach (Schoen 2005, 206–7). Among alternatives to commercial contraceptives, as suggested by birth control advocates, were concoctions that could be made by women themselves using ingredients found in their own kitchens. Marie Stopes recommended the use of

---

8   Interview with Lewit and Tietze, Family Planning Oral History.

cooking oil applied on a pre-prepared sponge or, if this was too expensive, on homemade cotton pads. Stopes claimed to have proposed the oil-sponge method in India as early as 1934, and found the method to be highly efficient when used correctly (Stopes 1952).

After WWII, 'homemade contraceptives' were enthusiastically promoted by Clarence Gamble. In the late 1940s and early 1950s, Gamble became increasingly preoccupied with the consequences of uncontrolled population growth, and transferred the focus of his activities to developing countries. At that time, Gamble strongly supported female sterilisation, an approach he called 'permanent contraception', and was also enthusiastic about 'eugenic sterilisation' (Gamble 1952, 1953a and 1953b). He was, however, aware of the difficulty of promoting, in non-Western countries, a technique which only a trained surgeon in a hospital setting could carry out. Gamble therefore turned his attention to the large-scale distribution of local contraceptives.

In the early stages of his intervention in developing countries, Gamble collaborated with local Planned Parenthood chapters and with IPPF, but in 1957 he founded his own organisation, the Pathfinder Fund. Initially, Pathfinder was a small enterprise, financed, operated and fully controlled by Gamble. Gamble hired women – usually single women or widows in their fifties – with some experience of charity or other administrative work, and sent them to developing countries to educate local people and dispense knowledge about contraception. Gamble's field workers, devoted to what he only half-jokingly called 'the great cause', were often overworked and underpaid. They were given only a minimal subsistence wage and were obliged to haggle with Gamble over every unplanned expense, however small. On the other hand, Gamble gave these women, many without formal training and bored with routine jobs, a unique occupational opportunity. As Pathfinder employees they travelled around the world and were free to organise their work as they wished. Gamble also took care of them if they became sick or depressed. Gamble's enterprise had clearly religious undertones, and field workers' tasks were modelled on that of Protestant missionaries. It is not surprising that those field workers who stayed with Pathfinder for a long time were, as a rule, fiercely devoted to Gamble.[9]

In the early 1950s, Gamble became interested in homemade contraceptives. Having experimented with a rice flour and salt jelly, he decided the rice was not really necessary, the best approach being to use a concentrated (20 per cent) salt solution on a sponge. Every woman could prepare such a solution in her kitchen, and use it successfully, if not to prevent pregnancies altogether, at least to space them considerably. The main issue was how to persuade women to apply the method every time they had sexual relations. Another issue was how to conserve plastic sponges: not only did they deteriorate in hot climates, cockroaches would destroy them.[10]

---

9   Mudd Emily. Interviewed by Reed James, 1974. Family Planning Oral History, Schlezinger Library.

10   Gamble to Marshall Balfour from the Rockefeller Foundation, 23.3.1951. Gamble papers, 205:3222. Gamble's notes on the rice flour jelly, Gamble's papers, 205:3230;

The idea of homemade contraceptives was strongly resisted by many birth control experts, who considered them inefficient and potentially risky. Mary Calderone explained that if one wanted a homemade method, withdrawal was at least as good.[11] Planning Parenthood activists were more sanguine. The founder of the Family Planning Association of India, Lady Rama Rau, argued that Gamble was promoting untested contraceptive methods in Asia that he would never have proposed for American women (Williams 1978). IPPF's staff accused Gamble not only of promoting ineffective methods, but also of lying to people: he distributed salt water, coloured and labelled to appear like a legitimate medication. Gamble's behaviour, his opponents claimed, was similar to that of Sunnen, the overzealous and uncritical promoter of Emko, with one important difference: Emko was a reasonably good contraceptive, while the salt solution did not work.[12] The conflict with IPPF surrounding the salt and sponge method was one of the main motivations behind Gamble's decision in 1957 to found his own organisation, Pathfinder.

The accusation that Gamble's collaborators enhanced saline to make it appear to be a medication was not entirely false. One of Gamble's field workers, Margaret Root, reported that in a Malaya clinic, a female doctor prepared a salt solution dyed with coloured vegetable dye, and sold it for a very small sum to her patients, who brought receptacles to fill.[13] Another contraception propagator, Mrs Erb from Singapore, coloured the salt solution, added perfume, put it in bottles with an official-looking label, and did not tell women it was merely salt and water until they started to use the method. There is no evidence that Gamble himself was in favour of such deceptive approaches. He nevertheless believed that, when used carefully and in a consistent way, the sponge-salt method was nearly as efficient as a diaphragm and strongly encouraged his field workers to promote this method, especially in rural settings. This was not always easy: health professionals were sceptical, while women complained about irritation, burning and other unpleasant side effects. Some women also resisted the use of a food stuff as a contraceptive.[14] Gamble, however, insisted that the salt solution was an ideal method for poor areas, as salt could be found in every household. He also believed the method

---

Gamble to his collaborator, Sue Pridle 28.2.1954. Gamble's papers, 206:3250; Gamble to Paul Reps, from Honolulu,12.12.1957. Gamble's papars, 209:3269; Bob McClure, from Ratlam Mission Hospital, India, to Gamble, 3.6.1958. Gamble's papers, 209:3282.

11   Interview with Mary Steichen Calderone, Interviewed by James Reed, 1974. Cambridge, MA: Schlesinger Library, Family Planning Oral History

12   Interview with Frances Hand Ferguson, president of PPFA (Planned Parenthood Federation of America), Interviewed by James Reed 1974, Family Planning Oral History.

13   Margaret Root. Notice on uses of simple contraceptives in Asia, 1954–1960. Undated, probably 1960. Gamble papers, 182:2870.

14   Edna McKinnon to Gamble, 17.11.1960. Gamble's papers, 184:2909; Gamble to Sarah Lewis, 2.9.1959, Gamble papers, 187:2935; McKinnon to Gamble, 17.11.1960, Gamble papers, 184:2909; McKinnon to Gamble, 19.11.1960, Gamble papers, 184:2909; Gamble to Margaret Root, 5.1.1962, Gamble papers, 182:2874; Gamble to Root, 15.8.1962, Gamble papers, 182:2876, Root to Gamble, 4.9.1962, Gamble papers, 182:2876.

should be made as simple as possible. Asking women to use boiled water added to the inconvenience of the salt and sponge method and, he suggested, should be omitted in places, except those where the water supply was truly problematic. Gamble was aware that women often preferred commercial preparations. In order to collect data on the efficacy and acceptability of the salt and sponge method, he explained, it should be introduced in places where women, 'do not know about other methods and will not be told about them by distributors of sponges'.

Opponents of the sponge and salt method claimed Gamble was 'trying to obliterate the dark races with a salt solution'.[15] But some of Gamble's field workers – Margaret Root for example – became enthusiastic converts to the use of salt as a contraceptive. Root continued to disseminate this approach in the early 1960s, a time when Pathfinder had become mainly interested in the distribution of intrauterine devices (IUDs). Women who refused IUDs or did not tolerate them well, she argued, could still benefit from a simple and efficient method of preventing conception. Root also claimed that the World Health Organization (WHO) had validated the efficacy of the salt-sponge method. Other Pathfinder field workers, such as Edna McKinnon, were more sceptical about the salt and sponge method, due to both its reported side effects and unproven efficacy, but also because Gamble's obstinate promotion of the method made cooperation with other organisations in the contraception arena difficult. Nevertheless, McKinnon found that in some places, such as Surabaja in Indonesia, women were pleased with the salt-sponge method. In Teheran, by contrast, all use of salt had been discontinued. Local health workers claimed that 'people here are so dirty, and they have so unhealthy vaginas, that the use of a poorly washed sponge with anything on it can be a source of their picking up more infection'.[16] Some women, apparently, were regarded as too backward to even use such an excessively simple contraceptive method.

Foam Tablets: A Panacea for Overcrowded Asia?

Gamble compared the efficacy of the salt and sponge method with the nearest commercially available alternative, foaming powder on a sponge. Such powders were developed in the 1930s and, unlike other female contraceptive preparations, were not greasy. They were tested by Hannah Stone, the medical director of the Margaret Sanger Research Bureau. Stone published the results of her first clinical

---

15   Gamble to Root, 25.9.1962, Gamble papers, 182:2876; Root to Gamble, 27.9.1962, Gamble papers, box 182:2876;Gamble to Root, 19.12.1962, Gamble papers, 182:2876; Gamble to Sarah Lewis, 2.9.1959, Gamble papers, 187:2935; Edna McKinnon to Gamble, 3.11.1960. Gamble's papers, 184:2909.

16   Margaret Root to Mary Bishop (who interviewed Root about her work with Pathfinder), 18.9.1968. Gamble's papers, 182:2888; McKinnon to Gamble, 7.8.1961. Gamble's papers, 184:2914; McKinnon to Gamble, 11.1.1961. Gamble's papers, 184:2912; McKinnon to Gamble, 8.2.1964. Gamble's papers, 184:2924.

investigations of foam powder in 1938 (Stone 1938). Margaret Sanger did not wait, however, for clinical test results before promoting the method. During her visit to India in 1935, Sanger attempted to persuade Gandhi that foaming powder would radically transform birth control, as it could be widely distributed by non-professionals and did not require a clinic visit (Schoen 2005, 31–3; Connelly 2008, 101). Sanger therefore promoted foam powder in Indian birth control clinics. The foam powder was a problematic contraceptive; many women complained of irritation, while others found the method unpleasant. In spite of Sanger's enthusiastic promotion of foam powder, the uptake of this contraceptive preparation in India remained very limited (Ahulwalia 2008, 65–9; Hodges 2008, 72–7).

Gamble became interested in the foam powder and sponge method in the 1930s, and participated in tests of the method in Florida (Ordover 2003, 255; Schoen 2005, 33). In the early 1950s, manufacturers of contraceptives began to market another, easier to apply contraceptive device: the foaming tablet. Such tablets, placed in the vagina immediately before sexual intercourse, acted like a sponge and foaming powder, but without the additional manipulation: dosing the powder on a sponge, correctly inserting the sponge, then retrieving it following intercourse. Foam tablets were relatively cheap, easy to store (usually in a glass bottle with a stopper), provided a reliable, fixed dose of the product, could be used in primitive living conditions (no bathroom was needed) and were reported to be stable in warm climates. In addition, the tablet could not be portrayed as a contraceptive destined for the 'dark races' alone: it was also sold in industrialised countries. Gamble became persuaded that foam tablets held the key to successful birth control in hot climates.

In the 1950s and early 1960s, Gamble's correspondence with his fieldworkers was often focused on the supply and distribution of foam tablets and foaming powders. Gamble frequently elected to distribute tablets manufactured in Asia, such as Contab produced in India, Sempori produced in South Korea, and Sampoon manufactured in Japan. These tablets were often cheaper than those produced in Europe or North America. On the other hand, Asian foam powders and tablets were thought less reliable by local populations with more interest in European or North American products. Margaret Root noted that in Ceylon (now Sri-Lanka) and South Korea, pharmacies sold only expensive foreign-produced tablets. When she asked why, she was informed that people did not trust local products. Birth control clinics often distributed foreign products as well, because they were obliged to pay for local tablets, but were frequently given tablets manufactured in the West.[17]

---

17 Gamble's materials for article on commercial contraceptive jellies and creams, secured in 1956. Gamble's papers, 213:3307; Gamble to McKinnon, 26.11.1961. Gamble's papers, 184:2915; Gamble's leaflet on simple methods of birth control, undated (probably 1955). Gamble's papers, 207:3255; Root to Gamble, 18.6.1962. Gamble's papers, 182:2875. Root to Gamble, 18.6.1962. Root to Gamble 18.9.1962. Gamble's papers, 182:2876.

Gamble had close contact with the mangers of Smith Stanistreet Ltd in Calcutta, the producers of the Contab tablet. He attempted to persuade the firm to improve the quality of their product through regular quality checks. When Contab failed to receive a marketing permit in the UK, Gamble suggested the Smith Stanistreet directors conduct tests of a new, improved formula for the tablet, which hopefully would gain UK approval. Such approval, Gamble felt, was important; its absence might also hamper the distribution of Contab in Asia. One of Pathfinder's field workers, Edna McKinnon, was involved in 1963 in an attempt to establish the production of a US foam tablet, Delfen, in Indonesia. The promoters of this project initially hoped to benefit from USAID (US Agency for International Development) funding. They discovered, however, that this was not possible as, at that time, USAID policy did not allow direct funding of birth control activities. Negotiations on the construction of a tablet-producing plant in Indonesia came to a halt. McKinnon proposed altering the definition of Delfen from a contraceptive to therapeutic agent, one which could protect women from venereal infections such as *Trichomonas vaginalis*. The US producers of Delfen tablets, she claimed, could provide proof their product actually reduced infection rates. However, USAID agents thought that Washington would view a redefinition of Delfen as pure subterfuge and, in all probability, the project would still be rejected. McKinnon mentioned a 'girlfriend' in Washington who might be able to intervene.[18] The 'girlfriend' was Leona Baumgartner, appointed in 1962 by President Kennedy to head the USAID Office of Technical Cooperation and Research. Baumgartner was credited with persuading President Johnson in 1965 to reverse the policy which forbade USAID to openly support birth control (Fowler 1991).

Foam tablets had a longer shelf life than 'traditional' spermicides, such as creams and jellies, but there were still serious problems surrounding their conservation in hot and humid climates. Contab tablets, Margaret Root complained, would sometimes swell, and could not be taken out of their glass bottles. Moreover, some doctors distributed tablets that appeared to be in a poor condition, greyish and crumbling. Gamble had discovered that the majority of foam tablets sold in India, including Contab, deteriorated after one to five months of storage. Only Sampoon and Sempori tablets were still active after a year on the shelf, but Gamble noted that these brands did not liberate much gas when placed in the vagina, and therefore might have a lower ability to prevent fertilisation (Gamble 1959). Another problem was that tablets were sometimes too expensive for distribution in cash-strapped birth control clinics. Foaming powders were usually cheaper, but it was necessary to teach women how to use them correctly.[19] An important

---

18 Gamble to Harvey, 25.5.1966. Harvey to Gamble, 9.9.1955. Gamble to Harvey, 3.10.1955. Gamble's papers, 207:3251; Gamble to Harvey, 3.10.1955. Gamble's papers, 207:3251; McKinnon to Gamble, 14.10.1963. Gamble's papers, 184:2923.

19 Margaret Root to Gamble, 6.10.55. Gamble's papers, 182:2860. Root to Gamble 22.2.1957. Gamble's papers, 182:2863; Gamble to Harvey, 15.1.1962. Gamble's papers, 214:3321; Edith Gates to Gamble, 8.10.1955. Gamble's papers, box 184, folder 2895.

proportion of the correspondence between Gamble and his field workers was dedicated to the comparison of prices and properties of different contraceptive preparations, evaluation of providers, attempts to secure gifts of contraceptives from manufacturers, and worries about shortages of tablets and powders in birth control clinics. For example, McKinnon and Gamble attempted to find the cheapest way of preparing the sponges distributed with foaming powder. They eventually decided to purchase large sheets of sponge, then cut them to the appropriate size with sharpened pipes, employed in a similar way to cookie cutters.[20]

The supply and distribution of tablets and foaming powders was only one side of the equation: another important issue was to ensure that women used the product, and could persuade their male partners not to resist such a use. Pathfinder started a home visit program in rural Indonesia, where houses were visited by a team of midwife and clerk. The results were not greatly impressive. Edna McKinnon believed that many women accepted tablets from house visitors because they did not want to be impolite, but either never used them or stopped after a short trial. The quantity of distributed tablets did not accurately reveal the number that would serve their purpose. In addition, many men objected to contraception, and women would often not dare to challenge their husbands. More education was needed, McKinnon argued, especially targeted at men.[21] In spite of the numerous obstacles to the successful distribution of foam tablets, Gamble was convinced the tablet was the right contraceptive solution for developing countries. In 1960 he informed C. A. Buxton, of the Smith Stanistreet Company, that an article on family planning in India, published in *Life* magazine on 23 November 1959, referred to foam tablets as the 'best method': 'this is quite a change since the time we first talked over the use of tablets in 1953, when you said that the company was doubtful of the value of continuing their manufacture'.[22]

The Competitive Market of Foam Tablets

Pathfinder did not intervene in India, probably at least partly because of the conflict between Gamble and the Family Planning Association of India. India was potentially a huge market for contraceptives, and the Indian brand of foam tablets, Contab, captured only a small segment. In the 1950s, two US producers of foam tablets began to compete on the Indian market: Fomos Laboratories (directed by Reuben Posner), and Durex Products. The owner of the latter company, Nathaniel

---

20   Gamble to Root, 20.6.1962. Gamble's papers, 182: 2875. McKinnon to Sunnen, 10.6.1963. Gamble's papers, 184:2918; McKinnon to Gamble, 1.3.61. Gamble's papers, 184:2913; Gamble to McKinnon, 16.6.1961. Gamble's papers, 184:2914; McKinnon to Gamble 14.3.1963. Gamble to McKinnon, 25.3.1963. McKinnon to Gamble, 28.5.1963. Gamble's papers, 184:2921.

21   Edna McKinnon to Hugh More, 21.11.1961. Gamble's papers, 184:2916.

22   Gamble to C.A. Buxton, 20.1.1960. Gamble's papers, 213:3312.

Elias, was married to the public health expert Leona Baumgartner (1902–1991). Baumgartner is best known for her tenure as Commissioner of Health of New York City (1954–1962) during which she made important contributions to improving the health of women and children (Fowler 1991; Malani 1991). In 1955, Baumgartner travelled to India, together with the demographer Frank Notestein, to advise the Indian government on family related issues, including contraception. This trip was funded by the Population Council.[23] During this visit Baumgartner and Elias discussed the possibility of the import and local production of foam tablets. Elias was also the main author of the 'Memorandum on Foaming Materials', annexed to the 'Report on Family Planning and Health Care', written jointly by Notestein and Baumgartner in December 1955.[24] This memorandum hailed preparations, such as Durafoam, that contained an active principle (alkyl phenoxy polyethoxy ethanol) long known to be efficient and safe, and criticised the Fomos tablet, because its active compound, hydroquinone, was less tested and thus potentially risky (Löwy 2011; Löwy 2012).

In 1955, advocates of the large-scale use of foam tablets in developing countries assumed the tablet would be efficient, but did not have proof this was the case. It was hoped that clinical trials conducted in Jamaica, Puerto Rico and India, would prove that foam tablets were indeed the right contraceptive for these countries. Initial reports of an early field trial of foam tablets (Volpar) conducted in Jamaica by Dr Lenwirth (Len) Jacobs were enthusiastic. This trial, however, was severely criticised by the demographer, Mayone Stykos, who claimed it was badly planned and executed.[25] In a memorandum to the Population Council, Stykos complained about the ignorance and amateurism of people who ran private programs of birth control in Jamaica: 'they tend to be foreigners or upper class locals who are imbued with the "lady bountiful" approach to social welfare. They ... fail to have a truly sensitive approach when dealing with lower classes. Instead of empathising with the patient they regard him (*sic*) as an inferior being who must be shown the light'. Stykos also criticised the absence of birth control propaganda targeting men, who, he argued, were the key to success in all efforts to limit population

---

23   Notestain to Baumgartner, 4.8.1955. Notestein's memorandum for the Population Council, 11.4.1956. Baumgardners's papers, 32: 1. Leona Baumgartner's papers, 1930-1970 Boston: Countway Medicine Library, Depository of Rare Books HMS c305, (subsequently, Baumgardner's papers), 41:5.

24   Leona Baumgartner and Frank Notestein, 'Report on Family Planning and Health Care', December 1955. Baumgardner's papers, 41:10; John Gordon, from Harvard Ludhiana project to Baumgartner, 21.2.1956. Baumgartner papers, 41:15. Baumgartner to Gordon, 1.3.1956. Baumgartner papers, 41:7.

25   'Jonas' (Reiner) to Elias and Baumgartner ('Leonat'), 20.2.1956. Baumgartner's papers, 41:10; Baumgartner to Notestein, 27.3.1956. Baumgartner's papes, 41:15. Notestein to Baumgardner, 2.4.1956, Baumgartner's papes, 41:5; Mayone Stykos to Notestein, 16.3.1956. Baumgartner's papers, 4:15; Notestein to Stykos, 19.3.1956. Baumgartner's papers, 41:15.

growth.[26] Elias, unsurprisingly, defended the Jamaican field trials, and claimed they demonstrated the efficacy of Durafoam.[27] During the 1960s, foam tablets continued to be employed in birth control clinics in Jamaica and many women had a positive opinion about them (Stykos and Back 1964, 60–63). However, in the late 1960s, the majority of the clients of birth control clinics on the island had switched to the contraceptive pill.[28]

Jamaica, a small British colony with a relatively well-developed medical infrastructure, was not, one might argue, a typical developing country. The results of clinical trials of foam tablets conducted in Puerto Rico were decidedly less encouraging. The pregnancy rate among couples that used foam tablets was 36 per 100 fertile couples per year. Emko foam was slightly more efficient: 29 per 100 fertile couples per year. The low efficacy of spermicides was attributed to their inconsistent use (Paniagua et al. 1961; Tietze et al. 1961). Nevertheless, couples who used the tablet had a lower fertility rate than those who did not use any contraceptive. The results of the most important clinical trial of foam tablets in a developing country, the India-Harvard Ludhiana population study in Khanna, Punjab, were even worse. The Khanna project, conducted by researchers from the Harvard School of Public Health, aimed to determine whether the distribution of foam tablets in Punjab villages would make a significant change in the rate of population increase. The project included detailed demographic observations and the controlled distribution of contraceptives to targeted families, but not the provision of medical care to local populations (Anon 1963; Connelly 2008, 171–3). The pilot phase of this project was conducted in 1955, with the definitive phase of the test scheduled to last from 1956 to 1960 (Rao 2004, 132–4). Manufacturers of foam tablets provided a supply without charge, hoping the Khanna project would demonstrate the efficacy of their products.[29] This, however, did not happen. The birth rate in the 'experimental villages' (where the tablets were distributed) was found to be higher than that in the 'control villages'. Only eight per cent of villagers became 'permanent acceptors', using the tablet for three months or more. The trial organisers concluded that, although people in Khanna claimed to want to limit their families to three children at most, they were not 'ready' to translate this

---

26   Memorandum from Mycone Stycos to Dudley Kirk and Robert (Bob) Snider, from Population Council, April 1958, Sleepy Hollow, New York: Rockefeller Archive Center (Population Council papers, subsequently Population Council papers), 11:149.

27   Elias to Tietze, 17.11.1958. Population Council papers, 75:1405.

28   Report of the Jamaica Family Planning Association for 1968. Harvard University, Schlesinger Library (Cambridge, MA), Emily Mudd Papers, M-103 (subsequently Mudd papers) 5:421.

29   Warren Nelson from Population Council to Gamble, 26.12.1956. Gamble's papers, 220:3397; R.P. Harvey to Gamble, 4.4.1955. Gamble's papers, 206:3251; John B. Wyon, from Harvard Ludhiana project to Leona Baumgartner, 29.5.1956. Baumgartner's papers, 41:15.

claim into concrete action (Anon 1963). This trial later became synonymous with inefficiency and scientific hubris (Connelly 2008, 171–2; Löwy 2011).

Christopher Tietze compared the low efficacy of foam tablets with the high efficacy of methods disseminated in the 1960s: hormonal contraception, IUDs and sterilisation.[30] Indeed, with the advent of these new contraceptive approaches, foam tablets and similar preparations lost much of their appeal. On the other hand, the trajectory of a drug is not defined exclusively by its 'technical efficacy': that is, its ability to produce specific physiological effects in ideal conditions of use. Relatively inefficient devices can still circulate, have effects, and generate income (Bonah et al. 2009). They can also find new uses.

The Second Life of Vaginal Spermicides: Prevention of Sexually Transmitted Diseases

In the 1960s, development of new products radically modified the contraception domain. Tietze wrote to Calderone in October 1961, stating that a study of the acceptability of the first hormonal contraception pill, Enovid, would be a waste of time (Ignaciuk, Ortiz-Gómez and Rodríguez-Ocaña, this volume; Thoms, this volume and references therein).[31] On the other hand, hormonal contraceptives were not problem-free drugs. The main difficulty, as promoters of the pill rapidly discovered, was the possible side effects (on its carcinogenic effect and woman movements in Germany, Stoff, this volume). The theoretical efficacy of the contraceptive pill was far higher than that of the older contraceptive methods, but its real-life efficacy depended on steady use. Condoms, diaphragms and local contraceptives were efficient each time they were used correctly. The pill was efficient only if taken every day. Clarence Gamble had noted that, 'one quarter of users stop because of undesirable effects, and when they do stop, pregnancy is often very prompt'.[32] The history of the pill in Western countries is one of permanent adjustments through the monitoring of adverse reactions. In addition, thanks to the diversification of products, women who found one kind of contraceptive pill problematic were able, with the help of their doctors, to switch to a different formula. The need for a medical surveillance of the pill's undesirable effects hampered the large-scale dissemination of oral hormonal contraception outside Western Europe and North America. The pill, initially conceived as a 'magic bullet' which would curb population growth in poorer parts of the world, actually had a relatively low impact in these countries (Watkins 1998; Marks 2001; Marsh and Ronner 2008).

Other new contraceptive methods became popular in the Global South in the 1960s: Depo Provera (a long lasting hormonal injection), IUDs, and sterilisation

---

30   Interview with Sarah Lewit and Christopher Tietze, 1975, Schlesinger Library, Family Planning Oral History.

31   Tietze to Calderon, 3.10.1961. NCMH papers, RAC, 81:1540.

32   Gamble to Ruth Martin, 25.9.1961. Gamble's papers, 188:2926.

(on IUDs see Tone 1999 and 2001). These contraceptive methods had two things in common: their implementation relied on health professionals, and they were 'user independent' – it was not necessary to apply them before each sexual intercourse and they could not be abandoned on a whim. Effects of a Depo Provera injection lasted several months; a woman had to see a health provider to have her IUD removed; and sterilisation was irreversible. Technology provided a solution to what was perceived as the major obstacle for the diffusion of birth control practices among women in non-industrialised countries (as well as poor women in Western countries) – the difficulty of transforming all women into 'faithful contraceptors'. Prior to the 1960s, the consistent use of a chosen contraceptive method, in spite of any possible drawbacks, was implicitly linked with the acceptance of middle class, Western values. User-independent methods, experts hoped, would be efficient without the need to make 'them' – women of colour; uneducated, poor, impulsive, unreliable, unruly – more like 'us' – white women; educated, affluent, reasonable, and capable of self control (Hartmann 1987). Tietze had already argued that the strong earlier preference for the (discrete) 'diaphragm-jelly' methods in birth control clinics, and the rejection of (vulgar and tasteless) condoms, reflected the middle class values of the organisers of these clinics.[33]

Some population control activists were aware of the risk of promoting IUDs, hormonal injections or sterilisation in the absence of an adequate medical infrastructure. Gamble explained in 1962 that IUDs should be distributed exclusively to gynaecologists with sufficient experience of their insertion. Tietze similarly insisted on the slow and careful introduction of IUDs. He feared that, 'if anything goes wrong, it would block the whole intrauterine program'. Margaret Root strongly disagreed:

> ... if there are some failures, even a death or two, it could NOT probably do real damage to the IUD case in the world. There would be 98 per cent successes which is good for any new thing. How many are dying over testing the Nuclear atom, tranquilizers, jets, etc, yet no one says 'wait 2-3 years'. Let us be sensible and sensitive to others. Let those whose thinking is ONLY West, not interfere in the EAST.[34]

Root expressed an opinion that prevailed over Tietze and Gamble's more prudent approaches, and which resonated with policies adopted in the 1960s by many international organisations (Weisz and Olszenko-Gryn 2010). Enthusiastic population controllers in the 1960s and 1970s, who propagated 'modern' contraceptive techniques in developing countries, frequently failed to pay sufficient attention to safety issues. Hurried insertions of IUDs, mass injections

---

33   Interview with Leavit and Tietze, 1975.

34   Gamble to Margaret Roots 12.9.62. Gamble's papers, 183:2876; Gamble to Roots, 22.10. 1962. Gamble's Papers, 183:2876; Roots to Gamble 30.10.62. Gamble's papers, 183:2876. Capitals in the text.

of Depo Provera, and accelerated sterilisation campaigns, produced harmful side effects, and in many cases led to rejection of the promoted contraceptive method (Hartmann 1987; Connelly 2008).

The distribution of 'modern contraceptives' in developing countries was facilitated by a change in US population policies. In 1965, the US President, Lyndon Johnson, declared that the multiplying problems of multiplying populations were the most profound challenge to the future of the world, and gave priority to programs designed to deal with that urgent issue. The result was an important increase in funds for population control, especially those channelled via the Population Bureau of USAID. The bureau's director, Reimert Ravenholt, came to hold remarkable power (Connelly 2008). Ravenholt employed charities and NGOs active in the population field to implement activities not permitted for a US governmental agency, such as direct distribution of contraceptives, diffusion of IUDs, sterilisation and abortion. USAID's new policy favoured an unprecedented growth of these organisations. In 1968, the Pathfinder Fund's budget was $271,900; 44 per cent of which ($119,400) was donated by USAID. In 1972, the fund's budget was $3,338,750; with 86 per cent ($2,887,850) coming from USAID. The predicted USAID donation for 1973 was $4,000,000.[35] USAID generously financed other organisations as well: thus, in the early 1970s it contributed more than 50 per cent of IPPF's budget. In 1973, nearly half of USAID's total allocation was dedicated to population control. With the changing attitudes to population control, the Population Council, originally an organisation dedicated to research and counselling, became increasingly involved in the supply of contraception (Warwick 1982, 44–67).

In the 1960s and 1970s, spermicides occupied a modest but non-negligible niche among contraceptives provided by USAID. Ravenholt believed the availability of non-prescription contraceptives such as condoms and spermicides, greatly increased uptake of these products. He was therefore in favour of the large-scale distribution of these contraceptive means in family planning clinics (Ravenholt 1977). Accordingly, in the early 1970s, three to five per cent of the USAID Population Bureau contraceptive budget was dedicated to women-controlled local contraceptives (Belsky 1975). In some places, the lower efficacy of these contraceptive methods was compensated for by the availability of abortion. For example, in Bangladesh, USAID promoted the distribution of spermicides, but also (via Pathfinder) 'menstrual regulation': an abortion performed up to ten weeks of amenorrhea without a pregnancy test by a paramedical Family Welfare Visitor; the visitor would then often propose the patient underwent sterilisation or accept an IUD.[36] Following Nathaniel Elias's death in 1964, USAID purchased Durex Products, Inc. In 1968, USAID shipped a large quantity of bulk Durafoam to Pakistan and Colombia. It was later discovered that the Food and

---

35 Pathfinder, 'In office memorandum on finances', 13.10.1972. Mudd's papers, 11:482.

36 Pathfinder's brochure, Bangladesh, 1981–1982. Mudd's papers, 11:493.

Drug Administration (FDA) had not approved the marketing of Durafoam as a contraceptive in the US. This was a problematic finding, since USAID's policy was to ship abroad only products with FDA endorsement.[37]

In the 1970s, there was a small revival of interest in chemical contraceptives in Western countries. Some Western women, dissatisfied with the pill and IUDs, returned to older contraceptive methods (Belsky 1975; for a feminist point of view see Bruce 1987). At that time, researchers observed a recrudescence of venereal diseases, attributed to the double effect of increasingly liberal sexual mores and the declining fear of these diseases. Spermicides, some investigators argued, could protect women from STIs. The argument that spermicides could prevent the transmission of venereal infections had been perceived in the early 1960s as a subterfuge to facilitate the import and production of contraceptives. In 1961, Nathaniel Elias proposed to Gamble that Durafoam tablets should be imported as a drug to combat *Trichomonas vaginalis*, then be distributed as contraceptives. Two years later, Edna McKinnon employed the same argument to enable the use of USAID funds to finance the manufacture of Delfen foam tablets in Indonesia.[38] In the 1970s, when spermicides had lost much of their importance as contraceptives, the argument that they might protect women from venereal disease led to renewed interest. Several research programs were established to test this hypothesis.

One of the leaders of investigations on STI prevention through the application of vaginal contraceptives was John Cutler (1915–2003). Cutler later became (in)famous for his early 1960s contribution to the Tuskegee syphilis experiment, in which Black patients in Tuskegee, Alabama, were denied access to efficient anti-syphilis medication, and his continued defence of this experiment, included in several public declarations (Jones 1993; Cutler 1993; Reverby 2000 and 2009).[39] In 2010, the uncovering of unethical human experiments by Cutler and his colleagues in Guatemala in 1947–1948, in which thousands of people, including psychiatric patients, were infected with venereal diseases without their consent, further harmed his reputation (Reverby 2011; Presidential Commission for the Study of Bioethical Issues 2011). In the 1970s, however, Cutler, who at that time was a professor of public health at the University of Pittsburgh and a respected expert on infectious diseases, received a five-year grant, 'Research services directed towards the development of a combined agent for disease prophylaxis and contraception, AID/csd contrat n° 2822', for 1970–1975, a total sum of $719,284. He and his co-workers tested the prophylactic properties of Conceptrol Creme (Ortho), a preparation based on Nonoxynol-9. Cutler had previously attempted to develop a local protection against syphilis for men (Mapharsen-Orvus), one

---

37   Raymond Belsky's report of 13.7.70. Princeton N.J.: Princeton University Library, Department of Rare Books and Special Collections Frank Notestein's papers, 1930–1977, Population Council Office Communications, 10:6.

38   Elias to Gamble, 10.2.1061. Gamble papers, 213:3315; McKinnon to Gable, 14.10.1963. Gamble papers, 184:2923.

39   Interview with Cutler in Nova TV documentary The Deadly Deception 1993.

of the main subjects of his 1947–1948 human experiments in Guatemala. With his colleague, Balwant Singh, Cutler investigated the prevention of STIs in women. From an epidemiological point of view, Cutler and Singh explained, one could see an unwanted pregnancy as a sexually transmitted condition. Hence the interest in a method that could prevent both conditions. A double epidemic of teen pregnancies and recrudescence of venereal infections increased interest in a 'pro-con' (prophylaxis-contraception) approach (Singh and Culter 1979). Cutler and Singh discovered that a wide range of commercial local contraceptives killed sexually transmitted pathogens in a test tube. These preparations also lowered the rates of gonorrhea and herpes infection in women (Cutler et al. 1973).

In the late 1980s, efforts to find a way to protect women from HIV were closely linked to an earlier search for vaginal preparations able to protect women from venereal infections. For example, Cutler and his colleague Richard Arnold, explained in 1988 that efforts to control AIDS should be grounded in approaches to limit the spread of STIs (Cutler and Arnold 1988). In the 1970s and 1980s, three US programs studied the intersections between the prevention of pregnancy and of STIs: the Program for Applied Research on Fertility Regulation (PARFR) at the Northwestern University Medical School, Chicago; Family Health International (FHI), a USAID supported organisation, at the University of Carolina at Chapel Hill; and CONRAD, also established with USAID funds at the East Virginia Medical School. The first director of Family Health International was Elton Kessel, an epidemiologist and the President and Executive Director of the Pathfinder Fund in Boston from 1966 to 1969. Kessel recruited another leading researcher from Pathfinder, Roger P. Bernard, author of one of the first studies of the efficacy of IUDs. In the late 1980s and the 1990s, FHI, PARFR and CONRAD were involved in the first attempts to develop women-controlled protection against HIV infection – an anti-HIV microbicide. The initial candidates for such a microbicide were contraceptive substances already tested for their anti-bacterial and anti-Chlamydia activity (Germain et al. 1992).

The 'official' genealogy of anti-HIV microbicides has often downplayed the continuities between earlier studies of venereal disease prevention in women and the search for women-controlled ways to prevent AIDS. The search for microbicides has been presented as an entirely new line of investigation, originating in the growing realisation that while men could use condoms, women had no way to protect themselves from HIV infection. Activists involved in microbicide research explained that this line of research originated in a felicitous encounter between scientists looking for ways to slow the spread of HIV, and feminists concerned by the exclusive focus on condoms – that is, on the goodwill of men – as a means of preventing AIDS (Stein 1990).

The 'official' history of microbicides usually begins in the 1990s, when a series of conferences, some financed by the Population Council, brought together activists and scientists interested in the development of a 'simple microbicide': a substance which, when applied locally, would diminish the frequency of HIV transmission. Anti-HIV microbicides were portrayed by their advocates as a women-controlled technology, despite the fact that some homosexual men were also interested in the use of microbicides as protection during anal intercourse. At first these women-centred programs had a relatively limited scope, but c2000 they gathered momentum, and mobilised important funds (Bell 2003). This historical presentation, while accurate so far as the activist-scientist alliance goes, fails to take into account the involvement of organisations such as FHI and CONRAD in microbicide studies, and the fact that the first candidate anti-HIV microbicide was nonoxynol-9, a spermicide extensively tested in the 1970s and 1980s for its microbicidal and virucidal properties. Nonoxynol-9 was elected as it already had a marketing permit (that is, it had been shown to be safe for vaginal application), had demonstrated anti-bacterial activity in earlier field trials, and had killed HIV in a test tube.

The high hopes for nonoxynol-9, however, were dashed. In the late 1990s, several clinical trials demonstrated that the product not only failed to protect women from HIV, but actually increased their vulnerability to this pathogen, probably because at concentrations needed to kill the virus it induced irritation of the vaginal mucosa (although it later did turn out to be effective, see Hillier et al. 2005; Vieira et al. 2008). This effect of nonoxynol-9 had already been indicated by a 1989 study; this study was, however, initially discarded as unreliable (Forbes and Heise 2000; Wilkinson et al. 2009). All other candidates for the role of 'simple microbicide' studied in the late 1990s and early 2000s also failed to demonstrate efficacy in clinical trials. With the demise of these trials, the focus of the search for an anti-HIV microbicide shifted to pre-exposure chemoprophylaxis, or PrEP: protection through the use of specific anti-retroviral drugs, such as Tenefovir. These drugs could either be taken orally, or applied locally, in a vaginal gel or a drug-releasing vaginal ring. In 2010, scientists announced the first successful prevention of AIDS through the local use of a PrEP. The use of Tenefovir in the CAPRISA trial was partly conducted by CONRAD (Abdool Karim et al. 2010; Krakower and Mayer 2011. The PrEP concept is grounded in the use of specific, high-tech pharmaceuticals; an endeavour that resonates with the development of a highly specific hormonal contraception. The latest attempts to find a simple solution to a complex reproductive health problem have been no more successful than previous ones. Moreover, as feminist promoters of anti-HIV microbicides have explained, clinical trials of these products also raise vexing questions on the extent to which advances in biomedical research can rectify longstanding inequities in access to global health resources (Heise, Shapiro and Slevin 2005; Nguyen 2010).

The tangled history – or rather, histories – of anti-HIV microbicides, 'simple products' designed above all to help women in the Global South, can be compared to the complex history of the promotion of 'simple contraceptives' in colonial and post-colonial countries. There is, however, an important difference between these two histories: the input of the feminist movement. Spermicides were distributed by population experts who often failed to notice the sex/gender of their 'targets'. Anti-HIV microbicides were energetically promoted by feminist activists, attuned to women's specific plight. On the other hand, multiple resonances between the trajectories of spermicides and microbicides reflect the persistence of problems that negatively affect women's health in the Global South: poverty, deprivation and a pervasive gender inequality. There is no simple 'technical fix' for these issues.

Acknowledgements

Archivists at Schlesinger Library, Harvard University, Depository of Rare Books, Countway Library, Harvard University, the Rockefeller Archive Center, Tarrytown, NY, and Mudd Manuscript Library, Princeton University, provided invaluable help with the location of archive material. This study was funded by ANRS grants 2009-919, 436 and 2010-375, in the framework of a larger study on the history and present uses of anti-HIV microbicides, conducted with Genevieve Paichler and Mathieu Caulier; I am grateful to both for stimulating discussions on the history of local contraception and the prevention of STDs in women, to all the participants in the workshop 'Gendered drug standards: historical and socio-anthropological perspectives' (Granada, 28–30 November, 2011) for their input, and to anonymous reviewers of this chapter for their extremely useful suggestions.

References

Abdool Karim, Q., Abdool Karim, S. S., Frolich, J. A., Grobler, A. C., Baxter, C., Mansoor, L. E., Kharsany, A. B., Sibeko, S., Mlisana, K. P., Omar, Z., Gengiah, T. N., Maarschalk, S., Arulappan, N., Mlotshwa, M., Morris, L. and Taylor, D. on behalf of the CAPRISA 004 trial group (2010), 'Effectiveness and safety of Tenofovir gel, an antiretroviral microbicide, for the prevention of HIV infection in women', *Science* 329:5996, 1168–74.
Ahulwalia, S. (2008), *Reproductive Restraints: Birth Control in India, 1877–1947* (Urbana: University of Illinois Press).
Anonymous (1963), 'India: The India Harvard-Ludhiana Population Study', *Studies in Family Planning* 1:1, 4–7.
Baker, J. R. (1935), *The Chemical Control of Conception* (London: Chapman and Hill).
Baker, J. R., Ranson, R. M. and Tynen, J. (1938) 'A new chemical contraceptive', *The Lancet* ii, 882–6.
Bell, S. (2003), 'Sexual synthetics: Women, science, and microbicides' in Casper, M. (ed.) *Synthetic Planet: Chemical Politics and the Hazards of Modern Life.* (New York: Routledge) pp. 197–212.
Belsky, R. (1975), 'Vaginal contraceptives: Time for reappraisal', *Population Reports* George Washington University Medical Center, January H:3.
Bonah, C., Masutti, C., Rasmussen, A. and Simon, J. (eds) (2009), *Harmonizing Drugs: Standards in Twentieth Century Pharmaceutical History* (Paris: Edition Glyphe).

Briggs, L. (2002), *Reproducing Empire: Race, Sex, Science and US Imperialism in Puerto Rico* (Berkeley: University of California Press).

Brodie, J. F. (1994), *Contraception and Abortion in Nineteenth Century America* (Ithaca: Cornell University Press).

Brown, R. L., Levenstein, I. and Becker, B. (1943), 'The spermicidal times of samples of commercial contraceptives secured in 1942', *Human Fertility* 7:3, 65–7.

Bruce, J. (1987), 'User's perspectives on contraceptive technology and delivery system: Highlighting some feminist issues', *Technology in Society* 9, 359–83.

Connelly, M. J. (2008), *Fatal Misconception: The Struggle to Control World Population* (Cambridge, MA: Harvard University Press).

Cowan, R. S. (1989), 'The consumption junction: A proposal for research strategies in the sociology of technology' in Bijker, W. G., Hughes, T. P. and Pinch, T. (eds) *The Social Construction of Technological Systems* (Cambridge, MA: MIT Press) pp. 261–80.

———— (2001), 'Medicine, technology and gender in the history of prenatal diagnosis' in Creager, A., Lunbeck, E. and Schiebinger, L. (eds) *Feminism in the Twentieth Century: Science, Technology and Medicine* (Chicago: The University of Chicago Press) pp. 186–97.

Cutler, J., Singh, B., Utidjan, H. M. D. and Arnold, R. (1973), 'Development of a vaginal preparation providing both prophylaxis against venereal diseases and contraception', *British Journal of Venereal Diseases* 49, 149–50.

Cutler, J. and Arnold, R. (1988), 'Venereal disease control by health department in the past: Lessons for the present', *American Journal of Public Health* 78:4, 372–6.

deVilbiss, L. A. (1938), 'The contraceptive effectiveness of the foam-powder and sponge method', *Journal of Contraception* 3:1, 7–9, 19.

Dingle, J. and Tietze, C. (1963), 'Comparative study of three contraceptive methods: Vaginal foam, tablets, jelly alone, and diaphragm with jelly or cream', *American Journal of Obstetrics and Gynecology* 85, 1012–22.

Eastman, N. J. (1949), 'Further observations on the suppository as contraceptive', *Southern Medical Journal* 42:2, 346–50.

Eastman, N. J. and Siebels, R. E. (1949), 'Efficacy of the suppository and of jelly alone as contraceptive agents', *JAMA* 139:1, 16–20.

Forbes, A. and Heise, L. (2000), 'What's up with nonoxynol 9', *Reproductive Health Matters* 8:16, 156–9.

Fowler, G. (1991), 'Leona Baumgartner 88 dies: Led New York Health Department', *New York Times*, 17 January.

Gamble, C. J. (1952) 'Population control by permanent contraception', *Annals of the New York Academy of Science* 54:5, 776–7.

———— (1953a), 'Preventive sterilization in 1948', *JAMA* 141:11, 773.

———— (1953b), 'Human sterilization and public understanding', *The Eugenic Review* 45:3, 165–8.

———— (1959), 'The durability of contraceptive foam tablets in warm and moist climates', *Calcutta Medical Journal* 56, 345–50.

Garvin, O. D. (1944), 'Jelly alone versus diaphragm and jelly', *Human Fertility* 9:3, 73–6.

Germain, A., Holmes, K., Piot, P. and Wasserheit, J. (1992), *Reproductive Tract Infections: Global Impact and Priorities for Women's Reproductive Health* (London and New York: Plenum Press).

Hartmann, B. (1987), *Reproductive Rights and Wrongs: The Global Politics of Population Control* (New York: Harper and Row).

Heise, L., Shapiro, K. and Slevin, K. W. (2005), *Mapping the Standards of Care at Microbicide Clinical Trial Sites* (Washington, DC: Global Campaign for Microbicides).

Hillier, S., Moench, T., Shattock, R. T., Black, R., Reichelderfer P. and Veronese, F. (2005), 'In vitro and in vivo: The story of nonoxynol-9', *Journal of Acquired Immune Deficiency Syndromes* 39:11, 1–7.

Himes, N. E. (1949) 'A decade of progress in birth control', *Annals of the Academy of Political and Social Science* 212, 88–96.

Hodges, S. (2008), *Contraception, Colonialism and Commerce: Birth Control in South India, 1920–1940* (Aldershot: Ashgate Publishing).

Jones, J. H. (1993), *Bad Blood: The Tuskegee Syphilis Experiment* 2nd edition (New York: Free Press).

Krakower, D. and Mayer, K. H. (2011), 'Promising prevention approaches: tenofovir gel and prophylactic use of antiretroviral medications', *Current HIV/ AIDS Reports* 8:4, 241–8.

Löwy, I. (2011), 'Sexual chemistry before the pill: Science, industry and chemical contraceptives, 1920–1960', *British Journal of the History of Science* 44, 245–74.

——— (2012), 'Defusing the population bomb in the 1950s: Foam tablets in India', *Studies in History and Philosophy of Biological and Biomedical Sciences* 43, 583–93.

Malani, P. (1991), 'Leona Baumgartner', *JAMA* 266:11, 1504.

Marks, H. (2000), *The Progress of Experiment: Science and Therapeutic Reform in the United States, 1900–1990* (Cambridge: Cambridge University Press).

Marks, L. (2001), *Sexual Chemistry: A History of the Contraceptive Pill* (New Haven: Yale University Press).

Marsh, M. and Ronner, W. (2008), *The Fertility Doctor: John Rock and the Reproductive Revolution* (Baltimore: Johns Hopkins University Press).

McLaren, A. (1990), *History of Contraception: From Antiquity to the Present Day* (Oxford: Basil Blackwell).

Meldrum, M. M. (1994), 'Departure from Design: The Randomized Clinical Trial in Historical Context, 1946–1970', Doctoral Thesis (New York: Stony Brook University).

——— (1996), '"Simple methods" and "determined contraceptors": The statistical evaluation of fertility control, 1957–1968', *Bulletin of the History of Medicine* 70:2, 266–95.

Millman, N. (1952), 'A critical studies of methods used to measure spermicidal actions', *Annals of the New York Academy of Science* 54, 806–24.

Nguyen, V. K. (2010), *The Republic of Therapy, Triage and Sovereignty in West Africa's Time of AIDS* (Durham, NC: Duke University Press).

Ordover, N. (2003), *Race, Queer Anatomy and the Science of Nationalism* (Minneapolis: University of Minnesota Press).

Paniagua, M., Piedras, R., Vaillant, H. and Gamble, C. J. (1961), 'Field trail of a contraceptive in Puerto Rico', *JAMA* 177:2, 125–9.

Presidential Commission for the Study of Bioethical Issues (2011), *Ethically Impossible: STD research in Guatemala, 1946 to 1948*, Washington, DC. Available at: http://www.bioethics.gov/ [accessed 28 September 2012].

Rao, M. (2004), *From Population Control to Reproductive Health: Malthusian Arythmethics* (New Delhi: Sage, India).

Ravenholt, R. (1977), 'The power of availability' in Gardner, J. S., Mertaugh, M. T., Micklin, M., Duncan, G. W. and Battle, W. A. (eds) *Village and Household Availability Contraceptives* (Seattle: Human Affairs Research Centers).

Reed, J. (1978), *From Private Vice to Public Virtue: The Birth Control Movement and American Society* (Princeton: Princeton University Press).

Reverby, S. (2009), *Examining Tuskegee: The Infamous Syphilis Study and Its Legacy* (Chapel Hill: University of North Carolina Press).

———— (2011), '"Normal exposure" and inoculation syphilis: A PHS "Tuskegee" doctor in Guatemala, 1946–1948', *The Journal of Policy History* 23:1, 6–28.

———— (ed.) (2000), *Tuskegee Truths: Rethinking the Tuskegee Syphilis Study* (Chapel Hill: University of North Carolina Press).

Schmalhausen, S. (1928), *Why We Misbehave* (New York: The Macaulay Company).

Schoen, J. (2005), *Choice and Coercion: Birth Control, Sterilization and Abortion in Public Health and Welfare* (Chapel Hill: University of North Carolina Press).

Siebels, R. E. (1944), 'The effectiveness of a simple contraceptive method', *Human Fertility* 9:1, 43–7.

Singh, B. and Cutler, C. (1979),'Vaginal contraceptives for prophylaxis against sexually transmitted diseases' in Zatuchini, G., Sobrero, A., Speidel, J. and Sciarra, J. (eds) *Vaginal Contraception: New Developments* (New York: Harper and Row) pp. 175–87.

Soloway, R (1995a), *Demography and Degeneration: Eugenics and the Declining Birthrate in Twentieth-Century Britain* (Chapel Hill: University of North Carolina Press).

———— (1995b) '"The perfect contraceptive": Eugenics and birth control research in Britain and America in the interwar years', *Journal of Contemporary History* 30:4, 637–65.

Stein, Z. (1990), 'HIV prevention: The need for methods women can use', *American Journal of Public Health* 80:4, 460–62.

Stone, A. (1952), 'Present day international trends in family planning', *Annals of the New York Academy of Science* 54:5, 769–75.

Stone, H. (1938), 'Clinical experiments with foam powder method', *Journal of Contraception* 3, 3–6.

Stopes, M. (1952), 'Birth Control in India', *The Eugenic Review* 44:2, 58.

Stykos, J. M. and Back, K. W. (1964), *The Control of Human Fertility in Jamaica* (Ithaca: Cornell University Press).

Tietze, C., Pai, C., Taylor, C. and Gamble, C. J. (1961), 'Family planning service in rural Puerto Rico', *American Journal of Obstetrics and Gynecology* 81, 174–82.

Tietze, C. and Gamble, C. J. (1948), 'A field study of contraceptive suppositories', *Human Fertility* 13:2, 33–6.

Tone, A. (1999), 'Violence by design' in Bellesiles, M. (ed.), *Lethal Immagination: Violence and Brutality in American History* (New York: New York University Press) pp. 373–92.

——— (2001), *Devices and Desires: A History of Contraceptives in America* (New York: Hill and Wang).

Vieira, O., Hartmann, D. O., Cardoso, C. M., Oberdoerfer, D., Baptista, M., Santos, M. A., Almeida, L., Ramalho-Santos, J. and Vaz, W. L. (2008), 'Surfactans as microbicides and contraceptive agents: A systematic in vitro study', *PloS One*, August 3:8, e2913.

Voge, C. I. B. (1933), *The Chemistry and Physics of Contraceptives* (London: Cape).

Watkins, E. S. (1998), *On the Pill: A Social History of Oral Contraceptives, 1950–1970* (Baltimore: Johns Hopkins University Press).

Warwick, D. P. (1982), *Bitter Pills: Population Politics and Their Implementation in Eight Developing Countries* (Cambridge: Cambridge University Press).

Weisz, G. and Olszenko-Gryn, J. (2010), 'The theory of epidemiologic transition: Origins of a citation classic', *Journal of the History of Medicine and Allied Sciences* 65:3, 287–326.

Williams, D. (1978), *Every Child a Wanted Child: Clarence James Gamble, M.D. and His Work in the Birth Control Movement* (Cambridge, MA: Harvard University Press).

Wilkinson, D., Ramjee, G., Tholandi, M. and Rutherford, G. (2009), 'Nonoxynol-9 for preventing vaginal acquisition of sexually transmitted infections by women from men: a review', *The Cochrane Library* 1, 1–18.

Woycke, J. (1988), *Birth Control in Germany 1871–1933* (London: Routledge).

Chapter 5

Managing Medication and Producing Patients: Imagining Women's Use of Contraceptive Pill Compliance Dispensers in 1960s America

Carrie Eisert

As the Pill enabled women to better control reproduction, physicians, pharmaceutical manufacturers and marketers scrutinised women's thoughts, behaviours, and mentalities concerning reproduction. Since taking the Pill entailed remembering to do something almost every single day, the very act of taking the Pill became a subject of interest, research and innovation. The Pill has long been considered unique in that it was intended to be taken by healthy women, not under the direct supervision of a physician, and for extended periods of time (Watkins 1998; Marks 2001). Thus, women and physicians were quite concerned with several main questions about the Pill: whether it was safe, what its side effects were, and what impact it would have on sexual behaviour and on society at large. The Pill challenged people to consider how much risk was acceptable for a drug that was not meant to cure anything, but to prevent pregnancy. Historians, too, have been drawn to these same weighty issues (see in this volume the chapters by Thoms, and Ignaciuk, Ortiz-Gómez, Rodríguez-Ocaña).

This broader prospect of treating the healthy with pharmaceuticals has drawn focus away from the more prosaic issue of how experts managed the transformation of healthy women into patients with an everyday pill-taking 'habit' (Neubardt 1967). This issue is particularly easy to overlook since prescriptions for chronic conditions, such as hypertension, were just coming onto the market in the 1950s and 1960s, and the pace of the pharmaceuticalisation of modern America has only accelerated since (Greene 2008; Tone and Watkins 2007). The concept of taking a medication every day has become more and more common, and therefore harder to see as something that was new and unusual. Physicians and those who designed packaging and advertisements for the Pill had an interest in making the Pill seem like a normal, and even a natural, part of life. Patient instruction manuals, Pill packages, popular books, and Pill advertising from the 1960s indicated that the 'how to' details of taking the Pill were seen as quite important. Physicians, in particular, understood their patients' adherence to treatment protocols as indicative of the reach of their authority.

The Pill is a special case with which to study the adoption of a medication regimen. The Pill was not always taken every single day, and each brand was defined by a specific regimen, which was individually and actively constructed. Pharmaceutical manufacturers and marketers used specific pill regimens and dispensers to define each brand of pill, and these attributes became each pill's defining characteristics (Tone 2006). In 1964, an engineer named David Wagner patented a special dispenser called a 'Dialpak' in order to help patients make sure that they adhered to their pill regimen. The iconic, round Dialpak dispenser was considered to be the first 'compliance package' intended to help patients remember to take a medication correctly (Gossel 2004).[1]

While forgetting the Pill was certainly a problem, this issue alone does not explain the scope, scale and complexity of material concerning remembering to take the Pill. I argue that the rhetoric surrounding compliance to the Pill regimen served greater functions. First, materials produced by pharmaceutical manufacturers and physicians served to make pill-taking seem like a normal and natural domestic occurrence in a time when the everyday taking of prescription medications was a novelty. Thus, pill-taking instructions and popular books focused on integrating the Pill into familiar, domestic routines, while playing on anxieties about the Pill's effectiveness. Second, Pill advertisements aimed at physicians stoked concerns about patient compliance and served to buttress physicians' sense of authority and control as patients learned to manage medication more autonomously. Taken as a whole, these materials reflected and reinforced prevailing psychological and psychoanalytic conceptions of women as ambivalent and immature with regards to sex and pregnancy. This chapter aims to explore representations of women's pill-taking by interpreting Pill packages, instructions and advertisements in relation to psychological notions of women's pill-taking. This study considered hundreds of pill packages and advertisements found in archival collections and in medical journals, but only a small sample of the most illustrative artefacts are discussed here.

The Pill, as a technology of liberation, came packaged in a 'technology of compliance', and required women to be motivated managers of their adherence to the new regime (Jones 2001). In exchange for a greater sense of freedom from unwanted pregnancy, women became more deeply embedded in a growing system of medical surveillance and supervision, as their experiences of the menstrual cycle were translated into the pill cycle. Women were active participants in this process, counting days, turning dials and managing their pills and periods with dispensers and calendars.

---

1 Patricia Peck Gossel was the Chair of the Division of Science, Medicine, and Society at the Smithsonian's National Museum of American History until her death in 2004. Gossel researched the Pill and helped amass a collection of artifacts for the Smithsonian's permanent exhibition 'Science in American Life'. The staff at the Smithsonian allowed me to access the materials Gossel collected in order to continue this line of research.

Research about whether or not women took the Pill as directed was contradictory, and studies did not corroborate one another or point to any clear conclusions. On top of this, concerns about 'ambivalence' (Lidz 1969, 762) and 'pill forgetting' (Bakker and Dightman 1964, 562) conducted by psychoanalytic psychiatrists and psychosomatic gynaecologists added a new level of complexity to the problem (Tourkow, Lidz and Marder 1973; Bakker and Dightman 1965; Zell and Crisp 1964; Meldman 1964). Beyond merely an issue of being unreliable, illiterate, uneducated or simply disorganised, forgetting to take the Pill was diagnosed as a potential sign of subconscious interpersonal conflict. Forgetting to take the Pill could be interpreted as a means of revenge against one's husband or a way of managing guilt surrounding the decision to not become pregnant. The experiencing or reporting of side effects was similarly seen as potentially psychosomatic and indicative of larger conflicts about a woman's femininity and family role.

According to psychoanalytic researchers, 'forgetting' the pill was just one of many possible side effects that plagued women who were conflicted over their freedom from the 'biological basis of the double standard' (Kistner 1969). Though psychoanalytic factors were usually not the only issues that physicians considered, the psychoanalytic logic surrounding the Pill was a pervasive undercurrent, making women's behaviours and reactions always seem suspect. These questions were never resolved through clinical trials, but instead they continued for many years under the rubric of research on contraceptive pill 'acceptance' (Wallach, Beer and Garcia 1967; Wallach, Watson and Garcia 1967). The concept of 'acceptance' encompassed both physical side effects and reasons for discontinuation with subjective psychological experiences and behaviours. Pill acceptance was a compelling subject of research in the field of population control, but it was also a subject of research for physicians concerned with their educated, white, middle-class patients, who made up the largest demographic group of pill-users in the 1960s (Westoff 1968).

Women interviewed in the 1965 National Fertility Study were quick to note that the Pill allowed them to avoid the pitfalls and drawbacks of earlier contraceptive devices. The Pill was remarkable in that it did not 'interfere with the sex act' by some messy, 'awkward process of protection' (Westoff 1968, 87). In exchange for these conveniences, women took on a new kind of challenge. The concept of memory entered in to the experience of contraception and became the explicit prerequisite necessary for the successful use of the Pill. Replacing the relatively bulky diaphragm or condom, which provided a concrete, physical barrier to conception, the 'thin white tablet' and the ability to remember to take it properly occupied the minds of women and the physicians who instructed them in adhering to the regimen. The thin white tablet was imbued with power both through its diminutive size as well as through its invisible mechanism of action. Since the tablet's power existed only through a woman's ability to take it correctly, the dispenser was able to take on the same importance and cachet as the pill itself.

Counting the Days of the Cycle

Prior to the oral contraceptive and its associated compliance packages, there was a well-established history of women keeping track of their menstrual cycles for the purposes of family planning (Viterbo 2004; Marsh and Ronner 2008). Research into the rhythm method, and later the Pill, helped to facilitate the process of making physicians and patients aware of the possibilities of controlling the menstrual cycle. Some physicians and clinics such as Planned Parenthood offered rhythm method services in which women could send in their information and receive their calculated safe and fertile periods by mail. For those who preferred to keep track of their own cycles, a variety of devices were developed in order to facilitate use of the method. The Rhythmeter, for example, was a complex device that took into account both the inconsistencies in the lengths of the calendar months of the year, and in the lengths and characteristics of women's menstrual cycles. In order to translate between 'calendar days' and 'cycle days', there were settings for regular months, short months, and of course, 'corrections' that needed to be made for the shortest and most difficult month due to the leap year, February (Tilbrook 1943). In controlling for variations in the menstrual cycle, there were settings to account for irregular days, missing days, and adjustable settings to account for the shortest and longest cycles.

Another rhythm method device, the Gynodate clock, is noteworthy because it bears some stylistic similarities to the birth control pill compliance dispenser that would come in the 1960s (Jaquet c1960, see Figure 5.1).

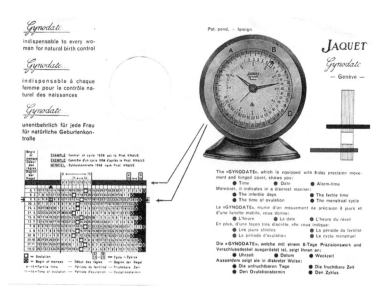

Figure 5.1   Gynodate Clock
Courtesy Jim Edmonson, Dittrick Medical History Center, Case Western Reserve University

The Gynodate clock was a rhythm method aid that at first glance resembled a sturdy brass table clock indicating the date and time precise down to the second hand. Upon removing a hinged cover, the user could find indicated, 'in a discreet manner', the infertile days, fertile time, time of ovulation, and menstrual cycle. What really set this device apart from the other methods of counting days was that the Gynodate was actually an alarm clock, capable of alerting the user to the beginning of the fertile period. Like the Gynodate, the birth control pill compliance packages purportedly took a more active role in reminding the user. The birth control pill compliance packages were also designed to be attractive and discreet, often appearing indistinguishable from common makeup compacts, mirrors and lipstick dispensers.

Much like the rhythm method devices, compliance packages assumed that women needed assistance in keeping track of the days of their menstrual cycles. A diverse array of devices and instructions were devised in order to make the contraceptive pill regimen seem easy, normal and natural to women. There was little consensus, however, on exactly what the contraceptive pill regimen should look like or what would be convenient for women to follow. Each new variation represented a trial and error attempt to construct a regulated, mechanised version of the 'natural' cycle. These regimens provide a rich source of information about how physicians and pharmaceutical manufacturers pictured the menstrual cycle, and how they imagined that women pictured their cycles. Many books and pamphlets promoting contraception in the 1960s lamented that women and men were woefully uninformed about reproduction (Neubardt 1967; Westoff 1968). This lack of information, attributed to guilt, shame, or immaturity, extended to knowledge of the menstrual cycle as well.

Despite the clear conceptual and medical connections between the rhythm method and the Pill, the longstanding existence of the rhythm method devices did not directly influence the initial design of the contraceptive pill dispensers. The design of contraceptive pill dispensers lagged behind, and did not build off of the design of rhythm method devices. The first contraceptive pill, Enovid, was released in 1960 as a simple brown glass bottle containing 20 white tablets. This meant that a woman had no way of easily knowing how many pills she had left to take or if she had missed one. In the early Pill regimens, there were not a set number of days in each cycle. Instead, women were told to count the beginning of their menstrual flow as 'Day 1', and then begin taking the first pill on 'Day 5'. Since a number of days elapsed between the last pill and the beginning of the next menstrual flow, this meant that the total number of days between cycles varied. An early set of instructions from Planned Parenthood for taking Enovid read:

> Mark the first day of your flow on a calendar. Count out 20 pills and keep them in a box. If you can't remember whether you took your pill look at the calendar, count the number you have left over and see if it tallies with the number you were supposed to have taken. If in doubt, it is better to take an extra pill than to make the mistake of missing a day. (Mount Vernon Planned Parenthood Center n.d.)

The regimen for taking Parke Davis' pill Norlestrin also did not rely on the menstrual cycle being a uniform number of days long. Instead, the instructions explained that the user should 'Take one tablet daily for 20 days, with a meal or at bedtime, starting on the fifth day (Day 5) after menstruation begins, and to continue though the twenty-fourth day' (Parke-Davis 1964). Though the number of pills was fixed at 20, ending on Day 24, there were an unspecified number of days at the end of the menstrual cycle between Day 24 and the beginning of menstruation. According to a 1964 package of Norlestrin, menstruation should start 'about three days after you have taken the last tablet', whereas a 1967 package allows a 'few days'. The instructions for what to do if 'no menstrual flow occurs' were also not set in stone. If no flow appeared, a new series of 20 tablets could be started on 'the 7th, or not later than the 8th day after taking the last tablet'.

In addition to the problem of not knowing how many pills were taken and how many were supposed to be left, some pill packages positioned the pills in arrangements that did not correspond to the days or weeks of a calendar. The Norlestrin tablets were arranged in four rows of five tablets each. Though superficially resembling a calendar, these rows did not match up to the seven days in a week, nor to the number of days in the variable menstrual cycle. The instructions recommended that women keep track of days, but the 'calendar' provided with the package was a simple row of boxes corresponding to neither calendar weeks nor months. The need for a package that allowed the day of the week to be adjusted to correspond to the correct pill became clear, but arriving at a solution was complicated by technical and legal concerns.

David Wagner and the Invention of the Dialpak

Historian and Smithsonian curator Patricia Peck Gossel chronicled the invention of the contraceptive compliance dispenser. Gossel conducted extensive interviews with the compliance pack's inventor, an Illinois engineer named David P. Wagner. Wagner found that 'there was a lot of room for error in whether "the Pill" was actually taken on a given day', and that he was 'just as concerned as Doris [his wife] was in whether she had taken her pill or not' (Gossel 2004). Wagner recalled that his wife became irritated with him constantly asking about whether she took her pill or not, and to resolve the problem, he arranged the pills on a piece of paper with the days of the week on their dresser. Wagner's arrangement of his wife's pills did 'wonders' for their relationship, but it was only 'about two or three weeks until something fell and scattered the pills and the paper all over the floor' (Gossel 2004, 106). Wagner then started sketching out ideas for a pill container that would prevent the pills from spilling, even if his wife carried them in her purse. Using simple materials, Wagner made some models of his dispenser, and filed for a patent with the help of a friend who was a patent attorney. The patent covered dispensers in which the pills were retained in a pattern and they could be adjusted in relation to an element having day-of-the-week identification.

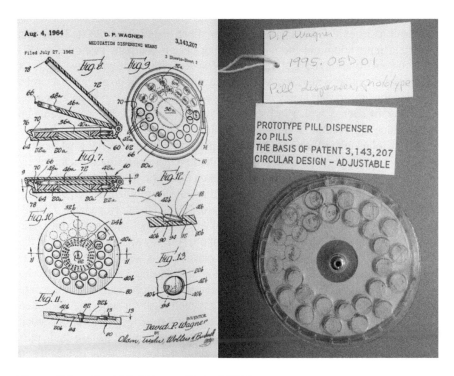

Figure 5.2   David P. Wagner Patent 1964
Courtesy Wagner Collection, Division of Medicine and Science, National Museum of American History, Smithsonian Institution

The dispenser was big enough for 20 pills to be arranged in rows of six, necessitating a system by which a piece of paper with the days of the week written out in rows of six had to be adjusted to match up to the correct pill (Wagner 1962). In retrospect, it seems strange that the pills are in rows of six instead of seven, since there are seven days in a calendar week, but such an assumption highlights the extent to which the pill regimen was not initially seen as something natural or tied to the calendar. There was also another variation of the patent in which the pills were arranged in a circular pattern rather than a rectangle (Figure 5.2).

Gossel argues that the various pill package designs were not merely cosmetic, but they had a significant pharmacological effect as newer designs increased the number of hormone-containing pills in the regimen. After Wagner realised that Ortho and G. D. Searle were copying his design, he threatened to sue. This encouraged G. D. Searle and other companies to come up with creative new designs that allowed them to circumvent the patent. G. D. Searle initially released the pill Ovulen in a circular dispenser that infringed upon Wagner's patent (Gossel 2004, 113). After paying royalties, G. D. Searle then decided to circumvent the issue by re-issuing the 20 pills in Ovulen as Ovulen-21, and

Enovid-E as Enovid-E 21. Increasing the number of pills from 20 to 21 was an important innovation and the most enduring design solution. Twenty-one pills could be easily arranged in three rows of seven pills each, and thus the user could start the pills on any day. Alternatively, the pills could be placed in a circle, allowing the user to start at any day of the week at a chosen location on the circle. The irony, of course, is that in seeking to evade a patent, G. D. Searle came up with a much more simple and elegant solution.

Mead Johnson's pill Oracon-28 added placebo pills so that the total number of pills was 28. Adding placebo pills simplified the patient instructions for taking the pills since a single pill could then be taken every single day. Advertisements explained that taking a pill everyday would eliminate the problem of 'forgetfulness' and eliminate the need for placebos, 'days off', and 'memory gadgets' (Parke-Davis n.d.). Patients were to expect a period when they took the placebo pills, and they were to begin taking the new package of pills the day after they completed the previous package. The introduction of the placebo pills was an interesting issue because it challenged the traditional definition of a placebo. Usually, for a placebo to work, a patient had to be unaware that she was taking a placebo. In the case of the Pill, however, the placebo served a psychological function and was often clearly labelled as a 'reminder pill'. Instead of acting covertly, patients understood that the purpose of the placebo was to help them remember to take their pills every day, through maintaining a pill-taking habit and keeping track of the pills in the pack. The very existence of a break between packs was maintained based on women's expectations, rather than physiological or pharmaceutical necessity. As one popular book explained:

> The purpose of stopping the Pill is to make the woman feel she is still undergoing her normal hormonal functions. If she didn't feel the habitual need to menstruate once a month, she could take a Pill every day and never bleed at all. (Westoff 1968)

The purpose of the withdrawal bleeding was to make the woman feel like she was still 'undergoing her normal hormonal functions', even if the normal functions in question were completely overridden by the synthetic hormones she was taking. Thus, the withdrawal bleeding was not 'real menstrual period' and performed no function other than satisfying a perceived feeling or need (Westoff 1968, 90). In sum, the variations in the pill regimens, and especially in the number of pills, were not initially justified by medical indications or reasoning, but were explained purely as a matter of what pharmaceutical companies thought patients would find convenient and easy to remember.

The compliance packs also represented a stark departure from the uniform, indistinct pharmaceutical packaging that had previously been standard. Most prescription drugs came in simple, plain glass bottles, and the biggest recent innovation in the early 1960s had been switching from glass to plastic as it was lighter, easier to ship, and resistant to breaking (New Role for Plastics 1964).

Though Ortho and G. D. Searle did not believe they needed what they considered promotional gimmicks, customised packaging quickly became a ubiquitous and very profitable marketing tool.

Advertising Pill Packages to Physicians

The interest in presentation was not limited to pharmacy owners and marketers aiming to impress patients. Advertisements promoting the compliance dispensers made frequent appearances in medical journals read by obstetricians and gynaecologists. Thus, while the compliance dispensers were supposedly designed with the patient in mind, the content in the advertisements was designed with the physician in mind. Many of the advertisements for the compliance dispenser promoted mechanical or behavioural readings of the package, suggesting that the package could watch over and even perform the work that the absent physician might wish that he could perform from afar. The language surrounding the dispensers imbued the devices with a sense of agency, allowing them to stand in for the physician. In the advertisements directed towards physicians, many ads took on a reassuring tone, convincing the physician that the pill package was overseeing or caring for the patient. The text of an Enovid-E advertisement from G. D. Searle illustrated the functions of the Compack in detail, explaining that it performed duties that served both the physician and the patient:

> The New Enovid-E Compack tablet dispenser DESIGNED WITH *HER* IN MIND
>
> Many years of physician experience with ENOVID and ENOVID-E have demonstrated the need for a better method of insuring strict adherence to the recommended dosing schedule. The New ENOVID-E Compack dispenser package has been developed to assist your patients in following your instructions. The highly feminine, highly fashionable ENOVID-E Compack suits the fancy of your patients. Easy to understand and use, yet appropriately inconspicuous, this new dispenser is clearly designed with *her* in mind.
>
> For *you*, there is the added assurance that your patient will take the medication as directed. The Compack removes the guesswork, makes the dosage regime 'unforgettable,' by providing a completely automatic record of her cycle and her 'pill' days. Push-button ease, crush-proof, individually sealed tablet protection, a built-in 'memory' mechanism *plus* the look and feel of a fashionable compact are the important reasons why you should specify Compack when you prescribe ENOVID-E. (G. D. Searle and Co. 1965)

The text of the advertisement explained how the dispenser would help the patient avert just about anything that could go wrong with taking the Pill – it was even 'crush-proof'.

Never to be outdone by G. D. Searle, an advertisement for the Ortho-Novin Dialpak 21 illustrated many of these same common themes. First, the advertisement mentioned that the Dialpaks 'remember for her' and there were no doubts because when the patient took a pill, 'the day is recorded' (Ortho n.d.). The ad also claimed that the packaging would insure that the patient would not miss any tablets as the 'Dialpak dosage insures the 100% method!' The ad showed an image of the pink Dialpak 'for her', but there was also a device intended for the physician himself. A 'watchstrap calendar keeps the date always to hand', so while the patient had control over her regimen with the Dialpak, the physician was also metaphorically overseeing the cycles of his patients by keeping his calendar in his control.

An Ovulen advertisement went one step further and suggested that the Pill could work as a tool to bring patients back to the physician. The text of the ad suggested that the physician: 'Prescribe with 5 Refills to bring your patient back on time for her six-month check-up' (G. D. Searle and Co. n.d.b). Not only was the dispenser meant to regulate the patient's pill-taking behaviour, but it was also a mechanism to regulate her visits to the doctor. The need for a 'six-month check-up', of course, originated with the Pill, and the number of refills acted to bring the patient back on time. The desire to obtain a prescription refill served as a powerful enticement to make another appointment and undergo additional breast and pelvic examinations (G. D. Searle and Co. n.d.a, 44). The need for regular check-ups presented an opportunity for gynaecologists to not only increase business at their practices, but to expand the boundaries of their profession.

Convenient and easy to understand packages also meant fewer questions from patients and less work for physicians. Wyeth capitalised on physicians' annoyance resulting from patients calling with questions about the Pill in an advertisement for Ovral. The text read 'Questions Questions Questions ... Oral contraceptives may prompt so many questions they'll give you "telephonitis"' (Wyeth 1967). All of the advantages of the drug were presented as assets because they would prevent patients from calling with questions. An advertisement for the British pill, Volidan 21, also shared this theme by asking doctors, 'Remember her? She was the one who asked all those questions', suggesting that the simplicity of the Pill would save the physician from having to field annoying questions (BDH Pharmaceuticals n.d.).

There were many variations among companies seeking to make their products unique. In 1965, Eli Lilly introduced C-Quens, the first sequential pill on the American market, which was supposed to more closely mimic a woman's natural shift in hormones throughout the month. Sequential pills included oestrogen-only pills in the first part of the cycle, but this was a short-lived enterprise since oestrogen-only pills caused increased side effects. In lieu of an innovative package design, the sequential regimen was pictured with flowers, marketed as being closer to nature. Because many users had suspicions that the Pill was in fact unnatural, framing one formulation as more natural than others was an asset. An advertisement for Oracon, a sequential birth control pill from Mead Johnson Laboratories, stated that it was 'so close to nature that it simulates the natural menstrual pattern'

(Mead Johnson n.d.). The 1965 patient instructional booklet that pharmacists dispensed with Oracon read, 'Your physician prescribed this product because it permits your body to closely simulate the normal menstrual cycle' (Mead Johnson n.d.). These advertisements focusing on the Pill as natural countered concerns about precisely the opposite; that using 'synthetic hormones to deceive the body into thinking it is pregnant' was unnatural (Westoff 1968, 90).

To allay fears and personalise the Pill, a number of advertisements tried to provide semi-personal portraits of hypothetical patients, providing examples like the young housewife, or the busy wife with children. Other advertisements addressed the issue of how the Pill fit in with nature and women's traditional roles. An ad for C-Quens asked 'Can Sara be herself on C-Quens?' The answer, of course, was a resounding 'yes', as Sara was shown on the next page smiling at home with her son. This advertisement presented a comforting, domestic picture that showed birth control as part of the domestic fantasy of the wife and mother fulfilling her roles; an image of domestic security so crucial during the Cold War years. Along with being traditional and domestic, the birth control pill was also construed as natural. An ad for Ovulen-21 from 1969 presented a peaceful view of motherhood, showing a mother resting with a baby accompanied by the text 'Ovulen-21 gives her time' so that she can care for her baby, her husband and herself (G. D. Searle and Co. n.d.b). Another Ovulen-21 advertisement used the slogan 'Ovuen-21 works the way a woman thinks by weekdays ... not "cycle days"' and shows thought bubbles emanating from a woman's head, illustrating which chores she associates with which days of the week.

An Australian advertisement for Eugynon ED explained that: 'The young housewife with children and the working wife are typical examples of busy women who have enough to think about without having to pay special attention to taking the pill' (Schering n.d). The advantage for the physician was that if there was less for the patient to remember, then there was less for the physician to explain. The theme of the harried, overwhelmed young housewife and other stereotypical portrayals of women were also used in ads for psychotropic medications (Herzberg 2009; Metzl 2003; Tone 2008). Matthew Hersch has shown how Smith Kline & French's antipsychotic Stelazine was marketed and successfully used to treat institutionalised patients diagnosed with schizophrenia, and at lower doses, the 'worried well' (Hersch 2008). Smith Kline & French advertised the use of Stelazine for regular, 'everyday' patients in a brochure entitled *Stelzaine in Everyday Practice*. The brochure illustrated a variety of regular patients, which Hersch describes as 'archetypes of superlative normality' (Hersch 2008, 142). One such archetype was 'the young mother'. With 'bills to pay, children to feed, house to clean', the young woman was overwhelmed and 'afraid of another pregnancy' (Smith Kline & French Laboratories 1965). Such a hypothetical patient might walk away from the physician with not just a prescription for Stelazine, but an oral contraceptive as well. Womanhood and motherhood in general, and fear of pregnancy in particular, became conceptualised as potentially pathological categories.

Also drawing upon the theme of domesticity, a British advertisement for Parke-Davis' pill Norlestrin 21 read, 'Many women have a regular and orderly existence. The pattern of their lives is governed largely by the demands of their families – meal times, domestic chores, shopping, to name a few' (Parke-Davis n.d.). In addition to routine housework, the ad also hinted at the woman's sexual role as another one of the family 'demands' that governed and shaped her life. The woman in the ad was pictured at home ironing in a frilly, lacy housedress with a bow in her hair and her head tilted provocatively to the side. Next to the flirtatious housewife were the lyrics to an English folk song about a man whose heart was stolen by a woman ironing her linen, 'dashing away with the smoothing iron'. The advertisement mentioned that the poem had been recited for years, highlighting both the repetitiveness of women's reproductive cycles as well as the repetitive nature of housework and women's duties in their families. In 1968, with speculation that the Pill was fuelling the sexual revolution, it was significant to place the Pill in the context of tradition and housework.

Surely, forgetting to take the Pill was a real problem that women faced, but the way the compliance package imagery was utilised suggests that it was perceived to hold a greater appeal to the physician. The forgetfulness imagery was embedded in representations of women's lives, transitions, and identities, representing women in specific female roles such as the 'newlywed', the working woman, the busy mother, or the 'housewife'. Thus, the conflict of remembering to take the Pill was presented to doctors not as a singular problem, but as embedded in the activities and meanings of women's roles. These deeply nuanced and contextualised scenarios presenting women's forgetfulness were compelling not because they represented the problem of remembering to take a pill, but because of the problems surrounding the complexities of what the Pill symbolised. They represented the uncertainties women and physicians were facing and with which they were struggling to come to terms. The problem of taking the Pill was not just about remembering, but about the enormous individual and cultural changes represented by the Pill.

Patient Instruction Booklets

While advertisements directed towards physicians made great use of the problem of forgetfulness, the instructions for women on how to take the Pill took this issue much more literally. Pill packages generally came with instructions on how to take them, while individual clinics and popular writers presented more general recommendations on pill-taking. Not only did these materials emphasise the importance of taking a pill every day, but they focused specifically on the time of day that the pill should be taken. Taking the pill at the same time every day was seen as important for the medication's effectiveness, but it was also crucial for integrating the Pill into the patterns of everyday life and promoting the concept of a compliant pill-taking patient. These materials became increasingly involved and elaborate towards the end of the 1960s and especially after 1970 when additional safety information was mandated (Watkins 1998; Junod 2007).

Materials directed towards patients usually emphasised the pill's effectiveness. In fact, the Pill was usually called 100 per cent effective, and most pregnancies were assumed to be failures on the part of the patient to take the tablets correctly. Therefore, pill packages walked a fine line between reassuring the woman that the product was effective, while simultaneously warning her that if the product failed, it was her fault. For example, a package for C-Quens read: 'This product has been found to be highly effective – but only when taken as directed. So do not fail to take each daily dose and keep a daily record.'

An instruction sheet for users of Enovid written by the Mount Vernon Planned Parenthood Center of New York was even more explicit: 'To obtain 100% protection you must follow these instructions EXACTLY. Please do not try to make your own rules' (Mount Vernon Planned Parenthood Center n.d.). These instructions seemed to suggest, in an amusing way, that the centre had experience admonishing patients who interpreted the rules in a creative fashion.

A 1970 booklet from G. D. Searle entitled 'Planning Your Family' was also rather explicit in explaining the need to take the pill 'regular as clockwork', and 'faithfully every "pill day"!' The booklet read:

> Take your pill at about the same time every day! You are probably wondering why the same time of day is important. By taking your pill at the same time every day it becomes a good habit and you are much less likely to forget. You may wish to keep your pills in the medicine cabinet near your toothbrush as a reminder to take them when you brush your teeth at night. (G. D. Searle and Co. 1970)

Similarly, *A Concept of Contraception*, a 1967 book for a general audience by a physician, encouraged patients to establish a daily 'pill habit' (Neubardt 1967). It did not matter if it was '8 p.m. on Friday night and 3 a.m. the following night', or even a daily habit in the morning or at lunch. The firm establishment of a habit was more important than the exact time.

The directions from the Mount Vernon Planned Parenthood Center also suggested that it was possible to take the Pill at any set time, 'but most women find it convenient to take it before retiring' (Mount Vernon Planned Parenthood Center n.d.). The instructions were framed in terms of what 'most women' found convenient, thus showing the premium Planned Parenthood placed on normalising the concept of taking a daily pill. The recommendation to take the Pill after eating or before going to sleep, however, probably did not originate from the experience of what 'most women' found convenient. Rather, the recommendation probably originated from the Planned Parenthood Medical Department. Some physicians believed that taking the Pill at night would reduce the chance of nausea, and other research indicated that nausea was often 'psychogenic', as it occurred just as frequently with placebos (Kallet 1962). Still, in order to circumvent the problem, suggesting that patients took the Pill at night meant that they were likely to sleep through any discomfort anyway.

Compliance Research

The struggles surrounding patients' adherence to treatment regimens were not going unnoticed by medical researchers and medical sociologists in the 1960s. In fact, the concept of 'compliance' was becoming a unique pathological entity, and a community of researchers concerned with non-compliance was beginning to stabilise (Greene 2004). Several historians and social scientists have focused on the concept of patient 'noncompliance' as a construction, ideology or category that increasingly became a concern of physicians and a subject of research (Lerner 1997; Trostle 1988; Greene 2004). Historian and physician, Jeremy Greene, links the development of the concept of compliance to a variety of trends, including a new pharmacopeia geared toward the treatment of chronic diseases as well as a Cold War 'ideology of social control' that allowed physicians to use the concept of noncompliance as a convenient way to shift blame to their patients (Greene 2004, 327). A focus on the ideology of patient compliance was used to bolster a 'flagging sense of physician authority' as the movements for informed consent and patient autonomy emerged (Greene 2004, 341).

The concept of noncompliance was also appealing to a younger generation of doctors beginning their careers after 1960, when the skills of epidemiologists were becoming more and more specialised and divergent from those of clinicians. In the 1950s and 1960s, methodological reformers persuaded medical researchers to adopt the techniques of double-blind randomised controlled trials, and the dominance of statistics facilitated a revolution that called for accurate and reliable data (Marks 1997). Though reform in the ethics and methods of clinical trials promised purer results that were better able to assess the safety and effectiveness of new drugs, medical knowledge still relied upon the cooperation of the patient.

According to sociologist Samuel Bloom's 1963 study of the doctor-patient relationship, physicians had a tendency to judge patients as 'good' or 'bad' based on how cooperative their behaviour seemed (Bloom 1963). Bloom found that during the course of medical school, physicians learned to 'judge patients on a moralistic basis', and these judgments stood in the way of 'understanding based on fact and reason' (Bloom 1963, 36). Getting beyond moralistic judgments could improve compliance to medical regimens, such as diabetes treatment, and uncover the underlying reasons why 'understanding and compliance on the part of the patient' was not always reliable (Bloom 1963, 44). Bloom's observation that physicians often made judgments about their patients was not limited to any specific context. Other social scientists have noted that the concept of patient compliance was problematic and loaded with value judgments. Anthropologist, James Trostle, has argued that compliance was essentially an ideology geared towards promoting the authority of medical professionals, emerging from the struggle of physicians to maintain control over infant-feeding technology (Trostle 1988).

Compliance research on family planning in the 1960s exemplified these themes. Researchers concerned with population dynamics shared clinical researchers' desire for reliable data, but their efforts to produce compelling data were plagued by value judgments and a lack of clarity about the terms and subjects of study. As such, statistics about patient compliance to Pill regimens were widely divergent. Elizabeth Whelan, a consultant for the Population Council, published a review of research on compliance with contraceptive regimens for the International Committee on Applied Research in Population (Cobb 1966, 565). Whelan found that comparing the results from different patient compliance reports was problematic because there was no single operational definition of noncompliance, and demographic differentials between the study populations also made comparison difficult (Whelan 1974). Beyond the challenges to compliance that plagued all medical regimens, there were additional characteristics unique to contraceptive compliance. Contraceptive 'acceptors' received no 'ongoing reinforcement' as they might if they had been taking an antibiotic to cure an infection, and furthermore, Whelan cited the 'general agreement' among psychologists and psychiatrists that 'decisions relating to pregnancy involve ambivalence' (Fawcett 1970; Sandberg and Jacobs 1971, cited in Whelan 1974, 249). Whelan also identified another challenge to compliance that resulted from the very existence of a choice of contraceptive methods. Knowledge of the existence of other methods of contraception made patients uncertain as to whether they had chosen the correct method, and this uncertainty was a cause of noncompliance.

Studies of patient compliance were conducted in a haphazard fashion so that results were difficult to compare, and different results could be deployed where it was politically useful. Though the results from studies of patient compliance were inconsistent, the studies were united by a desire to identify the characteristics of non-compliant patients, and to understand why some patients were more compliant than others. Young women, the most common users of oral contraceptives, were seen as already at a high risk of non-compliance by virtue of their age and sex, but again, without a clear way to measure compliance, psychological factors were persuasive explanations (Bakker and Dightman, 1964). Psychological theories such as 'willful exposure to unwanted pregnancy' (Lehfeldt 1959, 661) ambivalence, and immaturity were used as explanations (Tourkow, Lidz and Marder 1973; Lehfeldt and Guze 1966; Bakker and Dightman 1965; Barglow and Klass 1972; Sandberg and Jacobs 1971; Cullberg 1969).

Concerns over compliance were not limited to oral contraceptives. Physicians working in outpatient tuberculosis treatment programs used much of the same terminology that appeared in oral contraceptive advertisements (Jones 2001, 285). In fact, a large study of medication compliance on the Navajo Reservation in Arizona led to the invention of a radioactive pill clock intended to record whether or not patients took their pills as prescribed. Physician, Thomas Moulding, published a description of the rotating clock the same month that Wagner made his first 'Dialpak' model (Jones 2001, 297). While the Dialpak went on to become the most iconic pill dispenser in history, Moulding's invention did not spread far beyond the initial trial because it signalled too blatant an erosion of trust between doctor and patient.

Compliance to medication regimens would continue to remain a concern after the 1960s, though it took on different forms. As the scope of antibiotic resistance continued to expand over the 1960s and 1970s, resistant bacteria were a far greater cause of worry than a missed contraceptive pill. Furthermore, as Americans increasingly adopted daily medication regimens to prevent disease, the contraceptive pill's long-term daily dosing pattern ceased to be exceptional. The concept of compliance, too, was progressively replaced by the less judgmental term adherence (Lerner, Gulick and Dubler 1998). The failure to use contraception consistently would remain a concern for reproductive health, though it was eventually recast through the lens of feminist researchers (Higgins et al. 2008).

This chapter provides insight into the emerging concept of the contraceptive pill as a daily regimen that was integrated into women's lives with the help of pill dispensers, packages and patient instruction manuals. These materials provide a rich source of information about the way in which taking a pill every day became normalised, and how patients and medical experts oversaw and managed this shift. The information and advertisements directed towards physicians painted images of anxious and ambivalent women who were apt to forget to take the Pill and were generally in need of supervision. Representations of women's pill-taking, exemplified by the 'compliance package' invented for the Pill, reflected notions of deep-seated ambivalence evident in psychiatry research. Thus, popular perceptions of women's psyches were reflected in the way the Pill was packaged and marketed to physicians.

References

Bakker, C. B. and Dightman, C. R. (1964), 'Psychological Factors in Fertility Control', *Fertility and Sterility* 15:5, 559–67.
——— (1965), 'Physicians and Family Planning: A Persistent Ambivalence', *Obstetrics and Gynecology* 25, 279–84.
Barglow, P. and Klass, T. (1972), 'Psychiatric aspects of contraceptive utilization', *American Journal Of Obstetrics and Gynecology* 114:1, 93–6.
BDH Pharmaceuticals (n.d.), Volidan 21. *Remember her?* [advertisement] Syntex Collection of Pharmaceutical Advertising 1:25, Archives Center. Washington, D.C.: National Museum of American History, Smithsonian Institution.
Bloom, S. (1963), *The Doctor and his Patient: a Sociological Interpretation* (New York: Russell Sage Foundation).
Cobb, J. C. (1966), 'Oral contraceptive program synchronized with moon phase', *Fertility and Sterility* 17:4, 559–67.

Cullberg, J. (1969), 'The psychical and sexual adaptation of oral contraceptive users', *IPPF Medical Bulletin* 3:1, 1–2.

Eli Lilly (n.d.), *C-Quens*. [package] Contraceptive Collection. Washington, D.C.: National Museum of American History, Smithsonian Institution.

Fawcett, J. T. (1970), *Psychology and Population: Behavioral Research Issues in Fertility and Family Planning* (New York: The Population Council).

G. D. Searle and Co. (n.d.a), *Family Planning with the Pill: A Manual for Nurses* [booklet] Vertical Files. Washington, D.C.: American College of Obstetricians and Gynecologists.

———— (n.d.b), *Ovulen-21 Prescribe with 5 refills.* [advertisement] Patricia Peck Gossel files, Division of Science and Medicine. Washington, D.C.: National Museum of American History, Smithsonian Institution.

———— (1965), *Advertisement with Letter from Joseph G. Bond, Jr., Sales Manager at Searle to Staff Members, All Planned Parenthood Affiliates.* [manuscript] Sophia Smith Collection, Planned Parenthood Federation of America Records II, 68:71. Northampton, MA: Smith College.

———— (1969), *Ovulen-21 Gives her time* [advertisement] *Fertility and Sterility* 20:5.

———— (1970), *Planning Your Family.* [booklet accompanying pill pack] Ralph W. Hale, MD. Washington, D.C.: History Museum at the American College of Obstetricians and Gynecologists.

Gossel, P. P. (2004), 'Packaging the Pill' in Bud, R. et al. (eds) *Manifesting medicine: Bodies and Machines* (London: NMSI Trading Ltd) pp. 105–21.

Greene, J. A. (2004), 'Therapeutic Infidelities: 'Noncompliance' Enters the Medical Literature, 1955–1975', *Social History of Medicine* 17, 327–43.

———— (2008), *Prescribing by Numbers: Drugs and the Definition of Disease* (Baltimore: Johns Hopkins University Press).

Hersch, M. (2008), 'Calm but Still Alert: Marketing Stelazine to Disturbed America, 1958–1980' *Pharmacy in History* 50:4, 140–48.

Herzberg, D. L. (2009), *Happy Pills in America: From Miltown to Prozac* (Baltimore: Johns Hopkins University Press).

Higgins, J. A., Hirsch, J. S. and Trussell, J. (2008), 'Pleasure, Prophylaxis and Procreation: A Qualitative Analysis of Intermittent Contraceptive Use and Unintended Pregnancy', *Perspectives on Sexual and Reproductive Health* 40:3, 130–37.

Jaquet (c1960), *Gynodate Clock.* [clock] Courtesy of Jim Edmonson. Cleveland, Ohio: Dittrick Medical History Center, Case Western Reserve University.

Jones, D. S. (2001), 'Technologies of Compliance: Surveillance of Self-Administration of Tuberculosis Treatment, 1956–1966', *History and Technology* 17, 279–318.

Junod, S. W. (2007), 'Women over 35 Who Smoke: A Case Study in Risk Management and Risk Communications, 1960–1989' in Tone, A. and Watkins, E. (eds) in *Medicating Modern America: Prescription Drugs in History* (New York: New York University Press) pp. 97–130.

Kallet, A. to Guttmacher, A. F. (1962), *Draft of entry on oral contraceptives in The Medical Letter.* [manuscript] Sophia Smith Collection, Planned Parenthood Federation of America Records II, 111:26. Northampton, MA: Smith College.

Kistner, R. (1969), 'What the "pill" Does to Husbands', *Ladies' Home Journal* January, 66, 68.

Lehfeldt, H. (1959), 'Willful exposure to unwanted pregnancy', *American Journal of Obstetrics and Gynecology* 78:3, 661–5.

Lehfeldt, H. and Guze, H. (1966), 'Psychologic factors in contraceptive failure', *Fertility and Sterility* 17:1, 110–15.

Lerner, B. H. (1997), 'From careless consumptives to recalcitrant patients: The historical construction of noncompliance', *Social Science and Medicine* 45:9, 1423–31.

Lerner, B. H., Gulick, R. M. and Dubler, N. N. (1998), 'Rethinking nonadherence: historical perspectives on triple-drug therapy for HIV disease', *Annals of Internal Medicine* 129:7, 573–8.

Lidz, R. W. (1969), 'Emotional factors in the success of contraception', *Fertility and Sterility* 20:5, 761–71.

Marks, H. (1997), *The Progress of Experiment: Science and therapeutic reform in the United States, 1900–1990* (Cambridge: University of Cambridge Press).

Marks, L. V. (2001), *Sexual Chemistry: A History Of The Contraceptive Pill* (New Haven: Yale University Press).

Marsh, M. and Ronner, W. (2008), *The Fertility Doctor: John Rock and the Reproductive Revolution*, 1st Edition (Baltimore: Johns Hopkins University Press).

Mead Johnson (n.d.), *Oracon.* [package] Ralph W. Hale, MD. Washington, D.C.: History Museum at the American College of Obstetricians and Gynecologists.

Meldman, M. J. (1964). 'Behavioral Changes in the Husbands of Women Treated with Oral Contraceptives', *Psychosomatics* 10:5, 188.

Metzl, J. (2003), *Prozac on the Couch: Prescribing Gender in the Era of Wonder Drugs* (Durham: Duke University Press).

Mount Vernon Planned Parenthood Center (n.d.), *Directions for Taking Enovid.* [manuscript] Planned Parenthood Federation of America Records II, 111:25, Sophia Smith Collection. Northampton, MA: Smith College.

Neubardt, S. (1967), *A Concept of Contraception* (New York: Trident Press).

'New Role for Plastics in Drugs' (1964), *Modern Packaging* 37:5, 1000–1003.

Ortho (n.d.), *Ortho-Novin Dialpak 21. The important date always to hand* [advertisement] Syntex Collection of Pharmaceutical Advertising, Archives Center. Washington, D.C.: National Museum of American History, Smithsonian Institution.

Parke-Davis (n.d.), Norlestrin 21. *Many women have a regular and orderly existence.* [advertisement] Syntex Collection of Pharmaceutical Advertising, 2:2, Archives Center. Washington, D.C.: National Museum of American History, Smithsonian Institution.

————— (1964), *Norlestrin* [package] Ralph W. Hale, MD. Washington, D.C.: History Museum at the American College of Obstetricians and Gynecologists.

Sandberg, E. and Jacobs, R. (1971), 'Psychology of the misuse and rejection of contraception', *American Journal Of Obstetrics And Gynecology* 110:2, 227–41.

Schering (n.d.), *Eugynon ED The Young Housewife with Children.* [advertisement] Syntex Collection of Pharmaceutical Advertising 1:7, Archives Center. Washington, D.C.: National Museum of American History, Smithsonian Institution.

Smith Kline & French Laboratories (1965), 'The Young Mother', in *Stelazine in Everyday Practice, 24–25*. Smith Kline & French Laboratories, Klawans Collection, PSD:SZ 105, Philadelphia, PA: Chemical Heritage Foundation. Provided by Matthew Hersch.

Tilbrook, G. L. (1943), *Rhythmeter*. [device and patent] H MS c155. Cambridge, MA: Harvard Medical Library, Francis A. Countway Library of Medicine, Harvard University.

Tone, A. (2006), 'From naughty goods to Nicole Miller: Medicine and the marketing of American contraceptives', *Culture, Medicine and Psychiatry* 30:2, 249–67.

————— (2008), *The Age of Anxiety: A History of America's Turbulent Affair with Tranquilizers* (New York: Basic Books).

Tone, A. and Watkins, E. S. (eds) (2007), *Medicating Modern America: Prescription Drugs in History* (New York: New York University Press).

Tourkow, L. P., Lidz, R. W. and Marder, L. (1973), 'Psychiatric considerations in fertility inhibition' in *Human Reproduction: Conception and Contraception* (Hagarstown, MD: Harper and Row).

Trostle, J. A. (1988), 'Medical compliance as an ideology', *Social Science and Medicine* 27:12, 1299–308.

Viterbo, P. (2004), 'I got rhythm: Gershwin and birth control in the 1930s', *Endeavour* 28:1, 30–5.

Wagner, D. P. (1962), Prototype Pill Dispenser, David P. Wagner Collection. Washington, D.C.: Division of Medicine and Science, National Museum of American History, Smithsonian Institution.

————— (1964), US Patent 3,143,207 'Medication Dispensing Means'. Washington, D.C.: David P. Wagner Collection, Division of Medicine and Science, National Museum of American History, Smithsonian Institution.

Wallach, E. E., Beer, A. E. and Garcia, C. R. (1967), 'Patient acceptance of oral contraceptives I. The American Indian', *American Journal of Obstetrics and Gynecology* 97:7, 984–91.

Wallach, E. E., Watson F. M. and Garcia, C. R. (1967), 'Patient acceptance of oral contraceptives II. The private patient', *American Journal of Obstetrics and Gynecology* 98:8, 1071–9.

Watkins, E. S. (1998), *On the Pill: A Social History of Oral Contraceptives, 1950–1970* (Baltimore: Johns Hopkins University Press).

Westoff, L. A. (1968), *From Now to Zero; Fertility, Contraception and Abortion in America* (Boston: Little, Brown).

Whelan, E. M. (1974), 'Compliance with Contraceptive Regimens', *Studies in Family Planning* 5:11, 349–55.

Wyeth (1967), *Questions Questions Questions* [advertisement] *Fertility and Sterility* 18:1.

Zell, J. R. and Crisp, W. E. (1964), 'A Psychiatric Evaluation of the Use of Oral Contraceptives: A Study of 250 Private Patients', *Obstetrics and Gynecology* 23:5, 657–61.

Chapter 6

Doctors, Women and the Circulation of Knowledge of Oral Contraceptives in Spain, 1960s–1970s

Agata Ignaciuk, Teresa Ortiz-Gómez, Esteban Rodríguez-Ocaña

Doctor attacked for not prescribing contraceptives. Cardedeu (Barcelona). Local medical officer, Doctor José de Pelegrí Barberán, was attacked by a woman after he refused to give her a prescription for the contraceptive pill. The victim is suffering from a fractured rib, head injuries and general contusions, caused by a stone. The doctor asked the patient to leave his surgery, but she continued to hit Mr. Pelegrí Barberán until he lost consciousness. A passing policeman arrested the woman. Doctor Pelegrí was transferred to the nearby Granollers hospital, where he explained that the woman had been his patient for about ten years, but he had never believed she had symptoms [of illness] that required the use of anovulatory drugs. He also said he would file a claim [against the woman] in court. (*Abc* Sevilla 1975, 70)

This short story was published in *Abc*, one of the leading Spanish daily newspapers, in 1975, during the last months of the almost four decades of Franco's dictatorship. In November of that year, the leader's death triggered the beginning of the transition to democracy in Spain. The anonymous woman who violently confronted her doctor because he had refused her a prescription for oral contraception can hardly be considered representative of Spanish women of the time. However, the story raises several issues we will discuss in this chapter: namely women's demand for the pill and the reluctance of most medical professionals to prescribe it for contraceptive purposes prior to the mid 1970s, when it was still illegal to advertise or publicly display any contraceptive methods. A law prohibiting both abortion and contraception had been established in 1941 and remained valid, with only minor alterations, until 1978 (Ortiz-Gómez and Ignaciuk 2013).

In this chapter we focus on ideas held and practices carried out regarding the pill by male and female doctors, women users and campaigners, and on the ways the new drug acted upon and problematised established doctor-patient relationships. We address these questions through the analysis of medical publications (medical journals and textbooks), women's magazines and interviews with family planning activists. We examine the contexts within which information on the pill circulated, thereby revealing the roles played by doctors and health activists in these processes, and pay attention, not only to gender models and hierarchies contained within medical discourses on hormonal drugs, but also to ideas about femininity, maternity, fertility, women's health and social expectations of and for women. With this chapter, we complete our study of the circulation of knowledge on hormonal drugs and oral contraceptives in scientific publications (Rodríguez-Ocaña, Ignaciuk and Ortiz-Gómez 2012) and in the daily press during the Francoist regime (Ortiz-Gómez and Ignaciuk 2013).

Doctors and Anovulatory Drugs in Spain (1940s–1970s)

In Spain, as in other European countries, hormonal products became used extensively following the 'boom' in research on sex hormones and sex hormonal drugs that took place in Europe and the US during the 1920s (Oudshoorn 1994, 82–111; Gaudillière 2005). Through the 1940s and 1950s, information about new discoveries in the field kept pace with developments in major European countries, with local medical journals regularly reprinting articles on hormonal therapies published in the French, German, Italian, British and American press. Spanish authors also contributed to this knowledge with their own published research. Most authors were well aware of the contraceptive potential of the new synthetic hormonal drugs for women. However, as we have already suggested, given the legal and social Spanish context of the time, this crucial action was downplayed in favour of their therapeutic effect on some endocrinal and gynaecological diseases (Rodríguez-Ocaña, Ignaciuk and Ortiz-Gómez 2012).

The circulation of knowledge about newly introduced anovulatory drugs among Spanish medical professionals in the 1960s followed a similar pattern. When Schering launched *Anovial 21* onto the Spanish market in 1964, medical journals, especially those specialising in gynaecology and obstetrics, regularly published commercial advertisements for this and similar drugs, and the Spanish medical community began to debate whether these new pharmaceuticals should be called and considered anovulatories or contraceptives. 'Anovulatories' or 'anti-ovulatories' were the names commonly given to these drugs in medical publications, especially in the 1960s and early 1970s. At the end of the 1960s, there was still no consensus on whether 'anovulatory drug' was an exact synonym for 'contraceptive pill', mainly due to the strong influence of the Catholic Church and its opposition to contraception, an opposition echoed by the Spanish scientific community. Towards the mid 1970s, however, and for some years before and after Franco's death, public positions within the medical community diversified: many began to see contraception as a basic human and women's right.

Spanish Gynaecologists, Femininity and the Pill

Research in women's history has demonstrated how, in industrial societies, women's bodies have been configured as sites of political interest and intervention.

National states under both democratic and non-democratic regimes have considered women responsible for physically and symbolically reproducing productive citizens and the nation itself. Legal methods of regulating reproduction, abortion and contraception have therefore been implemented (Mayer 1999; Usborne 1992; Bock and Thane 1996). Doctors and medical systems have contributed to these policies and ideas, not only by supporting or complying with them, but by developing new discourses and knowledge about women's health. Although these discourses have changed over the nineteenth and twentieth centuries, they have essentially congregated along two lines: the tendency of the (middle class) female body to be sick, and motherhood as *the* female biological identity (Jagoe, Blanco and de Salamanca 1998; Ortiz-Gómez 1993; Sánchez 2002; Mitchell 2004).

During the twentieth century, Spanish gynaecologists, like their counterparts in other countries, came to be considered the most authoritative experts for defining the concept of 'woman', not only in medical terms, but also in relation to their social roles or position within the family (de Miguel and Domínguez-Alcón 1979, 9; Ortiz-Gómez 1993; Sánchez 1999). After 1939, in compliance with the ideological and political atmosphere of the time, many gynaecologists, defined woman in terms of her potential maternity, a potential understood to be her vital mission (Dexeus Font 1970, 121 quoted in de Miguel and Domínguez-Alcón 1979; Botella Llusiá 1966a and other works). As well as academic publications, a number of noteworthy Spanish gynaecologists also published texts targeted at the general public, in which they preached about women and their roles in marriage, family and society. These included discussions about contraception, and always followed the official guidelines of the Catholic Church (Clavero Núñez, several editions since the 1940s, 14th edition: 1968; Botella Llusiá 1966b; 1970; 1973; 1975a; 1975b; 1977). Professor José Botella Llusiá, one of the most prolific of these authors and an avowed Catholic, warned of the devastating effect that women's participation in paid employment could have on the family, perhaps even on the entire human species (Botella Llusiá 1966b, 22; 1970, 16–17). A firm believer in the traditional division of roles, he anticipated serious psychological problems for any woman who rejected the established gender order and wished to participate, like men, in the world beyond the household (Botella Llusiá 1975a, 26–8; 1970, 42–5). Regarding the education of women, he declared that:

> [she should receive] education the aim of which is not to make her a good citizen, but rather, a good wife and mother of a family, and in case she stays single, a person useful to others. (Botella Llusiá 1970, 30)

Sexuality was considered to be so closely related to procreation that Botella believed a childless woman could suffer from 'reproductive anxiety', the internal conflict being the inevitable result of denying her biological destiny (Botella Llusiá 1970, 45; 1975b, 102–18). He was very careful, however, not to discuss these theories explicitly in his work targeted at the medical community where, in an attempt of scientific objectivity, Botella Llusiá insisted anovulatory drugs were safe and their side effects transitory (Rodríguez-Ocaña, Ignaciuk and Ortiz-Gómez 2012).

These texts were being produced at a time when oral contraceptives were already available on the Spanish market. In Spain, as worldwide, the introduction of hormonal drugs presented doctors with both a challenge and an opportunity. In the broader context of the increasing medicalisation of female reproductive health, these medicaments provided gynaecologists with a subtle, effective and relatively harmless tool, with which they could 'normalise' women's physiology (Marks 2001, 133). Anovulatory drugs could be used to treat infertility and other gynaecological problems and to prevent conception, enabling doctors to reinforce their status and increase the social and moral control they could exert over women and their families. Some doctors advocated that oral contraceptives should only be prescribed to married women (Silies 2010, 89). Others employed anovulatory drugs only as therapeutic pharmaceuticals, particularly for a variety of menstruation-related 'problems' such as irregular or painful menstruation or pre-menstrual discomfort. This use was justified by the historical medical perception of the female body (especially that of a middle-class woman), whether menstruating or at other stages of the menstrual cycle, as something pathological which requires regulation and normalising. In absence of such 'symptoms of illness' they would refuse to prescribe the pill, as in our story from the daily *Abc*. Even when prescribed for a therapeutic purpose, gynaecologists did not necessarily inform their patients about the contraceptive 'side-effect'. In the 1960s, as in the US and the UK, most medical professionals found it difficult to accept the purely contraceptive use of these pharmaceuticals, as contraception was not generally considered a part of medical competence. At the beginning of the 1960s, many Spanish doctors rejected the use of any contraceptive method. A small poll conducted in Barcelona in 1963 revealed that 24.9 per cent of doctors interviewed were not willing to accept birth control in any case, 64 per cent considered it unnecessary to provide patients with more information on contraceptive methods, and 81.1 per cent declared that their religious beliefs influenced their medical practice considerably (del Campo 1968, 231–8). In medical journals published in Spain between 1965 and 1979, contraception in general was not an issue of great interest, appearing mainly in the context of a technical and moral discussion about the pill (Rodríguez Ocaña, Ignaciuk and Ortiz-Gómez 2012).

Towards the late 1960s, the pill as a prescription-only birth control method used under constant medical supervision, had helped to convince most British, American and German doctors that family planning was a legitimate medical activity (Marks 2001, 116–17; Watkins 1998, 34; Brockmann 2009, 104). However, Spanish doctors' acceptance of the contraceptive use of anovulatory drugs, and of birth control in general, took far longer. Open opposition was a regular feature of medical journals in the late 1960s, at a time when the General Council of the Spanish Medical Association pronounced itself against any measure of birth control (*Abc* Madrid 1967). The arguments put forward against using anovulatory drugs to control fertility in these professional medical journals, were similar to those expressed by doctors and moralists who opposed the pill in other countries: these drugs were unnatural, and harmful both to the female body, and the sexual act (de Soroa Pineda 1967; Nasio 1967). Some authors emphasised the negative 'physiological' influence of these drugs on the female body (Nasio 1967) while others employed 'psychological' arguments about 'defeminisation', ovulation being considered the basis of female identity (Horno Liria 1972; Polaino Lorente 1972). As a solution to these problems, those authors who accepted the practice of some kind of birth control recommended 'natural' contraceptive methods based on observation of the menstrual cycle (Horno Liria 1972; Polaino Lorente 1972).

In all countries, the introduction of anovulatory drugs obliged Catholic doctors to take a clear moral or ideological stand (Watkins 1998, 46). However, it must be remembered that the Catholic hierarchy and community, especially prior to the 1968 publication of the Encyclical *Humanae Vitae*, was not unanimous on the subject of contraceptive use (Felitti 2007). Before the publication of the Encyclical, which considered the pill and all contraceptive methods except those based on cycle observation illegitimate for Catholic married couples, a number of Spanish doctors took part in a moral discussion about possible cases in which the use of these drugs was appropriate (Abad Martínez 1964). They made a sharp distinction between acceptable 'indirect sterilisation' caused by the drug when the main purpose was not contraception, and unacceptable 'direct sterilisation', when contraception was the objective. Some cases, however, such as requests to guarantee adequate, 'natural' spacing between births, remained contentious. A number of authors, including both avowed Catholics (de Soroa Pineda 1967; Jiménez Vargas and López García 1973) and those who did not declare their ideological standpoint (Marqués Girault 1962) were opposed to any use of anovulatory drugs for contraceptive purposes. Others, wishing to appeal to international moralists, had difficulties in opting clearly for or against the pill (Abad Martínez 1964). At the same time, liberal gynaecologists, such as José María Dexeus, questioned the necessity for doctors to state their religious positions in publications on the medical aspects of anovulatories (*Dr. Doctor. Información Profesional y Administrativa* 1967, 55). After 1968, some doctors and moralists publically opposed the Encyclical *Humanae Vitae* (mentioned by Sánchez Carazo 1998, 478) and the idea of doctors imposing their own religious beliefs on patients (Carrera 1970; Cónill Serra 1974). However, extremely conservative positions identifying all contraceptive methods with abortion remained visible, particularly among doctors from the Catholic Opus Dei University of Navarra. For the female paediatrician and Opus Dei member, Ana María Álvarez Silván, the Encyclical *Humanae Vitae* was a valid reference, enabling both the interpretation of the concept of 'responsible parenthood' within the spirit of Catholicism, and the formulation of ethical arguments against the pill (Álvarez Silván 1971).

Doctor Álvarez Silván's discourse is a rare example of a female doctor's opinion on oral contraceptives and birth control, at a time when most Spanish doctors and gynaecologists were male. In 1960, female doctors constituted only 1.5 per cent of all Spanish doctors, a figure that had risen to 10.1 per cent by 1975 (Ortiz-Gómez et al. 2001, 128). A number of these belonged to the Spanish Medical Women's Association, which edited the journal *Actividades de la Asociación Española de Mujeres Médicos* (henceforth *Actividades AEMM)* from 1965 to 1971 (Ortiz-Gómez 2005, 89). Even though the association only managed to attract a small number of women doctors, most of whom were well established practitioners, its journal is a valuable source of medical women's opinions on the pill in the late 1960s and early 1970s, absent as they were from mainstream Spanish medical journals.[1]

In 1968, *Actividades AEMM* published extracts of conference papers presented by two Spanish representatives at the XI Congress of Medical Women's International Association, held in Vienna. Paediatrician, Lola Vilar, the association's founder and president, tackled the topic of the pill in relation to the leading congress issue: world famine. She acknowledged the great potential of the pill, which could be 'a redemption to the sexual slavery of women' (Vilar 1968, 53) and enable women to enjoy the same rights and opportunities as men. However, turning to Botella Llusiá's concept of 'reproductive anxiety', Vilar supported the claim that women undertaking professional careers and using contraception would result in disaster.

At the first and only national congress of the association in 1971, contraception and family planning was a key topic. Participants spoke openly about contraceptive methods, despite the presence of political authorities, such as the head officer of the National Public Health department (Director General de Sanidad, J. García Orcoyen, professor of gynaecology at the University of Madrid) and the president of the Women's Section of the National Movement (Sección Femenina de Falange, Pilar Primo de Rivera). A speech on the contraceptive pill given by Professor Botella Llusiá was later summarised and commented on in professional medical newspapers (*Tribuna Médica* and *Gaceta Médica Española*) and the women's magazine, *Ama*. Discussions took place about issues featured in medical journals and the daily press, such as the side effects of oral contraceptives (Álvarez Simó 1971; Álvarez Silván 1971; Gomis 1971), providing new, or at least uncommon, insights to the topic of the pill from women's perspectives. Although often referring to the Catholic Church's doctrine on family planning, these texts also echoed the arguments against the pill formulated by the feminist health movement in other countries. They criticised the commercial benefits pharmaceutical companies received from the pill (Álvarez Silván 1971, 33–4) and the coercive family planning programmes initiated in many developing countries

---

1   Through our search in the Índice Médico Español database (which contains articles published in Spanish medical journals after 1964) the only article authored by a woman between 1964 and 1979 was by Christine Imle (1970), 'Motivaciones contra el Uso de los Anovulatorios', *Folia Clínica Internacional* 20, 251–71 and 318–32, publication derived from her PhD thesis, in which she discusses contraceptive preferences of female patients at the University Gynaecological Clinic in Wurzburg with special focus on the pill.

(Meiggs 1971, 23). They also warned pill users against becoming mere sexual objects for their husbands (Álvarez Silván 1971, 33).

Prescribing the Pill: Ideal Women End Users

As with other medical drugs, prescription of the pill was at the doctor's discretion. To justify prescription, doctors could take both medical and social indications into consideration. In the 1960s and early 1970s there was a debate within medical literature on 'legitimate' indications for the prescription of anovulatory drugs. Opinions within this debate were heavily dependent on whether the author believed products such as Anovial 21 should be used as 'anovulatory' or 'contraceptive' drugs (Rodríguez-Ocaña, Ignaciuk and Ortiz-Gómez 2012). Having reviewed medical articles and books published in Spain between 1965 and 1979, we have found that indications felt to justify the prescription of these drugs fell into three categories: those relating to the female reproductive system; those relating to general health; and those taking social or personal motivations into account.

Most doctors approved the use of anovulatory drugs to treat irregularities of the menstrual cycle and other problems relating to the female reproductive system, such as 'menstrual alterations, endometriosis, [or] dysmenorrhea' (Caballero Gordo 1970, 341). The general health indicator implied a recognition of the contraceptive effect, as the drugs were often employed to prevent pregnancy 'after delivery, during breastfeeding or periodic irregularities when there is a high risk of pregnancy' (Novo 1969, 49) in women for whom a pre-existing illness or condition, such as varicose veins or heart disease (Morales Rodriguez and Trujillo Ramirez 1979) could be aggravated by a new pregnancy. These two indicator groups, the first in particular, could be accepted by doctors who, following the official position of the Catholic Church hierarchy on oral contraceptives, only approved of their employment if the main goal was not to impede conception or, in other words, if they produced 'indirect sterilisation' (Abad Martínez 1964). As for 'general health', in some gynaecological circles it was a wide enough concept to always justify prescription of hormonal contraceptives, such as at the outpatient family planning clinics created in the first half of the 1970s in some public hospitals, in cities such as Bilbao (Usandizaga and López Valverde 1978), Barcelona (Cónill Serra 1974; González Merlo 1979), Madrid (Fernández Penela 2010), Santa Cruz de Tenerife (Morales Rodriguez and Trujillo Ramirez 1979), Granada (Salvatierra, et al. 1978; Jiménez 2010) or Seville (de los Reyes 2009). As the gynaecologists at these clinics would admit after the legalisation of contraception, they included the third indication, the social and personal situation of the patient, within the general health label and therefore prescribed the pill to any healthy woman who requested it. These practices appear to have been at least partially clandestine before 1975, as so far we have only found one article openly recommending oral contraceptives for social reasons. This article, published in 1974 in a medical journal based in Seville, was by Enrique Solano Berral, a public health paediatrician who defended pill prescription to young women, single women and those with many children and little spacing between them, and to those facing economic difficulties or whose husbands had abandoned them (Solano Berral 1974, 741).

Gynaecologists were well aware of women's interest in the pill, with patients openly requesting information on oral contraceptives. In a 1958–1959 academic course inaugural speech before the members of the Spanish Gynecological Society, Professor Botella Llusiá officially introduced the ovulation-inhibiting potential of gestagens to Spanish scholars. Using a metaphor of a 'contraceptive bomb', Botella claimed the pill potentially as dangerous to the human race as the atomic bomb, but also referred to the its therapeutic properties, especially in treating infertility. He concluded the speech by recommending doctors inform themselves well about anovulatory drugs, as they would no doubt be facing 'female patients' questions' on the matter (Botella Llusiá 1959, 11; Rodríguez-Ocaña, Ignaciuk and Ortiz-Gómez 2012). This argument, extended to contraception in general, was also used by Professor Vicente Salvatierra in the 1973 edition of his textbook for medical students in Granada. In a chapter dedicated to 'Sexual problems and birth control,' he claimed that:

> Knowledge about [contraceptive methods] is useful, because in this course [gynaecology] we study the facts. The fact is that part of the population uses different methods, although there is a law which prohibits talking about them. So it is absurd for a doctor not to know them, and what to do in case of having to deal with their side effects. (Salvatierra 1973, 307)

Many doctors, regardless of their ethical stance, reported being asked by their patients about the pill. Gynaecologist, José Carrera, in a chapter on contraception in the 1970 gynaecology textbook edited by Santiago Dexeus Font, declared that doctors were obliged to provide information about contraception whenever there was demand, regardless of their personal opinion on the issue. The same idea had been expressed by Doctor A. Novo the previous year:

> The therapeutic aspect [on ovulation inhibitors] is beyond any doubt; however, the harsh problem still remains: which is its contraceptive use. We would like to escape from it, but we cannot avoid the fact that women ask for our advice, understanding, indulgence or complicity. Moral problems are individual, but we need to have some general, but flexible norms that can be adopted in every case. (Novo 1969, 49)

On the other hand, the religious or conservative argument was that such demands should be resisted and rejected by physicians, as in advice given to Opus Dei (an ultra-conservative catholic organisation founded in Spain in 1928) gynaecologists and GPs:

For some years now, all doctors face the problem of contraceptives daily. They [women] blatantly ask for prescriptions as if it was something they had the right to claim. At times, they ask indirectly, with some kind of excuse or pretence. He [the doctor] has to know how to say no. (Jiménez Vargas and López García 1973, 503)

Rather than merely rhetorical justification for doctors to legitimise and provide contraceptive drugs, the fact that doctors from all ideological points of view reported patients' demand for oral contraceptives can be considered proof this demand existed. It also indicates a shift in the doctor-female patient relationship. The fact that women were explicitly requesting a particular drug from their doctors is unusual in the history of the patient-doctor relationship (Watkins 1998, 39, 50; Marks 2001, 123). As Elizabeth Watkins has pointed out, the pill not only empowered doctors, it also empowered women as patients (Watkins 1998, 52). In Spain, during the 1960s and early 1970s, circulation of the pill helped reinforce the doctor's technical and gender power position, within an openly asymmetrical doctor-women relationship. Women, as users of the pill and other contraceptive methods, began to challenge this relationship from the mid 1970s onwards. During the Spanish transition to democracy, social and political changes initiated new spaces and new working styles, including family planning clinics run by gynaecologists within the state health system and private feminist family planning centres. At the same time as these new situations eased encounters between doctors and women seeking oral contraceptives, other contraceptive methods were starting to become part of gynaecological and general practice.

Women and the Pill

Access to Oral Contraceptives and Their Users

In spite of legal and ideological difficulties, the pill was available and used by Spanish women almost 15 years before its decriminalisation. Although use of the pill in Spain was considerably lower than in other European countries such as Britain, Germany or France, between 1964 and 1978 there was a steady rise in the sale of oral contraceptives (Ortiz-Gómez and Ignaciuk 2013). As in other European countries, the main channel through which the pill circulated among Spanish women was likely to have been medical prescriptions by gynaecologists and GPs (Marks 2001, 122; Silies 2010, 197). As we have discussed, prescription of oral contraception was legal where there were therapeutic indications. There probably also existed a degree of illegal circulation, and some women, especially unmarried ones, would certainly obtain the pill from friends who had travelled abroad (de Miguel and Domínguez-Alcón 1979, 143; Hernández 2010). Eva-Marie Silies has confirmed illegal circulation of oral contraceptives in West Germany, despite a lack of legal obstacles to the prescription or sale of these drugs.

This was instead the result of the relatively high price of the pill and, during its early days, difficulties some unmarried women found when attempting to gain access to prescriptions (Silies 2010, 89–90). As already discussed, after the mid 1970s in Spain, women could obtain contraceptives through the family planning clinics run by feminist activists and political parties. These received occasional support from the International Planned Parenthood Federation (Europe Region) and other foreign family planning groups, who provided sample boxes of oral contraceptives and other birth control methods, such as diaphragms, spermicides, condoms, cervical caps and IUDs (Jones 2010).

There is no data available for the period under study on exactly who pill users in Spain were. We suspect that, as in the West German case (Silies 2010, 113) young, urban, educated and probably also married women had easier access to oral contraceptives, having more opportunities to find a doctor willing to prescribe them (Jones and Toss 1987, 40). According to the sociologist, Amando de Miguel, these women could not only access prescriptions more easily, but also arrange an abortion abroad in cases of contraceptive failure. By contrast, lower class women were forced to use 'more primitive' and less secure methods (de Miguel 1973, 43). Literacy was also a key issue: information on the pill was circulated in the daily press and women's magazines but, in the 1960s especially, many rural women were illiterate and had no access to printed information. However, according to interviews we have conducted with feminist family activists and women doctors involved in the first family planning clinics, women from working-class neighbourhoods of large Spanish cities began to seek information on contraceptive methods and family planning services more actively during the second half of the 1970s (Jaime 2009; Galindo 2010).

Discourses on the Pill in Women's and Feminist Publications

Despite the difficulties discussed above, we can assume that, in general, women were aware of the existence of the pill. In Germany, where contraception was legal without restriction in 1965, four years after the introduction of Anovlar, 80 per cent of women knew of its existence. By the following year, almost all German women and men had some knowledge about oral contraceptives (Silies 2010, 94). In Spain, opinion polls conducted in the years 1970 and 1972 found the pill to be the best known contraceptive method among Spanish women and young people (Díez Nicolás 1973; Sánchez Carazo 1998, 251). In spite of its legal prohibition, and the apparent reluctance of many gynaecologists to share their knowledge with patients, there was a definite circulation of information about the pill among Spanish women, which potentially constituted the site of a clash between state-proposed models of femininity and women's individual interests in controlling their own fertility.

As has been suggested for other countries, Spanish women learnt about the pill from friends and trusted doctors, as well as from the mass media, (Sieg 1996, 139; Silies 2010, 99; Watkins 1998, 50). In the 1970s especially, there was considerable coverage in daily newspapers such as *Abc* and *La Vanguardia*, focusing mainly on the side effects of the drugs (Ortiz-Gómez and Ignaciuk 2013). Nevertheless, the information published was rather scattered and inconclusive, and Spanish doctors, like their German counterparts (Silies 2010, 208), often complained in professional journals about the low quality of information published in the daily press, and the fact that many news articles were overly sensational and unbalanced. During the 1960s and up until the mid 1970s, the last period of dictatorship, women's magazines played an important role in promoting the regime-supported ideal of femininity to Spanish women. The 1960s are considered a decade of successful development for these kinds of magazine, such as *Ama* or the Opus Dei-managed *Telva* (Sánchez Hernández 2009, 221). Following Franco's death in 1975, a new kind of women's magazine began to be published, such as *Dunia* which, although being a mainstream magazine, included frequent feminist approaches and proposals. The first exclusively feminist magazines were also founded at this time, the longest-published being *Vindicación Feminista*, established by the feminist activist and lawyer, Lidia Falcón, and printed in Barcelona between 1976 and 1979 (Larumbe 2009).

On the pages of the regime-oriented magazine *Ama*, the subtitle of which was 'a magazine for Spanish housewives', the pill became an explicit issue around 1968, with expectations and comments about the publication of the Encyclical *Humanae Vitae* (*Ama. Revista de las Amas de Casa Españolas* [henceforth *Ama*] 1968, 24–6). The first opinions about oral contraceptives had been published two years earlier, in the regular agony column, with answers and comments by a member of *Ama*'s editorial board, Carmen del Cid. Both the letters' authors and the journalist responsible for replying were opposed to the pill and all other forms of contraception, which were presented as immoral tools used to prevent the large families glorified by *Ama* (del Cid 1966a, 159; del Cid 1966b, 163; del Cid 1966c, 163). Even though the few publications on oral contraceptives published in this magazine before 1970 were highly critical of any contraceptive method, the presence of the pill in the section of readers' letters indicates social awareness of the existence of the drug and its contraceptive properties.

In 1970, *Ama* asked its young male and female readers to send the editors their opinions on various issues, such as love, friendship, freedom, divorce, homosexuality, God, and the role of priests. One of these issues was 'contraceptive procedures'. Opinions were published in several later issues of the magazine, and over half of those quoted were, surprisingly, in favour of contraceptives, with comments such as 'the best method to avoid [having] children, not a crime' (*Ama* 1970a, 38–9), or 'necessary' (*Ama* 1970b, 86–7) and something that 'should be authorised as they help to solve many poor families' problems' (*Ama* 1970c, 93). In the second half of the 1970s, during the democratic transition, *Ama* became more explicitly involved in the social debate around the legalisation of contraceptives. In 1977 it published the opinion of the president of the Spanish Women Lawyers' Association (*Asociación Española de Mujeres Juristas*), María Telo, on abortion and contraception. Telo considered the legalisation of contraception and the provision of family planning services by the state necessary to reduce the number of insecure clandestine abortions performed in Spain (Telo Núñez 1977). The magazine stated clearly that this was a personal opinion not shared by the editorial board. However, the fact that it was printed culminated this transition of the discourse on contraception and the pill in *Ama*. In 1978, the magazine reported the imminent legalisation of contraception (Calderón 1978) and printed an article on contraception in which a doctor endorsed the pill as a safe contraceptive method if used under medical supervision (Monedero 1978).

During the democratic transition, women's magazines such as *Dunia* and the feminist newspaper *Vindicación Feminista* discussed the pill to varying degrees. However, contrary to medical journals, where the pill was clearly the protagonist, in these magazines the oral contraceptive issue was raised within a broader context of the ongoing fight for women's rights, the legalisation of abortion and discussions surrounding new models of female sexuality.

Launched in 1976, shortly after Franco's death, *Dunia* was subtitled 'an intelligent magazine for a woman'. Before their official decriminalisation, *Dunia* published several articles and reports on contraceptive methods and the history, use and effects of the pill (*Dunia. Revista Inteligente para la Mujer* [henceforth *Dunia*] 1978a; 1978b; 1978c; 1978d; 1978e; 1978f). All of the mentioned articles plus others published in 1979, assigned sections of the magazine to medicine and health, in which oral contraceptives were discussed in a pragmatic way, with the side effects mentioned but not exaggerated. Doctors, especially gynaecologists, were quoted and portrayed as the main experts on the subject. The pill was depicted as a well-known and well-used drug, and the publications aimed to correct mistaken beliefs and stereotypes related to it, instead of advocating for the legalisation and increased availability of oral contraceptives. It could be assumed that the use of contraceptive drugs was so extensive, that the magazine preferred to focus on more urgent issues and claim reforms on abortion or family law (*Dunia* 1977, 76–7) rather than debate the legal status of contraceptives.

While in the general press and women's magazines the role of doctors remained indisputable, the longest published feminist magazine during the Spanish democratic transition, *Vindicación Feminista*, provided during three intense years (1976–1979) an alternative source of information produced by women and for women (Larumbe 2009).

Vindicación Feminista dedicated little space to oral contraceptives as an autonomous topic. As in *Dunia*, the feminist battle to legalise abortion seems to have been far more important to editors and contributors than the decriminalisation of contraceptives. Similarly to *Dunia*, oral contraceptives were discussed in *Vindicación Feminista*, only in the broader context of family planning in Spain. Journalist, Soledad Balaguer, in a report published in 1977, argued that the pill was used extensively in Spain despite negative media coverage of its side effects. She also emphasised that women were more likely to obtain prescriptions for the pill in private surgeries, where doctors were less opposed to the idea than those employed in the state health service (Balaguer 1977, 41). Women, especially unmarried ones, would visit pill-prescribing doctors whose names they had obtained through informal networks (Hernández, 2010). These doctors' motivations to prescribe the pill probably combined a commercial orientation with a practice less subject to external control and personal convictions in favour of women's and couples' right to family planning.

The idea that contraceptives, including the pill, could enable women to take control of their reproduction was described in the same issue of *Vindicación Feminista*, a concept championed by Spanish family planning activists (Jaime 2009), and raised in other countries, such as Germany (Sichtermann 1996; about pill rejection in Germany see Ulrike Thoms in this volume). The magazine also pointed out that women's choice of contraception was limited to the pill, due to the unavailability of other contraceptives in Spain, even if counter indications or side effects meant it was not the most suitable method (Oranich 1977, 45).

Other *Vindicación Feminista* articles published in 1977 focused on class and geographical inequalities in access to contraception in general, and for the pill in particular, with rural working class women reportedly being under the greatest influence of the Catholic Church, further complicating their access (Fagoaga, Vigil and Saavedra 1977, 36; Begoña 1977, 66). While in Spain the main axes that differentiated women's access to prescription of the pill were class and urban or rural residence, in West German feminist discourse on the issue of class inequalities in access to oral contraceptives, the focus was the high price of the pill and the benefits this generated for Schering AG and other pharmaceutical companies (Silies 2010, 385–9). In Spain during the second half of the 1970s, however, pharmaceutical companies often collaborated with young doctors in the early family planning clinics, sponsoring their participation in family planning meetings and conferences (Jiménez 2010; Villatoro 2010; Jaime 2009) and even providing oral contraceptive samples. While their goal was indisputably to increase the sales and circulation of their products, pharmaceutical companies played an important role in the proliferation of oral contraceptive knowledge throughout Spain (Sánchez Carazo 1998, 479–80).

In 1978, Leonor Taboada, an Argentinean feminist health activist who had resided in Spain since the mid 1970s, published a self-help health manual for women (Taboada 1978a), ideologically close to the American *Our Bodies, Ourselves* and the West German *Hexengeflüster*. In this book, and an article in *Vindicación Feminista*, Taboada echoed the feminist critiques of the pill that originated in the women's health movements of other countries. Both US feminists such as Barbara Seaman and German groups such as *Brot und Rosen* focused on the pill's side effects and criticised doctors for not providing enough information on the potential risks and counter indications for women taking these drugs (Seaman 1995 [1969]; Silies 2010, 385–9). In *Vindicación Feminista*, Leonor Taboada condemned the fact that 'women are made to swallow contraceptives with dangerous side effects', citing this as one of numerous demonstrations of the excessive medicalisation of the female body (Taboada 1978b, 38).

During the second half of the 1970s there was a considerable increase in the number of female students entering medicine and gynaecology in Spain. Some of these would later become involved in the new field of family planning and collaborate in the already mentioned outpatient clinics in some hospitals (de los Reyes 2009; Villatoro 2010; Jiménez 2010), or in the feminist family planning movement. The feminist family planning clinics were sites where doctors collaborated with health activists, formulating new ideas about the doctor-patient relationship which echoed those of the international women's health movement. They called for better communication between doctors and patients in a dynamic based on equality, in which women were considered not sick and passive patients but active participants, executing their newly recognised right to information about contraception and sexuality (Arnedo 1978; Ortiz-Gómez, et al. 2011). (Arnedo 1978; Ortiz-Gómez, et al. 2011). They also provided comprehensive information and advice on a variety of contraceptive methods, including the pill. This attitude became a model for medical practice in all Spanish family planning clinics developed in the 1980s, as well as the new primary health care model that was beginning to be implemented (Fajardo 2007).

Conclusions

During the 1960s and 1970s, Spanish doctors and their female patients shared a substantial interest in oral contraceptives. Their motivations, however, were quite different. While doctors focused on technical aspects of the pill, such as physiological mechanisms, therapeutic indications and side effects, women approached it as the most readily available method of avoiding an unwanted pregnancy.

The prohibition of the sale, advertisement and public exposition of contraceptive methods in Spain that lasted until 1978, accompanied by pro-natalist policies and the strong support of the Catholic Church, did not entirely prevent the circulation of knowledge about the pill among experts and the public. Discussions in the pages of medical journals reflect a broad range of positions regarding the pill, from complete opposition, through limited acceptance, to total approval. Although legal, social, political and religious factors contributed to the privileged position of conservative discourses, the political change triggered by the democratic transition following Franco's death in 1975, together with the increased presence of women within medicine and gynaecology, and the establishment and expansion of family planning clinics, all contributed to making favourable opinions of the pill visible. The introduction and prescription of anovulatory and contraceptive drugs was probably a source of internal conflict for many Spanish practitioners who, in order to decide whether and to whom to prescribe the pill, had to balance their religious beliefs and personal convictions, and the legal prohibition of providing oral contraceptives, against increasing patient demand.

Before the mid 1970s, women's access to the pill in Spain was considerably more difficult than in many other countries, but not impossible. While few women would be as determined to obtain a prescription as the patient of doctor Pelegrí Barberán described at the beginning of this chapter, their demand for the drug was an example of their increasing empowerment within society, and a doctor-patient relationship which was beginning to be challenged.

Access to the pill and to information about it initially varied considerably between urban and rural women. Married, urban, young and educated women certainly had much easier access to the pill in the late 1960s, but in the following decade, especially after Franco's death, knowledge of contraceptives in general, and the pill in particular, circulated freely among rural and working class women. As well as receiving information directly from sympathetic doctors, women could learn about the pill from the popular press and, in the 1970s, from family planning services. While knowledge of the pill circulated in a similar way as it did in the US and in other European countries, a particularity of the Spanish situation was the lack of a strong feminist opposition to the pill and the pharmaceutical industry. Despite feminists criticising doctors' control of access to oral contraceptives, they did not elaborate as harsh a critique of the medical profession as their late 1960s American and German counterparts. This lack of explicit criticism of pharmaceutical companies, which was viewed as crucial by US and German feminists, only appeared in the discourse of Catholic women doctors, to a limited extent, in the early 1970s.

Funding and Acknowledgements

This work is a result of two research projects: *La constitución de la planificación familiar en España durante los últimos años de franquismo y en la transición democratica* (Spanish Ministry of Science, ref. HAR2008-05809-HIST) and ASYS (Spanish Ministry of Economy, HAR2012-39644-C02-00). We are grateful to the participants in the workshop Gendered Drug Standards, held in Granada in November 2011, for their comments and suggestions and to Dennis Hubbard for copyediting early versions of this paper.

References

Abad Martínez, L. (1964), '[Revisión de conjunto] Las nuevas drogas anticoncepcionales. Puntos de vista deontológicos', *Revista Española de Obstetricia y Ginecología* 23:137, 317–26.

Abc Madrid (1967), 'Conclusiones de la XXI Asamblea Médica Mundial', 17 September, p. 79.

Abc Sevilla (1975), 'Un médico, agredido por no recetar anticonceptivos', 24 April, p. 70.

Álvarez Silván, A. M. (1971), 'Regulación de la natalidad', *Actividades de la Asociación Española de Mujeres Médicos* 4, 27–39.

Álvarez Simó, E. (1971), 'Anticonceptivos y acupuntura', *Actividades de la Asociación Española de Mujeres Médicos* 4, 15–21.

Ama: Revista de las Amas de Casa Españolas (1968), 'La Encíclica Humanae Vitae' 209, 15 August, 24–6.

———— (1970a), 'Chicos y chicas. Encuesta' 250, 1 May, 38–9.

———— (1970b), 'Chicos y chicas. Encuesta' 251, 15 May, 86–7.

———— (1970c), 'Chicos y chicas. Encuesta', 253, 15 June, 93.

Arnedo, E. (1978), 'Postura de la paciente cara a la Planificación Familiar' in *Comunicaciones al Tema Control de Natalidad e Inducción al Parto.*

Balaguer, S. (1977), 'Contracepción a la española: todas somos delincuentes (Reportaje)', *Vindicación Feminista* 7: 1 January, 41–3.

Barral, M. J. et al. (eds) (1998), *Interacciones ciencia y género. Discursos y prácticas científicas de mujeres* (Barcelona: Icaria).

Begoña (1977), 'Curas, maridos y anticonceptivos (Carta a *Vindicación Feminista*)', *Vindicación Feminista* 11, 1 June, p. 66.

Bock, G. and Thane, P. (eds) (1996), *Maternidad y políticas de género. La mujer en los estados de bienestar europeos, 1880–1950* (Madrid: Cátedra-Feminismos).

Botella Llusiá, J. (1959), *Sesión inaugural del curso académico 1958–59* (Madrid: Sociedad Ginecológica Española).

———— (1966a), *Endocrinología de la mujer*, 4th Edition (Barcelona: Editorial Científico-Médica).

———— (1966b), *Cuestiones médicas relacionadas con el matrimonio* (Barcelona: Editorial Científico-Médica).

———— (1970), *La mujer en la familia moderna* (Madrid: Alameda).

———— (1973), 'Nuevas perspectivas en la ciencia de la reproducción humana', *Tauta. Medicina y Sociedad* 8, 13–17.

———— (1975a), *Definición de la mujer* (Santander: Universidad Internacional Menéndez Pelayo).

———— (1975b), *Esquema de la vida de la mujer* (Madrid: Espasa-Calpe S. A).

———— (1977), *La contracepción* (Madrid: Cupsa).

Brockmann, U. T. (2009), *Die Debatte um die Pille in der Bundesrepublik Deutschland in ausgewahlenten Zeitschriften von 1961 bis 1968* (Saarbrucken: Dr Muller).

Caballero Gordo, A. (1970), 'Efectos colaterales de los contraceptivos orales. Sus peligros y contraindicaciones', *Acta Ginecológica* 21:5, 341–54.

Calderón, J. L. (1978), 'Pronto en España despenalización de anticonceptivos y planificación familiar', *Ama: Revista de las Amas de Casa Españolas* 442, 1 May, 29.

Carrera, J. M. (1970), 'Contracepción' in Dexeus Font, S. (ed.).

Clavero Nuñez, J. A. (1968), *Antes de que te cases* (Barcelona: Editorial Científico–Médica).

Comunicaciones al Tema Control de Natalidad e Inducción al Parto (1978), XV Reunión de Ginecólogos Españoles, 2–4 November.

Cónill Serra, V. (1974), 'La Planificación Familiar en la práctica hospitalaria', *Progresos de Obstetricia y Ginecología* 17, 29–36.

de los Reyes, S. (2009), Interview by Eugenia Gil García. Seville, December 15, 2009.

de Miguel, A. (1973). 'El mito del "Eterno Femenino"', *Tauta. Medicina y Sociedad* 14, 40–43.

de Miguel, A. and Domínguez-Alcón, C. (1979), *El mito de la inmaculada concepción* (Barcelona: Anagrama).

de Soroa Pineda, A. (1967), 'Puntos de vista del médico católico en un grave problema. Más consideraciones sobre la píldora anticonceptiva. ¿Justificación o capricho?', *Gaceta Médica Española* 51, 161–5.

del Campo, S. (1968), 'Los médicos ante el problema de la limitación de la natalidad' in *Cambios sociales y formas de vida* (Barcelona: Ariel) pp. 230–44.

del Cid, C. (1966a), 'Carta número 461', *Ama: Revista de las Amas de Casa Españolas* 159, 15 October, 163.

———— (1966b), 'Carta número 462', *Ama: Revista de las Amas de Casa Españolas* 159, 15 October, 163.

———— (1966c), 'Carta número 451', *Ama: Revista de las Amas de Casa Españolas* 159, 15 August, 159.

Dexeus Font, S. (ed.) (1970), *Tratado de ginecología* (Barcelona: Salvat).

Díez Nicolás, J. (1973), 'Actitudes de las mujeres españolas hacia los métodos de planificación familiar', *Revista Española de la Opinión Pública* 31, 27–59.

Dr. Doctor. Información Profesional y Administrativa (1967), 'Los médicos ante la píldora. Segundo coloquio de doctor', December, 49–57.

Dunia: una Revista Inteligente para la Mujer (1977), 'Realidad social y regulación jurídica del aborto' 11, March, 76–7.

———— (1978a), 'La primera enciclopedia de la píldora (4)', 29, 23 June–7 July, 39–42.

———— (1978b), 'La primera enciclopedia de la píldora (3)', 28, 9–23 June, 39–42.

———— (1978c), 'La primera enciclopedia de la píldora (2)' 27, 26 May–6 June, 35–7.

———— (1978d), 'La primera enciclopedia de la píldora (1)' 27, 12–26 May, 27–34.

———— (1978e), 'Hacer el amor sin miedo' 25, 28 April–12 May, 74–7.

———— (1978f), 'De dónde viene la píldora' 24, 14-28 April, 22–8.

Fagoaga, C., Vigil, M. and Saavedra, P. (1977), 'La revolución más silenciosa. Las agricultoras', *Vindicación Feminista* 11, 1 May, 29–39.

Fajardo, A. (2007), *El proceso de especialización en Medicina Familiar y Comunitaria en España. Cambios profesionales en Atención Primaria en la década de 1980* (Granada: Universidad de Granada).

Felitti, K. (2007), 'La Iglesia Católica y el control de la natalidad en tiempos del Concilio: La recepción de la Encíclica Humanae Vitae (1968) en Argentina', *Anuario IEHS 22*, 349–72.

Fernández, P. (2010), Interview by Eugenia Gil García. Madrid, November 11, 2010.

Galindo, E. (2010), Interview by Eugenia Gil García. Seville, January 17, 2010.

Gaudillière, J. P. (2005), 'Better Prepared than Synthesized: Adolf Butenandt, Schering AG and the Transformation of Sex Steroids into Drugs (1930–1946)', *Studies in History and Philosophy of Science Part C: Studies in History and Philosophy of Biological and Biomedical Sciences* 36:4, 612–44.

Gomis, C. (1971), 'Aspectos éticos de los anticonceptivos', *Actividades de la Asociación Española de Mujeres Médicos* 4, 41–9.

González Merlo, J. et al. (1979), 'Nuestra experiencia sobre planificación familiar', *Ginedips*, 525–32.

Hernández, R. (2010), Interview by Teresa Ortiz-Gómez. Granada, January 5, 2010.

Horno Liria, R. (1972), '"Anticoncepcionismo". Un problema de hoy, de Ayer, de Siempre', *Anales de Medicina y Cirugía* 52, 329–48.

Imle, C. (1970), 'Motivaciones contra el uso de los anovulatorios', *Folia Clínica Internacional* 20, 251–71 and 318–32.

Jagoe, C., Blanco, A. and Enríquez de Salamanca, C. (1998), *La mujer en los discursos de género. Textos y contextos en el siglo XIX* (Barcelona: Icaria).

Jaime, P. (2009), Interview by Teresa Ortiz-Gómez. London, July 26, 2009.

Jiménez, A. (2010), Interview by Teresa Ortiz-Gómez. Granada, January 12, 2010.

Jiménez Vargas, J. and López García, G. (1973), *Aborto y contraceptivos* (Pamplona: Ediciones Universidad de Navarra).

Jones (Hamand), M. (2010), Interview by Agata Ignaciuk. London, September 8, 2010.

Jones, M. and Toss, E. (1987), *Alternative Approaches to the Development of Family Planning Programmes* (Copenhagen: WHO).

Larumbe, M. A. (2009), '*Vindicación Feminista*: un ideal compartido' in *Vindicación Feminista: una voz colectiva, una historia propia. Antología facsímil de textos (1976–1979)* (Zaragoza: Universidad de Zaragoza).

López Beltrán, M. T. (ed.) (1993), *Las mujeres en Andalucía. II Encuentro Interdisciplinar de Estudios de la Mujer en Andalucía* (Málaga: Diputación Provincial).

Marks, L. (2001), *Sexual Chemistry. A History of the Contraceptive Pill* (New Haven and London: Yale University Press).

Marqués Girault, L. (1962), 'Consideraciones sobre la licitud en la administración de gestágenos durante el puerperio a fin de evitar la ovulación', *Revista Española de Obstetricia y Ginecología* 21:121, 31–6.

Mayer, T. (1999), 'Gender Ironies of Nationalism. Setting the Stage' in T. Mayer (ed.) *Gender Ironies of Nationalism: Sexing the Nation* (London: Routledge).

Meiggs, L. (1971), 'El control de la natalidad y la planificación familiar', *Actividades de la Asociación Española de Mujeres Médicos* 4, 23–5.

Mitchell, T. (2004), 'Authoritarian Medicalization and Gynephobia under Franco', *South Central Review* 21:2, 1–14.

Monedero, F. (1978), '[Medicina] La anticoncepción', *Ama: Revista de las Amas de Casa Españolas* 450, 1 September, 73.

Morales Rodríguez, J. and Trujillo Ramírez, F. (1979), 'Bases de Planificación Familiar', *Acta Médica de Tenerife* 40, 9–14.

Nasio, J. (1967), 'Los contraceptivos y el sentido moral en la investigación médico–científica', *Hispalis Médica* 24:278, 565–71.

(1970), 'Potencial humano de la República Argentina y el control de la natalidad', *Galicia Clínica* 43:3, 207–17.

Novo, A. (1969), 'Regulación de la natalidad', *Toko-Ginecologia Práctica* 28, 39–50.

Oranich, M. (1977), 'La anticoncepción: un medio para la maternidad libre (Reportaje)', *Vindicación Feminista* 7, 1 January, 44–5.

Ortiz-Gómez, T. (1993), 'El discurso médico sobre las mujeres en la España del primer tercio del siglo XX' in López Beltrán, M. T. (ed.).

—— (2005), 'Fuentes orales e identidades profesionales: médicas españolas en la segunda mitad del Siglo XX', *Asclepio* 57:1, 75–98.

Ortiz-Gómez, T., Fajardo, A., Gil García, E., Ignaciuk, A. and Rodríguez-Ocaña, E. (2011), 'Activismo feminista y movimiento asociativo por la Planificación Familiar en España' in Transmisión del conocimiento médico e internacionalización de las prácticas sanitarias: una reflexión histórica. *Proceedings of the XV Conference of the Spanish Society for the History of Medicine* (Ciudad Real: SEHM; Facultad de Medicina de Ciudad Real) pp. 141–5.

Ortiz-Gómez, T. and Ignaciuk, A. (2013), '"Pregnancy and Labour cause more Deaths than Oral Contraceptives": the Debate on the Pill in the Spanish Press in the 1960s and 1970s', *Public Understanding of Science* 19 November, 1–14.

Ortiz-Gómez, T., Távora Rivero, A., Delgado Sánchez, A. and Sánchez, D. (2001), 'Ser mujer y médico en la España de los años Sesenta', *Asparkía* 12, 125–33.

Oudshoorn, N. (1994), *Beyond the Natural Body. An Archaeology of Sex Hormones.* (London and New York: Routledge).

Polaino Lorente, A. M. (1972), 'Dimensiones psicológicas y antropológicas de la Planificación Familiar', *Galicia Clínica* 44, 357–76.

Rodríguez-Ocaña, E., Ignaciuk, A. and Ortiz-Gómez, T. (2012), 'Ovulostáticos y anticonceptivos. El conocimiento médico sobre 'la Píldora' en España durante el Franquismo y la Transición Democrática (1940–1979)', *Dynamis* 32:2, 467–94.

Salvatierra, V. (1973), *Apuntes de Ginecología* (Granada: Gráficas del Sur).

Salvatierra, V. et al. (1978), Experiencia en Planificación Familiar del Departamento de Ginecología de la Universidad de Granada, in *Comunicaciones al Tema Control de Natalidad e Inducción al Parto.*

Sánchez, D. (1999), 'Androcentrismo en la ciencia. Una perspectiva desde el análisis crítico del discurso' in Barral et al. (eds).

—— (2002), *El discurso médico de finales del siglo XIX en España y la construcción del género. Análisis de la construcción discursiva de la categoría la-mujer.* (Granada: Universidad de Granada).

Sánchez Carazo, C. (1998), *Introducción de los anovulatorios orales en España: Aspectos morales, sociales y médicos* (Madrid: Universidad Complutense).

Sánchez Hernández, M. F. (2009), 'Evolución de las publicaciones femeninas en España. Localización y análisis', *Documentación de las Ciencias de la Información* 32, 217–24.

Seaman, B. (1995 [1969]), *The Doctor's Case against the Pill* (Alameda: Hunter House).

Sichtermann, B. (1996), 'Die Frauenbewegung und die Pille' in Staupe and Vieth (eds).

Sieg, S. (1996), 'Anovlar – die erste europäische Pille. Zür Geschichte eines Medikaments' in Staupe and Vieth (eds).

Silies, E. (2010), *Liebe, Lust und Last: Die Pille als weibliche Generationserfahrung in der Bundesrepublik 1960–1980* (Göttingen: Wallstein).

Solano Berral, E. (1974), 'Planificación familiar. Métodos anticonceptivos', *Hispalis Médica* 31:362, 689–741.

Staupe, G. and Vieth L. (eds) (1996), *Die Pille. Von der Lust und von der Liebe* (Berlin: Rowohlt).

Taboada, L. (1978a), *Cuaderno Feminista. Introducción al Self-Help* (Barcelona: Fontanella).

——— (1978b), 'Cómo derribar la medicina masculina. El Self-Help o la descolonización de nuestro cuerpo', *Vindicación Feminista* 20, 1 February, 38–40.

Telo Núñez, M. (1977), 'La española ante la Ley. El adulterio. El aborto', *Ama: Revista de las Amas de Casa Españolas* 413, 15 February, 40–41.

Usandizaga, J. M. and López Valverde, M. (1978), 'Lo que la Mujer nos ha contado acerca de la "pastilla" en seis años de Recetar anovulatorios', in *Comunicaciones al Tema Control de Natalidad e Inducción al Parto*.

Usborne, C. (1992), *The Politics of the Body in Weimar Germany: Women's Reproductive Rights and Duties* (Ann Arbor: University of Michigan).

Vilar, L. (1968), 'La explosión demográfica y su control. Medidas preventivas: aspectos religiosos, psicológicos y educacionales', *Actividades de la Asociación Española de Mujeres Médicos* 1, 53–7.

Villatoro, A. (2010), Interview by Teresa Ortiz-Gómez. Madrid, May 19–20, 2010.

Watkins, E. S. (1998), *On the Pill: a Social History of Oral Contraceptives, 1950–1970* (Baltimore: Johns Hopkins University Press).

Chapter 7

The Contraceptive Pill, the Pharmaceutical Industry and Changes in the Patient-Doctor Relationship in West Germany

Ulrike Thoms

In 1961, the first contraceptive pill was marketed in West Germany, prompting fierce debates over morals and ethics, the nature of sexuality in general and relationships between men and women in particular. Overall the pill was a catalyst for social change as it enabled new life choices and lifestyles (Silies 2010; Watkins 2012). Moreover, it had a massive impact on gynaecological practice. Women had formerly visited a gynaecologist's office for medical complaints and advice in pregnancy. Now healthy women came in, wanting a prescription for a pharmaceutical substance that should prevent pregnancy. The majority of doctors were somewhat overwhelmed by this development; even more so because of the growing impact of media influences on medicine and the new grassroots medicine, which deeply challenged the professional identity of gynaecologists and the relationship between gynaecologists and women.

In this chapter I will analyse how pharmaceutical companies assessed these changes, how they adjusted their marketing strategies accordingly and, in particular, how they established contact with the women who ultimately had to swallow the pill. Utilising the rich sources held in the business archives of the German firm, Schering, I will examine how the firm's marketing campaigns reacted to changes in the doctor-patient relationship and address how the firm actively shaped these relations for the sake of sales. Due to the very different history of the pill in the context of the socialist-planned economy of East Germany, I will limit my analysis here to West Germany.[1]

1   This chapter originates from the French-German research collaboration, GEPHAMA (From Advertisement to Marketing. Pharmaceutical Enterprises, Patients, Physicians and the Construction of Medical Markets), funded by the German Research Foundation and Agence National de Recherce between 2009 and 2012, from the German part, located at the Institute for the History of Medicine, Berlin. The author wishes to thank Thore Grimm from the Schering business archive for his support.

Introducing the Pill to Patriarchical-Structured West German Medicine in the 1960s: The Story of Anovlar

The introduction of the pill in the Federal Republic of Germany was a somewhat risky undertaking for Schering. The firm had had the pharmacological knowledge to produce it since the 1940s, but legal restrictions dating from the Nazi era, social, religious, ethical and, last but not least, political reasons, had so far made it unthinkable to publicly promote oral contraception. German gynaecologists believed their task was to assist women in pregnancy and birth, not prevent them. Hoping to detect change, the firm observed developments and undertook an opinion poll among gynaecologists (Laengner 1981). Having tested the waters in Australia, the board of trustees finally dared to introduce Anovlar in Germany in June 1961.

The introductory campaign followed the usual strategy. Doctors were seen as the main partners in the business; thus promotion was strictly limited to the sphere of medical experts. In a pre-marketing phase the pill had been made known to leading gynaecologists by including them in clinical investigations, spreading the news to opinion leaders. In the second phase, Anovlar was introduced to known specialists and gynaecologists through an informative letter, a product brochure and a sample. Advertisements in leading journals followed to maintain interest. Later, the promotion was extended to general practitioners.

How reluctant the firm was to spread news to the public is well illustrated by the panic that arose after the well-known popular journal, *Stern*, reported on the coming introduction, before Schering had informed doctors. Schering, fearing doctors might be upset (Dietrich 1994), immediately ordered their pharmaceutical representatives to inform gynaecologists the article had not been published on the firm's initiative (Schering AG Berlin 1961). Moreover, it sped up the informational campaign for practitioners, who were sent a letter explaining that the firm had not initiated the article nor known about it (Schering AG Berlin n.d.). These activities demonstrate how eager the firm was to protect the illusion that firm and physicians were close partners.

The situation was complicated further by many doctors refusing to prescribe the pill (Silies 2010, 190–96; regarding Spain see Ignaciuk, Ortiz-Gómez, Rodríguez-Ocaña in this volume). In tribute to the doctors' expert status, while presenting itself as acting upon a purely scientific basis, Schering actively declined to comment on any public discussions, advising their representatives not to mention these debates when visiting doctors (ibid.). The firm did not even dare to speak openly about contraception. Instead, the product brochures spoke vaguely of the 'ovarian rest' as an effect of Anovlar, thus leaving the doctor to determine the drug's uses (Anovlar 1961). Only since the fourteenth edition of the brochure, published in October 1968, did the title openly indicate the purpose of the drug to be a hormonal contraceptive (Anovlar 21 1968). At this time, Schering had relinquished its hesitation about promoting contraception in Germany and portrayed itself as the leading firm in the field. Every marketing campaign that followed underlined the firm's experience and innovativeness, qualities which enabled it to produce a constant flow of newly developed contraceptives (Dietrich 1994).

The firm created a very detailed program of how the drug should be presented to doctors – and constantly learned from their experiences, as representatives reported feedback (Besprechungsprogramm 1962). Staff and representatives were provided with scientific information by the in-house 'Anovlar-Bulletin'. Going through at least 17 editions, this bulletin provided promotional tips.[2] 'Scientific Information on Anovlar 21', containing abstracts and extracts from scientific articles, together with special prints from scientific articles, was sent out to doctors (Wissenschaftliche Informationen zum Anovlar 21 n.d.). The firm thus paid tribute to doctors', and even practitioners', scientific knowledge. In fact, doctors knew very little about pharmacology in general, let alone contraceptive practices (Marks 2001, 119–37; Silies 2010, 186–221; Amendt 1985; Pacharzina 1975). As Schering realised, if they wanted to sell their pills at all the firm had to educate doctors. A closer look at the brochures and publications reveals that many served the needs of doctors who ran busy practices and had little time to read. They concentrated on the main problems and had a design that allowed doctors to easily grasp the most important content (Was leistet Anovlar? n.d.), and the distributed extra prints summarised scientific articles in four pages. All these publications were written in a down-to-earth-language to ensure the texts would be properly understood, despite the overall illusion of a scientific conversation.

A systematic vocational training of physicians in contraception began late in West Germany, the first courses taking place in Giessen in 1967, in close cooperation with the German family planning association, 'Pro Familia' (Dose 1989, 69; Ärztlicher Fortbildungskurs 1968). This association and a few health insurance companies were the first to provide the public with systematic and neutral information (Jaentsch-Zander 1981, 5.1–5.3). Although many conferences on family planning took place during the late 1950s and early 1960s in other countries, and discussions about the use of hormones for contraception took place at a number of gynecological conferences from 1961 onwards, the lack of debate in Germany endured due to the German Society for Gynaecology and Obstetrics being dominated by surgically-orientated traditional physicians (Lauritzen 1986, 259).

Another factor was the strong tradition within Germany of a patient-doctor model which identified women as 'help-seeking' and doctors as 'advice-giving' authorities, a situation reflected in the few advertisements from these early years. They depict couples, or women with children in their arms, listening to the doctor, an elderly, expert adviser, and trusting his experienced advice on contraception (see Figure 7.1). In later times, there was not a single advertisement for any of the newer pills that presented the doctor physically, only the product and the women.

Following the introduction of the pill, other firms entered the German market. Four years after Schering had marketed the first oral contraceptive in Germany

---

2   See S1-348-4. Schering Archiv, Bayer AG.

Anovlar 21 erleichtert Ihnen die Beratung junger Mütter

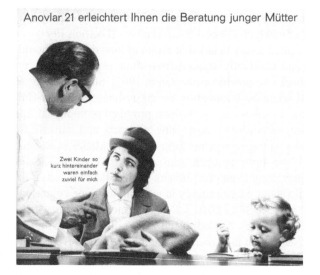

Zwei Kinder so
kurz hintereinander
waren einfach
zuviel für mich

Figure 7.1   Advert for doctors: 'Anovlar 21 makes counseling of young
mothers easier for you. "Two children so shortly after each other
were simply too much for me.'"
Source: S1-347, Schering Archiv, Bayer AG

there were 20 products from different firms on the market, with their number
continuing to rise. In order to keep track of developments, Schering began to
make extensive use of market research and finally established a market research
department ('Anovlar im Brennspiegel der Marktforschung' 1965). Moreover, it
began to buy expensive market data from the Institute for Medical Statistics (IMS).

Opinion researchers had studied contraception since 1949, when the
important 'Institute for Demoscopy' had requested information about opinions
on contraception, the resulting study finding roughly two thirds of the population
accepted it (Silies 2010, 94; Prill 1966, 95). A number of other actors, including
the journal *Stern*, the German government and pharmaceutical companies,
initiated similar polls. Schering itself ordered one in 1965, in connection with
the integration of its new marketing department. It commissioned Marplan, a
well-known institute for opinion research that opened its first German office
in 1959, to gauge the level and source of knowledge about the pill. Two years
later it financed a second, comparative study, with its competitor, Heyden
(Imle 1968, annex).

What does this mean? Although Schering maintained the pretence of limiting its
marketing activities to doctors, the firm was increasingly aware of womens' active
role in demanding prescriptions for certain products. Research clearly showed that
women's knowledge was based largely on articles in the popular press. In a 1965
poll, at least 64 per cent of women cited the press as their main source, rising to 70
per cent two years later, with only 8 per cent having been informed by their doctors.

Interestingly, 90 per cent wished to be informed about the pill by their physicians (Imle 1968, 64). Schering also discovered that physicians had refused to prescribe the pill to 14 per cent of their patients, and that a third of this group would probably use oral contraceptives if the need for prescription was lifted (ibid.). Schering was therefore concerned that doctors' lack of communication with their patients was hindering the pill's introduction. An unsatisfactory relationship between doctor and patient was seen to endanger compliance, the basis of hormonal contraception efficacy. Experiences in Puerto Rico had clearly demonstrated that the safety of any contraceptive method, and women's satisfaction with it, depended less on the method itself than on the relationship between doctor and patient, success rates being highest where communication took place in a friendly and relaxed atmosphere (Angrist 1966; Nijs 1972). In contrast, bad relations between doctors and patients reduced compliance and success rates. A doctor's behaviour could damage trust in the pill's safety, and therefore harm the firm's reputation and reduce sales. The 1967 enquiry also revealed that two thirds of the early pill users had in fact switched to other methods, often due to perceived risks. Schering therefore took measures to increase compliance, one such move being the introduction of the so-called month pack, with 21 pills in a blister package, allowing women and doctors to easily monitor if the pill had been taken (Die Spezialpackung schützt weitgehend vor Einnahmefehlern 1964; about US pill dispensers see Eisert in this volume). Moreover, it began to provide women with informational material, explaining how the drug worked plus when and how it had to be taken (Peck Gossel 1999).

Female Rebellion and the Marketeers' Reaction

Recent studies have analysed the pill's contribution to the medicalisation of female sexuality and pregnancy, in which doctors dominate the relationship with their patients (Watkins 1998, 50–52; Marks 2001, 117). Doctors welcomed the fact that pharmaceutical companies recommended a medical check up before prescription and regularly during medication. This ensured women visited their office regularly and also allowed for regular cancer screening (Bekanntgabe des wissenchaftlichen Beirats' 1970; Marks 2001, 125).

Although gynaecologists claimed the right to decide on the necessity of any therapeutics and prescriptions, they were increasingly confronted with women demanding a prescription for the pill. If a doctor was not willing to prescribe, many women knew how to obtain the pill anyway: by sending a friend to get a prescription, buying it on the grey market or smuggling it from countries where the pill was freely available, such as Czechoslovakia (Sillies 2010, 89–91).

Gynaecologists also had to compete with family planning institutions (Marks 2001, 118) like 'Pro Familia' and marriage counseling institutions run by health insurance companies, such as the *Allgemeine Ortskrankenkasse* (AOK) in Berlin, or charity organisations like the Catholic *Caritas*. Although these organisations were not allowed to prescribe the pill themselves, they could employ doctors to do so.

Unlike doctors, who viewed the pill as the safest and most recommendable medication, these institutions also informed their clients about other methods of contraception (Kepp 1970). Although nominally leaving the choice to women themselves, they clearly encouraged the use of the temperature method or mechanical devices, considered by many doctors to be uncomfortable, unaesthetic or unsafe. Many practitioners, however, prescribed the pill without ever examining women, not being fully aware of possible side effects, and did not explain the risks at all (Marks 2001, 125; Pacharzina 1978).

Although initially welcomed by many women, public discussions about the risks associated with the pill produced some scepticism, which was amplified by feminist journals. The *Grande Dame* of German feminism, Alice Schwarzer, raged violently against the pill, claiming it would result in the patriarchic claim of women's constant sexual availability (Schwarzer 1977). It would also tie women to a medical system dominated by male doctors, and to the predominately male pharmaceutical industry (Schwarzer 1984). Her radical views were not shared by the majority of women, but a strong grassroots movement emerged during the 1970s: female health journals like *Clio* appeared and alternative medical handbooks were published, such as translations of the famous American book, *Our Bodies, Ourselves* (Davis 2007), and its German counterpart, *Witches Whispers* (*Hexengeflüster* 1975). Women's Health Centers also emerged (Berg 1999), which focused heavily on questions of sexuality, contraception and birth. These developments impacted on the pill's use among German women between 15 and 44 years of age. The number of pill-users had almost stagnated between 1971 and 1974, increasing only among women over 40 and less than 19 years, who had formerly been excluded from contraception for medical reasons ('Das Unbehagen' 1977). The percentage of pill users peaked at 33 per cent in 1975, but decreased by 5 per cent between 1976 and 1977, only reaching the 30 per cent mark again in 1987 (Unger and Lachnit-Fixson 1991, 970).

Viewing the pill as a signifier of medical and even social progress, scientists and gynaecologists could not understand why women had become so sceptical that Schering's sales decreased by 10 per cent (Richter 1977, 57–60). Instead of critically assessing their contribution to this situation, they blamed the public press for fearmongering, exaggerating the true level of risk (Unger and Lachnit-Fixson 1991, 986; 'Abschlussdiskussion' 1977). Schering's marketing department did not believe the relatively small number of about 20 articles had created these fears, but had merely brought these changes to light. Women were obviously tired of the pill. They said this to their doctors, who reported the development in scientific publications, and from there it crossed over to the public press. One should not underrate the significance of such debates. They are at the heart of fights over scientific expertise, as scientists often accused journalists of having massively contributed to unreasonable fears, despite not having grasped the scientific facts properly. Remarkably, in this context, it was a male journalist who opposed the scientists' view during an event organised by Schering. He criticised the experts for wanting the public to accept their scientific view instead of recognising their right to interpret things differently and make up their own minds (Waldner 1977, 60).

The relationship between gynaecologists and their patients was at stake: women's journals such as the very popular *Brigitte* refused to see contraception as an affair of women who – very conveniently for men – were expected to automatically choose the pill any longer. Consequently a series of articles on alternative methods called on men to take up their share of responsibility, inconvenience and risk.

Schering recognised the need to know more about the doctor-patient relationship in order to halt the decline in sales. For a long time their direct business partners had been doctors, but they now realised that women's complaints about bad doctor-patient relations endangered their sales figures. Therefore they developed a twofold strategy: they adjusted product information to better suit doctors' needs, and they ordered a detailed inquiry.

Exploiting the Doctor-Patient Relationship

In the late 1960s, sociologists and psychologists had begun to investigate the relations between doctors and patients (Imle 1968; Pacharzina 1978; Amendt 1982). In 1977 women's journals joined the debate. *Brigitte*, for example, conducted a survey among its readers, which was then conceptualised and evaluated by Ruth Höh from the Institute for Medical Sociology at Hamburg ('Wie gut sind Frauenärzte' 1977). This revealed that women reported twice as many negative things about their gynaecologists, such as time pressure during visits making it difficult to have questions answered and problems explained, than positive aspects. Other points were made about doctors being rude and impolite, having judgemental and moralistic attitudes, and women feeling that doctors did not take them seriously (ibid.). While *Stern* issued a similar enquiry five years later, *Brigitte* undertook a follow-up among 10,000 readers in 1982, which was published under the heading 'Bad marks for gynaecologists' ('Schlechte Noten' 1983; 'Eine Eins in Überheblichkeit' 1983; 'Das müssen Frauen' 1983; Höh 1983). Gynaecologists' performances had obviously not improved. Half the women consulted complained about judgemental and moralistic attitudes, about being made to feel vulnerable and shameful during their visits, and about being reduced to their organs and their pathological function. So far, the only noticeable change was in the female patients, who had found more self-confidence ('Schlechte Noten' 1983). For the journal editors, who had campaigned for information on the side of the doctors and the women alike, these results were rated as discouraging and alarming. In 1977, every sixth woman had felt she received insufficient information from her doctor; six years later every fifth woman felt this way.

Schering monitored the female press carefully and was therefore aware of the problematic relations between gynaecologists and their female patients.[3] In order to help doctors give adequate information to their patients, the firm thoroughly researched the doctors' needs and the appropriateness of the firm's information strategy. In 1970 it had already conducted an opinion poll among doctors in the run up to the marketing campaign for the newly introduced Neogynon. Though its impact should not be overestimated, the resulting report emphasised some important facts. Schering's representatives interviewed 1000 doctors about their opinion on the information for its new pill Neogynon. As expected, it found doctors wanted to be informed about the advantages of the new product in comparison to already existing contraceptives. To its surprise, however, the company learned that only 38 per cent of gynaecologists and 21 per cent of practitioners wished for more in-depth information about the chemical composition of the drug. As the safety of Neogynon was a matter of course for the firm, it was equally surprised that 50 per cent of doctors explicitly requested the drug, whereas only 11.5 per cent wanted to know about side effects (Schering AG Berlin 1970).

In other words, the reality of doctors' wants and needs differed from their self-portrayal as scientists, to which the company's marketing had so far been addressed. Obviously doctors did not want detailed information, but basic and applicable knowledge. Schering's report concluded that informational brochures should stick to general information ('pauschale Angaben') instead of going into great detail. The development of product brochures clearly illustrates this new policy. By 1969, they had expanded to a length of 49 pages and included a growing list of literature. Arguing that these lists were only bulking up the brochures, after 1973 they were simply left out, bringing the brochure size down to 28 pages. Seven years later the brochures were reduced to four-page flyers: but there was no uproar from doctors.[4]

This contrasts with the increasing segmentation of the pill market. Segmentation is the usual answer to increasing competition in a mature and almost saturated market, allowing sales to continue increasing by including clients at the margins of consumer groups. In pharmaceutical marketing the most important way of achieving this is to widen the indication to as many target groups as possible and address them differently. In Schering's case this policy led to the development of a family of different products to meet the different needs of different women ('The Problem' 1972; Eine neue Möglichkeit 1972). This went far beyond addressing different lifestyles in consumer advertising, as well as far beyond changing visualisation strategies (Malich 2012), because this classification was purposefully constructed in scientific publications and included in promotional material. Picking the right drug was therefore made a scientifically based activity of doctors, who were presented with a list of side effects and the corresponding pills and recommended to use these as pointers to finding the right pill (Golob n.d.).

---

3 See clippings, S1/280, Schering Archiv, Bayer AG.
4 See Anovlar brochures, S1-347. Schering Archiv, Bayer AG.

This once again confirmed the doctor's expert position, to themselves as well as to outsiders (Döring 1970), while creating the impression the choice was only made possible by the firm's outstanding innovative power and restless scientific efforts.

In the end a kind of system was formulated that offered solutions for every hormonal type: Diane, for example, was introduced in 1975 for the 'masculine' type of women with acne and greasy hair. Microgynon (1973) was established as the contraceptive of choice for older women (Neu von Schering 1975; Schering AG Berlin 1974), with Sequilar (1974) recommended for younger women (Sequilar n.d.; Schering AG Berlin 1975) (Figure 7.2). Microlut, a one-phase pill that was very low in estrogens, was introduced in reaction to the discussion about side effects of the pill in 1972. It was never intended to replace the older drugs, but to complete Schering's spectrum of pills. The most important supporting argument for Microlut was that it could be prescribed for those women who could not take the other pills due to medical reasons; it was therefore named the pill for 'the other women', or the pill for 'special cases' ('Sonderfälle') (Eine neue Möglichkeit 1972). Other firms followed similar strategies, resulting in around 40 different pills being on the market in the early 1970s. Schering used the confusion which might have arisen from this situation to develop a new marketing strategy. It presented the variety of pills as a system, which, as an advertisement said, offered the perfect way out of the labyrinth of pills (Der Weg aus dem Labyrinth 1975; Seqilar für die jüngere Frau n.d.). When the company introduced Ediwal in 1976, in response to the decline in sales of Eugynon and Neogynon which had targeted the average, 'normal' woman, they promoted it for women with irregular cycles and spotting, creating the impression of an orchestrated system of contraceptives in order to stabilise Schering's market share (Horn n.d.). The large number of different contraceptives massively complicated information provision. It also increased promotional activities and costs, as Schering had to develop promotional material for every one of these pills. As information provision became more complex, the

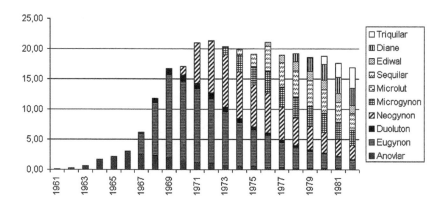

Figure 7.2   The sale of different pills by Schering (1961–1982)
Source: B1-285-3, Schering Archiv, Bayer AG

firm responded with a whole set of informational media for doctors, including symposia, medical and psychological seminars, economic, legal and computer seminars and, last but not least, informational material for patients.

This was more than public relations material and a friendly service for patients. It was also a service for doctors. Many had neither the time nor the energy to discuss contraception or the reasoning behind the choice of a certain contraceptive with their patients. Schering was aware of this fact. The 1966 marketing campaign for Schering's second contraceptive, Eugynon, directly argued that Eugynon's low hormone dosage 'virtually eliminates the need for trial and error selection of products'. Thus it would relieve the doctor of time-consuming patient complaints (Schering AG Berlin 1966, 11). The distribution of informational material from industry to patients shifted the task of basic information-gathering from the doctor and his office to the patient in the waiting room. A well-informed patient would save the doctor time, or at least allow discussions to begin at a higher level. Moreover, the doctor would have the opportunity to point to the weighty evidence of the written word.

Schering was eager to produce such patient leaflets from early on. In 1965 it had produced the brochure 'What you should know about Anovlar 21', containing basic information on the action of Anovlar ('Was Sie wissen sollten über Anovlar 21' 1965). Three years later it brought out 'The Pill in Questions and Answers', which is a very interesting case. This brochure had originally been distributed to doctors in 1962 as a basic form of information on the ground-breaking new product, Anovlar (Döring 1970). It was later replaced by a newly written leaflet for doctors that pretended to discuss all arguments (Schering AG Berlin n.d.; Schering AG Berlin n.d. [c1969/1970]), with the brochure then distributed to women. This nicely demonstrates how Schering realised and appreciated that women had left behind their status of innocence and had gained the level of knowledge formerly held by physicians.

Schering reinforced its efforts to produce informational literature for patients during the years to come. In 1979 it issued the brochure 'What a man and a women want to know about contraception today', which referred directly to the newest scientific progress and experiences from practice (Was ein Mann und eine Frau n.d.) (Figure 7.3).

As basic and banal as this brochure may appear today, its production was taken very seriously by the company. In order to assess their needs, 160 women had been interviewed about the pill and contraception, before the Cologne advertising agency McCann developed the brochure with scientific advice from Prof. Döring and Dr Frick-Bruder. Once it was printed, pharmaceutical representatives were informed of the leaflet's aims and instructed on how to introduce it to doctors: the explicit aim of the brochure was to maintain or – even better – increase the acceptance rate of contraceptives by informing patients about the pill and stressing its outstanding safety (Schering AG Berlin 1979). From 1984 onwards, the dissemination of this brochure was further broadened as Schering offered it to pharmacists, who could order it for distribution to their customers (Schering AG

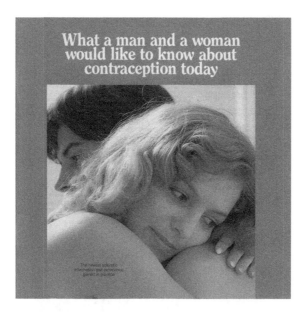

Figure 7.3   Brochure by Schering, 1979
Source: B1-285-3, Schering Archiv, Bayer AG

Berlin 1984a). The same year, another brochure was issued that addressed young girls and gave information about their first visit to the gynaecologist – the barrier to a pill prescription (Schering AG Berlin 1984b) (Figure 7.4).

Overall, we can conclude that pharmaceutical companies like Schering worked not only on their relationship with doctors, but also on their relationship with patients. It was important for them to generate consumer satisfaction with its products. But even when addressing the patient, it also reached out to the doctor, enabling him to perform his job quicker and more efficiently on a better-informed patient. As doctors profited from this, they had reasons to be thankful to Schering, definitively strengthening the bonds between them and the industry.

Femovan: 'The New G-Class of the Pill' – and the New Role of Consumers in Schering's Marketing Concepts

The 1987 campaign for Femovan advanced this general trend. It emphasised Schering's achievement of once again reducing the hormone dose through the development of its active principle, the substance gestoden. The firm's marketing strategy for Femovan was as new as the substance itself. Schering commissioned the Frankfurt advertising agency Lintas to develop an entirely new and integrated concept for the introduction of Femovan. This campaign targeted doctors as well as the intended consumer group of girls between 14 to 20 and their mothers.

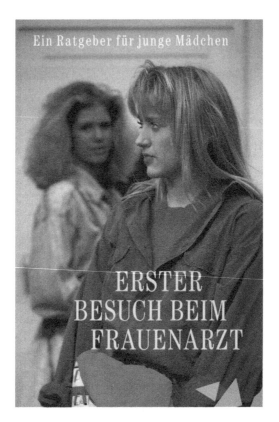

Figure 7.4   'A guide for young girls. The first visit to the gynaecologist.'
                Brochure by Schering, 1984
Source: B1-285-3, Schering Archiv, Bayer AG

Differing from former campaigns, it did not use Schering's company colour, a deep green, in the promotional material. Instead a newly developed brand sign was introduced, consisting of orange and pink stripes. These colours were thought to better suit the intended target group of young girls. Moreover, these colours are usually associated with feminity and emotions ('Rosa [Farbe]' 2012).

In fact, the firm established new standards with regard to the dimensions of its campaign. On 5 May 1987, 1500 doctors were invited to a conference which took place in Berlin, Düsseldorf and Munich simultaneously. Well-known TV moderators led these local events. At certain points, the three events were connected via video conference which, at this time, was rather a spectacular and expensive communication channel. Attached were press conferences with around 80 journalists, at which Femovan was presented as the beginning of a new era for the pill (Femovan-Einführung 1987).

Although the campaign used the usual channels in addressing doctors, by pretending to put the girls' needs for information and their need to be protected from too-early pregnancies at the centre of the campaign, it provoked paternal feelings in the doctors (Schering AG Berlin 1987). The firm was very well aware this strategy was on the margins of the legally permissible, as consumer advertising was not allowed for prescription products. But by using the slogan 'We set standards' (Schering AG Berlin n.d. [c1988]), Schering not only presented itself as the major player in the field by once more proving its innovative power in the field of hormones, but insinuated in a very subtle and ambiguous way that its innovativeness included the ability to push marketing to a new level by taking the needs of consumers and their right for information into account. Consequently Schering claimed to make them 'more enlightened in health matters' and to improve the relationships between doctors and patients (ibid.).

Even before this event Schering had managed to launch articles on the new pill to come, in women's journals like *Für Sie, Freundin, Petra* and *Brigitte*, as well as in the yellow press, which named Femovan the super-pill without risk ('Die neue Superpille 1987'). It also placed adverts in journals for girls, such as *Mädchen*, and the famous youth journal, *Bravo*. For youngsters the latter was an important source for knowledge on all aspects of sex. Especially important was its letters section, in which readers asked all kinds of questions about sex, questions they would hardly dare ask their parents.

Once Femovan had been officially introduced, this bi-weekly journal published image adverts for Schering in every second issue. These did not directly advertise the product, but presented some information while mentioning the firm's name. These adverts were placed in close proximity to, or in the direct neighborhood of articles on such questions as 'Do you talk about contraception?' ('Bravo-Umfrage' 1987), close to the page 'Love, Sex and Tenderness' ('Liebe, Sex und Zärtlichkeit' 1987) or to articles reporting on such catastrophic events as the fact that teen star Nino de Angelo would soon become a father ('Nino de Angelo' 1987).

Though not mentioning the product, these adverts were in the Femovan colours and design. They depicted girls on the left, with a text block in the centre addressing the problems adolescent girls typically faced, such as the first visit to a gynaecologist, sex education and how to be prepared for sexual intercourse.[5] The tone of these adverts was non-moralistic, down-to-earth and soothing (Claus 1987). The same adverts appeared in *Für Sie* and *Brigitte*, now addressing mothers ('Was heißt Urlaubsvorbereitung' 1987; 'Mit 14 schon zum Frauenarzt' 1987). Again, the adverts were embedded within surrounding articles on sexual problems and different methods of contraception ('Spirale' 1987; 'Wann ist es sinnvoll' 1987; 'Kondome' 1987; 'Verhütung' 1987). These image adverts were accompanied by a horde of other public relation activities, such as discussion and information circles for youngsters. Schering had also produced a cassette with information on application and dosage which doctors could hand to their patients. This strategy also included boyfriends, who were invited to take part in the

5   The adverts were published in *BRAVO* (1987) 25, 19; (1987) 28, 51; (1987) 31, 43; (1987) 38, 32; (1987) 42, 17; (1987) 48, 18; (1987) 50, 19.

public events. The overall strategy, however, was to convince girls and their mothers that it was never too early for a visit to the gynaecologist. The gynaecologist was portrayed as someone who would be extremely cautious during examination and give advice in a friendly manner. At the same time, doctors and mothers were warned with statements like 'At 14 she makes up her own mind. But she cannot decide everything yet' or 'For the mother she is still a child. For the boyfriend she is already a woman'. Doctors were presented as gatekeepers who, by prescribing the pill to girls, gave them more active responsibility and protection against pregnancy. Equally important is the fact that the doctors were always addressed as those who knew, who consciously made the (right) decisions, who were objective and acted responsibly, and sometimes even alluding to fatherly feelings.[6]

By commissioning a sociological and psychological study from the well-known Sinus Institute at Heidelberg, Schering had attempted to put the doctor-patient relationship on a more solid footing. Psychological studies of subgroups of consumers had become standard tools when planning marketing campaigns for consumer goods and even drugs. However, companies usually kept their results a secret, while using them to determine market segments and consumer groups. Schering went in a completely new direction, presenting the results of this investigation to the public, thus positioning itself as a socially responsible company, offering services to people who then might be better able to solve their problems (Schrödel 1988). The entire study was intended to determine the thoughts and emotional landscape of young gynaecological patients. It contained two parts: a pilot study focused on the relationship between patients and gynaecologists, and a typology of girls developed as a kind of consumer typology, as had been used from the early days of market and consumer research (Liebe-Sexualität-Verhütung 1988; Nowack 1988; Bauch and Claus 1988). From today's point of view and marketing practice, this strategy seems appropriate, especially as the women were to take lifestyle medicaments and had the right to be properly informed (Siegel-Watkins 2012). But for those involved, especially the physicians and pharmacologists, this was totally unacceptable and an intolerable violation of borders.

Surprisingly, it was not the obvious traditional and paternalistic doctors who were upset by this strategy. In fact it was Ulrich Moebius, one of the editors of the leftist and critical *arznei-telegramm* who was most active, establishing a press campaign against Schering. He did not argue that existing advertising law had been violated by the addressing of patients. This would have had little effect, as the adverts had not mentioned the product name, so were to be regarded as mere image campaigns. Moebius did not comment on Schering's efforts to inform women and girls either, but instead criticised the pill from a purely scientific and medical perspective, raising questions about pharmacological problems and the dangers of its main substance, Desogestrel. Doing so, he cited a study that had been commissioned by Schering itself and conducted by the endocrinologist Herbert Kuhl at the university clinic in Frankfurt. Ironically, Schering had chosen

---

6   See folder S1-348-2. Schering Archiv, Bayer AG.

Kuhl to undertake this examination because he was known as a particularly critical scientist. Kuhl and his co-authors had found a concentration of Desogestrel in the blood which was not lower than the older pills, as the ads argued, but in fact higher (Kuhl, Jung-Hoffmann and Heydt 1988). Comparing Femovan to the competing product, Marvelon, from Wyeth, Moebius claimed this hormone concentration posed a severe risk to patients and accused Schering of misleading advertising, in which it had been claimed the product had the smallest hormone content ever. Moreover, he suspected Femovan could provoke thrombosis and cited the case of an English woman who had died after taking Femovan ('Dokumentation' 1995).

Moebius did not take any social aspects into account, not even mentioning patients' wishes or situations. Positioning himself as a scientist, he systematically undermined Kuhl's and Schering's credibility by using only pure scientific, medical and pharmacological arguments. Restlessly traveling from one TV and radio station to another, he gave countless interviews on the subject.[7] He also collected incriminating data on the assumed dangerous effects of the drug and published them in the *arznei-telegramm* ('Dokumentation' 1995), while leaving Schering to prove the accusations unfounded. Overall this strategy was very effective, although the English authorities, who had been alarmed by the case of the woman's death and had investigated the drug, had found no reason to ban the product. Even Kuhl's statements that the described effect of gestodene was only of scientific interest and probably had no or only very little clinical importance were not heard (Kuhl 1989b). On the contrary, Herbert Kuhl reported that the events had damaged his scientific reputation, causing many of his colleagues to treat him as an outlaw or traitor (Kuhl 1989a).

This campaign against Schering has to be seen in the context of the activities of the highly political SCHan-network. Against the background of the emerging leftist green movement in Germany, this network attacked Schering as a producer of chemicals which would massively contribute to air and environmental pollution. These arguments were mixed with accusations about Schering's role in developing countries (Mathews 1992; Redebeitrag der Aktionärsvertreterin Jungmann 1992), where the firm would trial drugs it would then market in rich countries (Jungmann 1989, 66; Jungmann, Redebeitrag 1989).

The campaign proved to be effective: the Berlin health authorities judged that the Femovan cassette was indeed a misleading advertisement of prescription medicines to laypeople and prohibited its further distribution ('Dokumentation' 1995). Sales of Femovan had skyrocketed in 1987, making it the second most popular contraceptive throughout the world; they now dropped by 50 per cent. Schering attempted to influence reports in the public press, but in fact its only choice was to commission more expensive studies in order to prove the substance's harmlessness. It is interesting that Moebius and his friends were

---

7   See the notes from the magazine 'Gesundheit' from 15 April 1989, in S1-280, Schering Archiv, Bayer AG, and the notes on three other interviews on SAT 1, Südwestfunk I and RIAS 2. Schering's publicity department's comment demonstrates that the firm tried everything to influence public reports.

so upset. Obviously this was not just because of the new substance and its properties. Articles in renowned newspapers assumed the critics had been waiting for a chance to attack Schering with whatever argument they could find (Mackenthun 1989a). The journalist, Gerhard Mackenthun, criticised Moebius's strategy as rampant male(!) fact-checking which was both misleading and irrelevant. For Mackenthun, the real problem was not the facts about the pill, but the widespread uneasiness of women with it. Pharmacological studies had limited their perspective to phenomena they could count, such as the occurrence of spottings. Women who came to the doctor's office complaining about weight gain or mood changes were not taken remotely seriously. Alluding to discussions about hysteria and to the dominance of emotions in women, German gynaecologists indicated their expert status and treated women's complaints as mere psychosomatic effects. Mackenthun rightly accused his fellow males of leaving women alone with contraception and exposing them to a paternalistic medical system and pharmaceutical industry, which only answered their fears with figures and rated their complaints as negligible instead of taking them and their wishes seriously (Mackenthun 1989b; Bräutigam 1989).

Others accused the activists of being in search of publicity, rather than concerned with the interests of women (Feldmann 1989; Westhoff 1989). The initiators of the *arznei-telegramm* were indeed men with very 'masculine', confrontational conflict strategies. They acted, and still act, from the professional position of physicians and pharmacologists and claim to always base their judgments on pure scientific pharmacological facts; despite it being well known that scientific facts are always socially constructed and that most doctors had neither the knowledge nor the interest to understand the problem, nor were they willing to think about it. In fact it had been exactly this position that created part of women's problems with the pill.

Conclusion

Schering's marketing activities for the pill in Germany provide an interesting case study. It demonstrates that pharmaceutical firms paid tribute to the fact they relied on doctors' willingness to prescribe certain drugs. They therefore tried to stabilise this relationship and avoided anything doctors might see as a violation of their professional expertise and status. Accordingly, the status of doctors as the decisive authorities was always honoured. Nevertheless, the firm had to realise that many doctors had no solid pharmacological knowledge and, specifically, no knowledge on contraception, which until the 1970s did not form part of the medical curriculum. Against the background of an increasingly competitive market, Schering reworked its marketing strategies, aiming at market segmentation by establishing different types of pills for different types of women. This application of consumer typology clearly demonstrates the quick change of the pill into a lifestyle medicament.

Schering noted this change and instrumentalised it for marketing purposes. Through market and social research, the firm learned that relations between female patients and doctors were the decisive elements in drug prescription. It therefore extended its informational campaigns. Though still concentrating on doctors, it began targeting the consumer via the instrument of the doctor, with informational material for their patients. Doing so circumvented the limitations of German drug advertising law, which strictly prohibited drug advertisement to patients. As long as these materials did not mention drug names or allude to certain products, this strategy worked well and did not lead to any criticism. But in 1984, when the firm employed a more offensive and visible strategy when promoting Femovan to young women, critics of the pharmaceutical industry responded strongly. Against the background of the rising green movement in Germany with its reservations about the chemical industry, and driven by the furor over the violation of doctors' expert status, these critics managed to temporarily put a halt to such marketing practices and exert a negative influence on sales figures.

This story is historically significant because it demonstrates that the German pharmaceutical industry has attempted to connect with consumers since the late 1960s. Much like the consumers themselves, the industry saw and displayed pills as part of a modern lifestyle. In contrast, pharmacologically-orientated critics did not accept this view: they did not pay tribute to the positions, wants and needs of women. Their perspective was limited to the 'facts' of pure science and their claim to be the decisive experts. Thus, they took the stance of scientific truth, disregarding the fact that science is socially constructed and that scientific results are always negotiated in the context of the concrete historical situations of societies. From their outdated patriarchcal position, they reduced the discussion on the pill to a clash of expert positions and limited its discussion to male-dominated scientific circles, in which consumers had no voice at all. By provoking the fierce struggle between doctors and patients during the 1970s, they definitively drove forward the establishment of the patient movement. Ironically, there is still no solid basis for productive cooperation between doctors and patients, as doctors often deem a visit by a well-informed patient a harrassment, as such a patient questions their expert status and – above all – demands a lot of time-consuming discussion and information.

References

'Abschlussdiskussion' (1977), in Deutsche Gesellschaft für Bevölkerungs-wissenschaften (ed.), *Orale Kontrazeption. Medizinische und gesellschafts-wissenschaftliche Aspekte*, Symposium, (Berlin) pp. 57–60.
Amendt, G. (1985), *Die bevormundete Frau oder Die Macht der Frauenärzte* (Frankfurt: Fischer Taschenbuch Verlag 1985) [1st edition 1982 under the title: *Die Gynäkologen* (Hamburg 1982)].
Angrist, S. S. (1966), 'Communication about birth control', *Journal of Marriage and Family* 28, 284–6.
Anovlar (1961), [brochure] S1-348, Schering Archiv, Bayer AG.
'Anovlar im Brennspiegel der Marktforschung' (1965), *Scheringblätter* 1, 2.

Anovlar 21 (1968), Zur vorübergehenden Ruhigstellung des Ovars, 14th edition [Berlin] October, S1-347. Schering Archiv, Bayer AG.

Ärztlicher Fortbildungskurs der Medizinischen Fakultät der Justus-Liebig-Universität Gießen über Fragen der Kontrazeption (1968S1-285), Deutsche Gesellschaft für Familienplanung Gießen 1 (1967) (Stuttgart: Thieme).

Bauch, W. and Claus, W. (1988), Schering Presseinformation: Junge Mädchen, Erwartungen und Erfahrungen [manuscript] 6 September 1988, Sch-A, B1-285. Schering Archiv, Bayer AG.

'Bekanntgabe des wissenschaftlichen Beirates der Bundesärztekammer: Leitsätze zur Verordnung oraler Ovulationshemmer' (1970), *Deutsches Ärzteblatt* 29, 2267–8.

Berg, L. (1999), 'Eine ereignisreiche Phase in der Medizingeschichte. Das Berliner Feministische Frauengesundheitszentrum ist 25 Jahre alt geworden. Von der Selbsterfahrungsgruppe zum Infocenter, in: *Berliner Zeitung online* 8.9.1999' http://www.berliner–zeitung.de> [accessed 4 November 2011].

Besprechungsprogramm (1962), 1 January, S1-348-4. Schering Archiv, Bayer AG.

Bräutigam, H. H. (1989), 'Erbitterter Streit um die Mikropille. Viel Lärm um nichts. Ein Kampf um Marktanteile wird ohne Rücksicht auf die Frauen ausgetragen', *Die Zeit* 12, 94.

'Bravo–Umfrage der Woche: Sprecht Ihr über Verhütung?' (1987), *BRAVO* 24, 11.

Claus, M., (1987), 'Einführungskampagne für die Pille Femovan. Neues Konzept – voller Erfolg', *Scheringblätter* 8, 8.

'Das müssen Frauen nicht mitmachen' (1983), *Brigitte* 12, 169–73.

'Das Unbehagen an der Pille' (1977), *Der SPIEGEL* 6, 38–49.

Davis, K. (2007), *The Making of Our Bodies, Ourselves. How Feminism travels across Borders* (London and Durham: Duke University Press).

Der Weg aus dem Labyrinth der Pillen (1975), [leaflet] October, S1-237. Schering Archiv, Bayer AG.

'Diaphragma und Kondom – alte Mittel werden neu entdeckt' (1977), *Brigitte* 9, 96–102.

'Die neue Superpille – sichere Verhütung ohne Nebenwirkungen' (1987), *Neue Revue* 1.

'Die Pille für den Mann' (1971), *Stern* 8, 174.

Die Spezialpackung schützt weitgehend vor Einnahmefehlern (1964), [brochure], S1-347. Schering Archiv, Bayer AG.

Dietrich, W. (1994), Zur Geschichte der oralen Kontrazeption oder – wie der Volksmund kurz sagt – der Pille [manuscript], undated, B1-285-1. Schering Archiv, Bayer AG.

'Dokumentation. Acht Jahre Femovan/Minulet' (1995), *arznei–telegramm* 5, 62–5.

Döring (1970), Die Pille in Frage und Antwort, ed. by Schering AG, Berlin/Bergkamen. [brochure], S1-285-5-3. Schering Archiv, Bayer AG.

Döring, G. K. (1970), 'Differenzierter Einsatz von Ovulationshemmern', *Deutsches Ärzteblatt* 67, 1360–62.

Dose, R. (1989), *Die Durchsetzung der chemisch-hormonellen Kontrazeption in der Bundesrepublik Deutschland* (Berlin: Wissenschaftszentrum Berlin).

Dürr, Klaus (1972), 'Microlut – keine Konkurrenz für die "Pille"', *Scheringblätter*, no. 2, 18.

'Eine Eins in Überheblichkeit' (1983), *Brigitte* 11, 119–23.

'Eine neue Möglichkeit der hormonalen Kontrazeption für Sonderfälle' (1972), *Medizinische Mitteilungen Schering* 2, Special Issue.

Feldmann, H. U. (1989), 'Kampagnen', *Gyne* 3, editorial.

Femovan-Einführung (1987), Diskussion per Video-Konferenz, May, S1-280. Schering Archiv, Bayer AG.

'Für manche Frauen die beste Lösung: das IUP' (1977), *Brigitte* 8, 134–8.

Golob, E. (n.d.), Ergebnis verantwortungsbewußter Forschung. Die Ovulationshemmer von Schering. Eugynon. Neogynon, Schering Wien [manuscript], SchA, B1/285-5-3. Schering Archiv, Bayer AG.

Hexengeflüster. Frauen greifen zur Selbsthilfe (1975), (Berlin: Selbsthilfeverlag).

Höh, R. (1983), *Brigitte Fragebogenaktion 'Wie gut sind Frauenärzte?' Zusammenfassung der vorläufigen Ergebnisse, nebst: Frauenärzte – haben sie dazugelernt?; Ergebnisse einer Fragebogenaktion 1982 und 1983 (*Hamburg: Gruner + Jahr).

Horn, R. (n.d.), Pharma Deutschland Marketing: Entwicklung des neuen oralen Kontrazeptivums Ediwal in Deutschland innerhalb der ersten 6 Monate und Zukunftsaspekte der Bewerbung [manuscript], S1-242. Schering Archiv, Bayer AG.

Imle, C. (1968), *Motivation für die Ablehnung der Ovulationshemmer (im Rahmen einer psychologischen Studie über Empfängnisverhütung)*, Medical Dissertation (Würzburg: ph. Diss.).

Jaentsch-Zander, W. (1981), 'Erste Erfahrungen mit der hormonalen Kontrazeption in der gynäkologischen Praxis', *Die Pille wird 20. Von Anovlar zu Triquilar. So begann es ... und da stehen wir heute. Symposium* Berlin (Berlin: Schering Pharma Deutschland) pp. 5.1.–5.3.

Jungmann, B. (1992), 'Maxidisput um Mikropille. Der Femovan–Skandal' in Mathews H. (ed.), *Schering Schering – Die Pille macht Macht. Berichte über die Geschäfte des Schering-Konzerns* (Stuttgart: Schmetterling-Verlag).

Kepp, R. (1970), 'Ovulationshemmer für junge Mädchen. Zu den Leitsätzen der Bundesärztekammer in Heft 40/1970, S. 2907' *Deutsches Ärzteblatt* 3, 679.

Kirchhoff, H. and Haller, J. (1959) 'Konzeptionsverhütung durch oral wirksame Gestagene', in *Deutsche Medizinische Wochenschrift* 84, 2189–92.

'Kondome'. Wie werden sie verwendet? Und wovor schützen sie wirklich? (1987), *Freundin* 8, 117–19.

Kuhl, H. (1989a), 'Wirklich viel Lärm um nichts? Über einige Schwierigkeiten im Umgang mit der Pille', *Das Wissenschaftsjournal Forschung und Praxis der Ärzte-Zeitung* 8:74, I, VIII.

——— (1989b), Interview, 'Warnungen vor Antibabypillen'. [manuscript] March, S1-280. Schering Archiv, Bayer AG.

Kuhl, H., Jung-Hoffmann, C. and Heydt, H. (1988), 'Alterations in the serum levels of gestodene and SHBG during 12 cycles of treatment with 30 micrograms ethinylestradiol and 75 micrograms gestodene', *Contraception* 38:4, 477–86.

Laengner, H. (1981), '20 Jahre Schering-Kontrazeptiva – von Anovlar zu Triquilar', in *Die Pille wird 20. Von Anovlar zu Triquilar. So begann es ... und da stehen wir heute. Symposium Berlin 1981* (Berlin: Schering Pharma Deutschland), pp. 6.1–6.5.

Lauritzen, C. (1986), 'Geschichte der gynäkologischen Endokrinologie des deutschen Sprachraumes von 1935 bis zur Gegenwart' in Beck L. (ed.) *Zur Geschichte der Gynäkologie und Geburtshilfe. Aus Anlass des 100jährigen Bestehens der Deutschen Gesellschaft für Gynäkologie und Geburtshilfe* (Berlin: Springer Verlag).

Liebe – Sexualität – Verhütung (1988), Erwartungen und Erfahrungen junger Mädchen heute. Zusammenfassung einer Studie des SINUS-Instituts, Heidelberg, im Auftrag der Schering AG [manuscript] Sch-A, B b1-285. Schering Archiv, Bayer AG.

'Liebe, Sex und Zärtlichkeit, Frau Dr. med. Keppler antwortet' (1987), *BRAVO* 25, 20 and 48, 17.

Mackenthun, G. (1989a), 'Streit um Mikropille ein Sturm im Reagenzglas. Mit Statistiken wird der Kampf um Marktanteile ausgetragen', *Berliner Ärzteblatt* 102, 301–3.

———— (1989b), 'Der Streit um die Mikropille scheint ein Sturm im Wasserglas zu sein. Keine gravierenden Unterschiede bei einzelnen Präparaten mit niedriger Hormondosis', *Frankfurter Rundschau*, 22 April.

Malich, L. (2012), 'Vom Mittel der Familienplanung zum differenzierenden Lifestyle-Präparat. Bilder der Pille und ihrer Konsumentin in gynäkologischen Werbeanzeigen seit den 1960er Jahren in der BRD und Frankreich', NTM. Zeitschrift für Geschichte der Wissenschaften, Technik und Medizin 20, 1–30.

Marks, L. V. (2001), *Sexual Chemistry. A History of the Contraceptive Pill* (New Haven and London: Yale University Press).

Mathews, H. (ed.) (1992), *Schering – Die Pille macht Macht. Berichte über die Geschäfte des Schering-Konzerns* (Stuttgart: Schmetterling-Verlag).

'Mit 14 schon zum Frauenarzt' (1987), [advertisement] *Freundin* 11, 123.

Neu von Schering (1975), October [leaflet] S1-237. Schering Archiv, Bayer AG.

Nijs, P. (1972), *Psychosomatische Aspekte der oralen Antikonzeption* (Stuttgart: Enke).

'Nino de Angelo. Er wird Vater' (1987), *BRAVO* 42, 18.

Notes from TV-magazine 'Gesundheit' (1989), 15 April, S1-280. Schering Archiv, Bayer AG.

Nowack, D. (1988), Liebe – Sexualität – Verhütung. Erwartungen und Erfahrungen junger Mädchen heute. Zusammenfassung, [manuscript] Sch-A, S1-285. Schering Archiv, Bayer AG.

Pacharzina, K. (1975), 'Sexualmedizin der Allgemeinpraxis II: Die Wissenslücken', *Sexualmedizin* 4, 535–42.

———— (1978), *Moralwächter im weißen Kittel. Zur Sexualmedizin in der Allgemeinpraxis, Med. Diss.*, Lollar.

Peck Gossel, P. (1999), 'Packaging the Pill' in Bud, R., Finn, B. and Trischler, H. (eds) *Manifesting Medicine. Bodies and Machines* (Amsterdam: Harvard Academic Press) pp. 105–21.

'Pillenmüde?' (1977), *Brigitte* 7, 133–40.

Prill, H. J. (1966), 'Motivation und Einstellung der Frau zur Kontrazeption' in Kepp R. und Koester H. (eds) *Familienplanung. Erster ärztlicher Fortbildungskurs der Medizinischen Fakultät der Universität Gießen über Fragen der Kontrazeption am 24./25. Juni 1966* (Stuttgart: Thieme Verlag) pp. 94–104.

'The problem of the "other women"' (1972), [brochure] Sch-A, S1-233. Schering Archiv, Bayer AG.

Redebeitrag der Aktionärsvertreterin Beate Jungmann auf der Schering Hauptversammlung (1989), [manuscript] 14 June, S1-280. Schering Archiv, Bayer AG.

Richter (1977), 'Abschlussdiskussion' in *Deutsche Gesellschaft für Bevölkerungswissenschaften* (ed.) *Orale Kontrazeption. Medizinische und gesellschaftswissenschaftliche Aspekte, Symposium* (Berlin: Schering AG) pp. 57–60.

'Rosa' (Farbe) (2012), Available at: http://de.wikipedia.org/wlkl/Rosa_(Farbe) [accessed 10 July 2012].

Schering AG Berlin (1961), Rundschreiben Nr. 16/61 an die Herren wissenschaftlichen und kaufmännischen Mitarbeiter, 22 June, S1/348-6. Schering Archiv, Bayer AG.

———— (1966), Medizinisch-Wissenschaftliche Abteilung Ausland, Sales Conference 1966. Eugynon. [Lecture Notes], 13 September, S1-227. Schering Archiv, Bayer AG.

———— (1970), Informationsdienst 69/70, betr. Auswertung der Fragebogen zum Neogynon 21/28.29. September 1970, S1-228. Schering Archiv, Bayer AG.

———— (1974), Letter to doctors, March, S1-237. Schering Archiv, Bayer AG.

———— (1975), Letter to doctors, June, S 1-237. Schering Archiv, Bayer AG.

———— (1979), Rundschreiben an die Damen und Herren des Außendienstes Nr. 26/779, 13 June, B1-285-5-3. Schering Archiv, Bayer AG.

———— (1984a), Letter to pharmacists, March 1984, B1-285-5-3. Schering Archiv, Bayer AG.

———— (1984b), Erster Besuch beim Frauenarzt. Ein Ratgeber für junge Mädchen. [brochure], Berlin: Schering AG, B1-285-5-3. Schering Archiv, Bayer AG.

———— (1987), Presseinformation, Zu viele Kinder werden Mütter [press information], 3 May, S1-280. Schering Archiv, Bayer AG.

———— (n.d.), Letter to doctors, S1/348-6. Schering Archiv, Bayer AG.

———— (n.d. c1988), Neueinführung von Femovan. Wir setzen Zeichen [Letter to doctors] S1-280. Schering Archiv, Bayer AG.

———— (n.d. c1969/1970), Medizinisch-wissenschaftliche Abteilung, Letter to doctors, B1-285-3. Schering Archiv, Bayer AG.

'Schlechte Noten für Frauenärzte' (1983), *Brigitte* 10, 100–108.

Schrödel, R. (1988), Motivation, Ziele und Aufgaben einer psychosozialen Studie, erstellt im Auftrag der Schering AG, München, 6 September [manuscript] S1-280. Schering Archiv, Bayer AG.

Schwarzer, A. (1977), 'Penetration', in *EMMA* 1, 4.

———(1984), 'Immer nur schlucken? Wir Frauen haben mit ihr die Verantwortung. Aber auch die Kontrolle', *Emma* 3, 20–22.

Sequilar (n.d.), Die Pille mit dem natürlichen Rhythmus [leaflet] S 1-237. Schering Archiv, Bayer AG.

Sequilar für die jüngere Frau (n.d.), [order card] S1-237. Schering Archiv, Bayer AG.

Silies, E. M. (2010), *Liebe, Lust und Last. Die Pille als weibliche Generationserfahrung in der Bundesrepublik 1960–1980* (Göttingen: Wallstein).

'Spirale: Was Ärzte heute Frauen empfehlen' (1987), *Freundin* 3, 60–61.

'Und wann kommt die Pille für den Mann?' (1977), *Brigitte* 11, 105–8.

Unger, R. and Lachnit-Fixson, U. (1991), 'Case F: Die Entwicklung der Pille (Oral Contraceptive)' in Albach, H. (ed.) *Culture and Technical Innovation. A Cross-Cultural Analysis and Policy Recommendations, (Berlin and New York: de Gruyter).*

'Verhütung. Alle Methoden. Ihre Vorteile. Ihre Nachteile' (1987), *Freundin* 12, 124–5.

Waldner, (1977), 'Abschlussdiskussion' in Deutsche Gesellschaft für Bevölkerungswissenschaften (ed.), *Orale Kontrazeption. Medizinische und gesellschaftswissenschaftliche Aspekte, Symposium* (Berlin: Schering AG) pp. 57–60.

'Wann ist es sinnvoll, die Pille zu wechseln' (1987), *Freundin* 25, 126–8.

'Warnungen vor Antibabypillen sind reine Vorsichtsmaßnahmen' (1987), Main-Echo, Aschaffenburg, 4 March.

Was ein Mann und eine Frau heute über Empfängnisregelung wissen möchten (n.d.), Alles über die neuesten Erkenntnisse der Wissenschaft und Erfahrungen aus der Praxis [brochure] B1-285-5-3. Schering Archiv, Bayer AG.

'Was heißt Urlaubsvorbereitung' (1987), [advertisement] *Freundin* 31, 34.

Was leistet Anovlar? (n.d.), [brochure] S1-348a. Schering Archiv, Bayer AG.

'Was Sie wissen sollten über Anovlar 21'[brochure] (1965), S1-347b. Schering Archiv, Bayer AG.

Watkins, E. S. (1998), *On the Pill. A Social History of Oral Contraceptives 1950–1970* (Baltimore/London: Johns Hopkins University Press).

——— (2012), 'How the pill became a lifestyle drug: the pharmaceutical industry and birth control in the United States since 1960', *American Journal of Public Health* 102, 1462–72.

Westhoff, J. (1989), 'Marketing oder Medizin? Hintergründe des Streits um die Risiken der Mikropille', *Tagesspiegel*, 14 March.

'Wer läßt sich sterilisieren – sie oder er?' (1977), *Brigitte* 10, 204–13.

'Wie gut sind Frauenärzte' (1977), *Brigitte* 17, 66–8.

Wissenschaftliche Informationen zum Anovlar 21 (n.d.), [brochure] S1-347. Schering Archiv, Bayer AG.

PART III
Users and Abusers Then and Now: Discourses and Practices

Chapter 8

Women, Men, and the Morphine Problem, 1870–1955

Jesper Vaczy Kragh

Recent scholarly work on the history of opiate addiction has drawn attention to a gender shift that occurred during the late nineteenth and early twentieth centuries. Over the course of this period, the image of the typical drug abuser was transformed from an educated upper-class woman into an unskilled working-class man (Courtwright 2001; Campbell 2000; Kandall 1996; Strausser and Attia 2002; Acker 2002, 1–2). Contrary to today's conception of drug abuse as a primarily male problem, morphinism, or morphinomania, was originally primarily associated with women. As David Courtwright has stated, in his extensive study of the history of opiate addiction in America, 'the outstanding feature of nineteenth-century opium and morphine addiction is that the majority of addicts were women' (Courtwright 2001, 38). Estimates of the number of American addicts suggest that between two-thirds and three-quarters of the total were female (Kandall 1996, 15). British historians have similarly pointed to a link between morphine use and women (Zieger 2005; Seddon 2008; see also Kohn 1992). According to these studies, medical practice in the late nineteenth century was the main reason for this predominance of women among the addicted population. Women were seen as less capable of managing painful conditions than men, and therefore as being in greater need of opium and morphine, which was liberally dispensed to them by male physicians. As has been noted by Mara L. Keire, doctors injected women with morphine 'to numb the pain of 'female trouble', or to turn the wilful hysteric into a manageable invalid. Up through the turn of the century, morphine was a literal prescription for bourgeois femininity' (Keire 1998, 809; see also Palmer and Horowitz 1982).

The claim that the majority of morphinists were female, however, might require further scrutiny. Late nineteenth-century physicians did not universally agree that women were more likely to become morphine habitués, and quantitative studies conducted at the time point in different directions. Even though contemporary medical writing in countries such as England placed an emphasis on female drug abusers, according to Virginia Berridge, this might not 'bear much relation to reality' (Berridge 1999, 148–9). Berridge points out that British prescription books reveal that morphine was prescribed to as many men as women, and admission statistics of asylums such as Bethlem, confirm there was no prevalence of females among morphine users. A similar point regarding French drug history has been put forward by Jean Jacques Yvorel (Yvorel 1993, 106).

This essay investigates the issue of gender and class in morphine addiction. By exploring German, French, and Danish sources, I will argue that morphinism was most frequently linked with men in the late nineteenth century. I will argue, furthermore, that of the morphine users who received treatment for drug abuse, well-educated upper-class women did not overshadow all other groups of patients. Male physicians, in fact, appear to be the most prominent demographic group among morphine addicts in this period. There is a dearth of historical research, however, regarding how the existence of these morphine-addicted doctors influenced drug policy in various countries.[1] By focusing on events in Denmark, I will contend that health authorities sought to address the problem internally and remained quiet about it in public. It was not until the late 1940s and early 1950s that drug addiction appeared in Danish public discourse. When it did, however, it became a heated topic, although it was not addicted male physicians who became the centre of media attention, but primarily the lower classes. Thus, the shift in gender distribution appears to be the opposite of that which occurred in America, as Danish sources indicate a higher number of female addicts in the early twentieth century than in the late nineteenth century.

Archival Sources

The fact that historians have not written a great deal about addicted physicians may, in part, be due to problems accessing certain archival sources. The main source for information on patients treated for drug abuse is the records of mental hospitals. In some countries, the confidentiality and privacy of psychiatric patient records is an obstacle to accessing such information, while in others, mental hospital records have simply not been preserved. In Denmark, however, the Danish State Archives have collected all records of patients at the state mental hospitals, and permission to use these can be obtained.

Patient records offer a wealth of information about the social position of inmates. Psychiatrists collected information from general practitioners, close relatives, the school system, employees, and the legal system. This information could then be used to analyse the social background of patients. Case notes were made at a time when it was only psychiatrists who had access to records; consequently, they often contain personal comments and observations. In addition, transcripts of conversations between psychiatrist and patient, questionnaires and patients' letters – the latter intercepted by psychiatrists – also appear, providing

---

1   No in-depth studies of drug-addicted physicians have been carried out, although the issue is often mentioned in works touching upon the history of addiction; see, for example, Courtwright 2001, 41/49; Berridge 1999, 269–70; Davenport-Hines 2002, 80–81; Milligan 2005, 541–53.

extra information about patients' experiences. As has been noted in studies of patient records, however, case notes do not give the researcher access to 'what really happened', and only partly and incompletely describe what was said and done (Braslow 1997, 8; on patient records see also Ackerknecht 1967; Risse and Warner 1992; Noll 1994; Edwards 1998; Gillis 2006). In addition, patient records do not provide a complete picture of the total population of drug users in society. A number of morphine users never had interactions with the mental health system. As with all historical sources, medical records must be evaluated carefully and, furthermore, compared to other available sources. In order to attain a broader understanding of drug addiction, I have therefore examined other forms of information from health authorities and police archives, as well as annual reports of hospitals, surveys, academic textbooks and contemporary articles in journals and newspapers.

Early Opiate History

The properties of opium had been known to the Sumerians, the Assyrians and the Persians for centuries, but the concept of drug addiction is a more recent phenomenon (Hickman 2004; Berridge 1979). In classical antiquity, opium was praised by poets and priests – even the medical authority of the Roman Empire, Galen, had nothing to say on the dangers of addiction. Whereas excesses in alcohol use were well known and often punished in Rome, opium was not linked with criminal or immoral behaviour (Dormandy 2012, 17–22; Booth 1999; Hodgson 2004). Opium lost its position in the Western world for a time, following the fall of Rome in 476 AD. The tradition of using the drug for medical and recreational purposes, however, continued in the Muslim world. Holy warriors brought opium back to the Continent during the Crusades, and by the sixteenth century, opium was well established within Western European medicine. With the 1660s introduction of Thomas Sydenham's laudanum, a combination of opium and alcohol, opium became widely available to people of various backgrounds. Addiction was recognised but rarely discussed in this period, and gained little public attention until the early nineteenth century, when medical interest in opium eating and its potential dangers increased (Dormandy 2012, 91–103; De Quincey 1821–1822). With the isolation of morphine by the young German apothecary's assistant, Friedrich Wilhelm Sertürner, a method he first published in 1805, and made important additions to in 1817, the issue of opiate misuse gained a new dimension (Maehle 1999, 189–93). In the 1820s, commercial production of morphine began in the UK and Germany, and by the 1840s the drug was accepted, and often preferred, within medical practice (Davenport-Hines 2001, 48; Berridge 1999, 138). In Denmark, morphine first appeared in *Pharmacopoeia Danica* in 1840, along with directions on how to isolate morphine from opium, as well as the first information on the acetate of morphia (Collegium Sanitatis 1840, 188).

With the invention of the hypodermic syringe, Sertürner's new drug gained wider acceptance. The French doctor, G. V. Lafargue, developed a procedure for introducing morphine under the skin using a lancet dipped in the drug in 1836. Other experiments were conducted by the Dublin-based physician, Francis Rynd, who described how he had cured a patient of neuralgia by administering subcutaneous injections of morphine, and Alexander Wood, of Edinburgh, who devised the technique of hypodermic injection in 1853. London-based doctor, Charles Hunter, further advanced the technique and coined the word 'hypodermic' in the late 1850s (Howard-Jones 1947; Berridge 1999, 139). As Norman Howards-Jones has noted, it was first assumed that the hypodermic injection of morphine would circumvent the habit-forming property of orally-ingested opiates, and few warnings about the risk of addiction were issued in the 1850s and 1860s. Morphine was hailed as a potent drug that could be used to treat a wide range of disorders and diseases: neuralgia, sleeplessness, headache, dysmenorrhoea, asthma, anxiety – to name but a few (Courtwright 2001, 48; Kandell 1996, 23–32). The first articles on hypodermic injections to appear in Denmark were published in 1860, and mention experiments conducted by Alexander Wood and others, along with Danish hospital reports on hypodermic or subcutaneous injections (Anonymous 1860, 193–4; Schou 1959). In the late 1860s, frequent reports on the hypodermic injection method were published in Danish medical journals but, as in other European countries, a need for restraint in administering repeated doses of morphine to a patient was rarely expressed. Morphine, and its prescription, initially raised the prestige of doctors who administered it, through the alleviation of a wide range of painful conditions (Norm et al. 2006; Berridge 1999, 142; Davenport-Hines 2001, 69).

Morphine Problems

Early cases of the repeated use of morphine were reported in Germany in 1864 but did not arouse much interest at the time. The issue was only given serious consideration when Heinrich Laehr, at an 1871 meeting of the Psychiatric Organisation in Berlin, made a presentation on the misuse of morphine injections (on Laehr's work see Erlenmeyer 1897, 402–10; Faust 1900, 6; Jakob 1925, 87–96). Laehr described a 28-year-old woman experiencing severe pain after a surgical operation who was given morphine injections. She began to request and use morphine daily, and Laehr compared this desire for the drug with alcoholism. He recommended that such patients be treated in a 'well-ordered hospital', and not in their homes, where their families would have difficulties preventing them from taking the drug (Laehr 1872, 352). Laehr's paper was followed by an article, 'Ueber den Missbrauch subcutaner Morphium-Injectionen' ('On the misuse of subcutaneous morphine injections') by the Dresden-based doctor, Carl Ludwig Fiedler, who described five patients – four men and one woman – suffering from a new disease (Krankheit) caused by the repeated use of morphine. Fiedler cautioned that the moment the layman got a syringe in his hand and learned how to use it, it would lead to his ruin. Even though the drug user 'eagerly fights against the force of habit' he 'can no longer exist without morphine' (Fiedler 1874, 231).

The first large-scale study to garner wide recognition, however, was Eduard Levinstein's 1877 book, *Die Morphiumsucht.* An English translation, *Morbid Craving for Morphia,* was published the following year; a French version appeared in 1880 (Levinstein 1877, 1878, 1880). The book was based on Levinstein's own experiences in the institutional treatment of addiction in Berlin, and was instrumental in defining morphinism as a disease (Parssinen and Kerner 1980, 278–9; Berridge 1999, 142–3; Padwa 2012, 42–4). Levinstein studied 110 morphinists, 82 of whom were male. As he noted in his book, he did not believe men were 'predisposed' to misuse morphine (Levinstein 1883, 7). It was instead their occupational position and the importance of maintaining the ability to work that led men to resort to morphine. According to Levinstein, 'every person, whether of a strong or of a weak constitution' has 'a tendency towards morbid craving for morphia', and once they had started using the drug, they could not stop:

> … the craving for morphia increases daily, the vicious circle draws closer around them, until, at last, all power of resistance having failed, they succumb under its action. (Levinstein 1878, 5–6)

Like Laehr, Levinstein emphasised that morphinists should be treated in institutional, hospital-based settings. The chief principle of Levinstein's treatment was 'sudden deprivation' of the drug. The patient was locked in a room, where he or she would stay for a period of 8 to 14 days until the withdrawal symptoms had disappeared. The patient was allowed alcoholic stimulants – champagne, port wine, and brandy – as well as hypnotics and anaesthetics – such as chloral hydrate or chloroform – and was constantly watched by two nurses (Levinstein 1878, 113–14).

Even though Levinstein's views were highly influential among doctors working with drug abusers, some physicians considered his treatment to be cruel and dangerous (Krafft-Ebing 1893, 596). The Bendorf-based physician, Albrecht Erlenmeyer, author of *Die Morphiumsucht und ihre Behandlung* ('On the treatment of the morphine habit'), opposed Levinstein's abrupt method, instead recommending a gradual reduction of morphine over a period of one to two weeks (Erlenmeyer 1883). A third method was introduced by the Bonn-based doctor, Rudolf Burkart, who increased the treatment period to three to four weeks, leading to fewer withdrawal symptoms than the more abrupt methods. In addition to gradual drug reduction, Burkart also used opium as a substitute for morphine (Burkart 1880). Although Burkart's views on the treatment of morphine abuse differed from Levinstein's, he made similar observations regarding the gender distribution of morphinists. In an 1883 study, he reported that, of 115 morphinists, 85 were male (73.9 per cent) (Burkart 1883).

German physicians were pioneers in the emerging field of addiction medicine, but doctors from other countries quickly followed suit. Shortly after the reports by Laehr and Fiedler had been published, the first French monograph on the topic was published by Lépold Calvet (Calvet 1876; see also Rodet 1897, 1–9; Bachmann and Coppel 1989; Retaillaud-Bajac 2009). In the 1880s, French newspapers such as *Le Temps*, *Le Gaulois* and *Le Figaro* published lots of articles on the subjects, claiming that morphinists 'tend to be female' (Yvorel 1993, 106). These claims, however, were not supported by statistical analyses. In an 1884 article, 'Morphine et morphinomanie' ('Morphine and morphinomania'), the French doctor Rambaud maintained that only 25 per cent of morphinists were female, and physicians such as Paul Regnard, Paul Sollier and Oscar Jennings arrived at similar figures (Yvorel 1993). Georges Pichon found a higher percentage of morphinists to be female; nevertheless, men still comprised the majority – 66 of 120 (55 per cent) – in his study (Pichon 1889). Comparable surveys were not conducted in the UK during the late nineteenth century, but admission statistics of inebriant's homes and mental hospitals do not reveal a disproportionately large percentage of women among morphinists (Berridge 1999, 149; Foxcroft 2007, 131). Quantitative studies from other countries, however, were in line with the German and French findings. Professor Heinrich Obersteiner of Vienna reported in 1883 that men accounted for 73 per cent of his patient base (Obersteiner 1883; see also Obersteiner 1879–1880 and 1882–1883). In a large survey of morphinism cases reported in literature from various countries, Paul Rodet established that 65 per cent of 1,000 morphinists were male (Rodet 1897, 37).

These late nineteenth-century morphinism statistics also highlighted a high rate of addiction among physicians. Obersteiner stated that, among morphinists, 'no other profession is more frequently represented than the medical profession'; Erlenmeyer declared that all contemporary observers agreed the majority of morphinists were found among the ranks of medical professionals; French physician, Ernest Chambard, expressed similar views (Obersteiner 1883, 63; Erlenmeyer 1883, 3; Chambard 1890, 38). Burkart studied 115 morphinists, 45 of whom were medical doctors; Levinstein included 32 physicians among his 110 patients; and Obersteiner found 67 doctors out of 194 patients. In the extensive survey conducted by Rodet, 28.7 per cent of morphinists were physicians. Even more startling figures were presented by Jennings, who claimed that 'one medical man out of four is a drug-habitué, and most often a morphinist' (Jennings 1910, 193; on Jennings, see Malcolm 1999). Women married to physicians were also well-represented among morphinists. Medical professionals such as nurses, members of the allied health professions, as well as pharmacists and dentists, also accounted for significant shares of the total addict population (Table 8.1).

Medical experts on drug abuse did not ignore the fact that physicians played a major role in the spread of morphinism. As one expert noted, not only did physicians fall victims to morphine themselves, they also caused addiction through their medical treatment (iatrogenic addiction):

... if medical men are charged; and it is to be feared, justly, with the propagation of this disease, owing to their carelessly, or for mere convenience sake, leaving morphia and a subcutaneous syringe with the patient, it may be regarded as their punishment that the demon morphinism finds among them his favourite victims. (Mattison 1883, 621)

Table 8.1   **Early German, Austrian and French morphinist studies, 1883–1897**

	Cases	Men	Women	Doctors	Doctors' wives
Levinstein 1883	110	74.5%	25.5%	38.2%	10.9%
Burkart 1883	115	73.9%	26.1%	40.8%	5.2%
Obersteiner 1883	194	73.7%	26.3%	34.5%	-
Pichon 1889	120	55%	45%	20%	10%
Rodet 1897	1000	65%	35%	28.7%	3.5%

Emil Kraepelin was in no doubt that physicians were responsible for the rise of addiction and declared frankly that 'there would be no morphinism if there were no doctors' (Kraepelin 1896, 398). According to Kraepelin, morphinism was a disease of doctors – who had easy access to the drugs – and well-educated, affluent people, who could afford the habit and had learned how to use morphine via careless physicians. Apart from those from the medical professions, military men – especially officers – business men and lawyers were also often mentioned in work on morphine habitués. The largest groups among female morphinists were doctors' wives and nurses (Levinstein 1883, 4; Erlenmeyer 1883, 4–5; Cambard 1890, 38).

Danish Studies of Morphinism

Warnings about morphine abuse reached Denmark in 1876–1877, when editorials in medical journals called attention to Levinstein's work and recommended stricter control over the prescribing of morphine. The first large Danish study was published in 1883 by Knud Pontoppidan, psychiatrist at the Municipal Hospital in Copenhagen. The results supported the French and German findings that morphine users were predominantly affluent, as Pontoppidan noted in his monograph, *Chronic Morphinism*:

> It is almost exclusively from the upper class or the well educated middle class
> that the morphinists are recruited, and it is an exception if we see morphinism in
> working class communities. (Pontoppidan 1883, 16)

According to Pontoppidan, this was because people of lower social classes could not afford morphine – at least not enough to use it regularly – therefore alcohol remained the working class drug of choice. In Pontoppidan's study of 25 morphinists, 32 per cent were medical doctors, and 60 per cent were male. He attributed the higher percentage of men to social factors. As family providers, it was more important for men to be able to work. Physicians who had easy access to drugs and demanding jobs were consequently more inclined to use morphine to overcome daily stress and fatigue. People with intellectually demanding jobs would generally prefer to use morphine, which improved their working ability without the stupefying effects of alcohol.

Pontoppidan remained uncertain, however, as to whether specific mental dispositions favoured morphinism. He presumed that large numbers of patients disposed to mental disorders did become chronic morphinists, but considered it a hypothesis for psychiatrists to prove in future studies (Pontoppidan 1883, 25). Like his contemporaries across Europe, Pontoppidan linked morphinism with painful chronic disorders, melancholia, overstrain and, to some extent, hysteria and nervous weakness. He considered disabling disorders – such as neuralgia, migraines and peptic ulcers – to be the main cause of chronic morphinism.

When it came to the treatment of chronic morphinism, Pontoppidan had initially used Levinstein's abrupt method. While this was found to work well in some cases, he discovered that a number of patients might experience a 'serious collapse' in the course of treatment, which could lead to death. This was referred to as 'the Achilles heel' of Levinstein's cure (Pontoppidan 1883, 76). Pontoppidan found that Burkart's slow withdrawal treatment, on the other hand, prolonged the morphinists' suffering. Pontoppidan consequently suggested a middle way, a quick withdrawal therapy that should be carried out in five days. After the patient endured the withdrawal therapy, however, a longer stay in hospital was necessary to prevent the patient from falling back into drug abuse. Ideally, Pontoppidan recommended a hospital stay of around half a year; other psychiatrists advised an even longer hospitalisation period. In the experiences of many doctors, morphinists relapsed into drug abuse shortly after leaving hospital. At least 16 of Pontoppidan's 25 patients relapsed, and several of his European colleagues also reported negative results with their patients. As Erlenmeyer noted, the morphinist's prognosis was 'highly unfavourable', and most patients were expected to resume using drugs (Erlenmeyer 1883, 204).

Pontoppidan dominated the field of morphinist studies, and Danish psychiatrists routinely referred to his work when the topic arose. His study was not followed up by other medical researchers, however, and the issue gradually receded from public consciousness. It was not until the 1940s that chronic morphinism again caught the public eye. This lack of attention, however, was not attributable to a decline in the number of morphinists admitted for treatment. On the contrary, hospital records show a constant increase in the number of cases in the period from the late nineteenth century to the 1940s.

Mental Hospital Records

At the time of Pontoppidan's publication on chronic morphinism, the Danish mental hospital system consisted of three state hospitals, a municipal mental hospital in Roskilde and the Copenhagen psychiatric department where Pontoppidan was employed. In the late nineteenth century, this psychiatric department was the only receiving unit for the entire city, and most psychiatric patients from Copenhagen were admitted to this facility (Schulsinger et al. 1975). Pontoppidan's department had approximately 130 beds in the 1880s, the state hospitals slightly more than 400 each and the institution in Roskilde around 1,000 (Beretninger 1886).

This psychiatric hospital system, however, was greatly expanded in subsequent decades. In the early twentieth century, a total of seven state mental hospitals were managed by a directorate within the Ministry of the Interior. Providing between 7,000 and 7,500 beds out of a total of about 11,000 psychiatric beds, these institutions housed the largest number of psychiatric patients in Denmark (see Figure 8.1). Apart from the state mental hospitals, the municipal mental hospital in Roskilde and four psychiatric clinics in Copenhagen provided the additional 3,000 beds. The private psychiatric sector of the Danish mental health system remained small, providing only one mental hospital, Filadelfia, with just under 200 beds. In 1950, these private, municipal and state institutions were expected to address the needs of a population of approximately 4.2 million (Sundhedsstyrelsen 195, 125–5; Vaczy 2010, 51–2). Most such hospitals were run by a senior consultant and a small staff of doctors and nurses. For the treatment of approximately 1,000 patients there would usually be six to seven psychiatrists, therefore day-to-day contact between psychiatrist and patient was limited. It was in these psychiatric institutions that long-term treatment of drug addiction was carried out in the late nineteenth and early twentieth centuries. During the period 1880–1955, a few private clinics opened, but none survived long and they did not play an important role in the treatment of morphinism.

Patient records from the mental hospitals support the studies by Pontoppidan and others, showing that the majority of morphinist patients were male. These records, however, do not provide an accurate picture of all Danes who used morphine on a regular basis. Obviously, not all morphine users were treated for drug abuse, and many Danes avoided institutional treatment even though their families or health authorities regarded them as morphinists. In order to gain a more thorough understanding of the issue, I have compared patient records with other primary sources.

The state mental hospital in Vordingborg (Southern Zealand), founded in 1858, received a substantial percentage of all patients treated for drug abuse. Patients of all

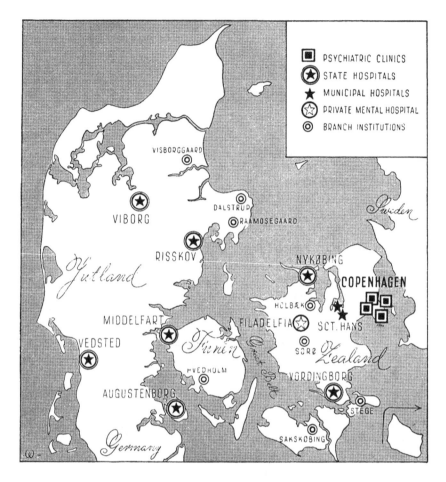

**Figure 8.1   Map of Denmark showing psychiatric institutions in 1952.
The branch institutions for elderly psychiatric patients were
placed under the control of the state mental hospitals.**
Courtesy Medical Museion

ages and from every stratum of society entered this approximately 400 bed hospital
in the 1880s; the hospital was expanded to 850 beds in the 1950s. In the records
of 4,683 patients a total of 56 were assigned the diagnosis chronic morphinism, or
abusus medicamentorum, in the period 1890 to 1930.[2] In the late nineteenth century
a large majority of these patients were middle-aged males, the average age being 41,
and the most prevalent group was that of physicians (comprising 39 per cent

---

2   There were some variations in terminology. The terms most frequently used in
hospital records were 'chronic morphinism', 'morphinismus', 'abusus medicamentorum'.

of all morphinists). Among the female patients, doctors' wives and nurses were predominant (40 per cent of all female patients). Like the male morphinists, female patients tended to be in middle age when admitted to the Vordingborg hospital, the average age being 39 years (the youngest being 26 years and the oldest 63). Most of the women had begun using morphine after receiving medical treatment for painful disorders such as neuralgia, rheumatism, and various postpartum problems. Only two patients had been introduced to morphine by non-physicians. In addition to physical ailments, psychiatric disorders were mentioned in a number of case notes: depression (four patients), neurosis (four patients), psychopathia (four patients), hysteria (two patients), and neurasthenia (one patient). In the records of ten female patients, however, no psychiatric comorbidity was mentioned.

Among the male morphinists, physicians were the dominant group (70.9 per cent). Of these patients, general practitioners were the largest subgroup. Psychiatrists, who had easy access to morphine, were also well-represented. Psychiatrists with a drug problem were usually permitted to enter a mental hospital situated in a different part of the country. The same procedure was employed for the top physicians at university clinics in Jutland. In order to avoid potential scandals, these physicians were admitted to hospitals in Zealand where they were less well-known. The second largest group of morphinists were apothecaries, who made up 12.9 per cent of male patients. Although patients with working-class backgrounds and smallholders were admitted to the hospital in Vordingborg, none were diagnosed with morphinism. Similarly to the female patients, physical ailments were given as the primary reason for the male patients' use of morphine. Psychiatric disorders such as depression (seven patients) and psychopathia (three patients) were only mentioned in just over one-third of records.

**Table 8.2   Patients' gender and profession, the state hospital in
Vordingborg, 1880–1930**

	Cases	Doctors	Doctors' wives	Health professionals
Women	25	-	28%	12.5%
Men	31	70.9%	-	-

Source: The Danish State Archives: The Mental Hospital in Vordingborg, Archive number HE-510, patient records males and females, 1880–1930

Physicians with a drug problem were rarely admitted of their own volition and – as in the case of a 45-year-old consultant – it was often the patient's wife who had notified the health authorities about the drug abuse. According to his own statement, the chief physician had begun using morphine because of long work hours, attendant health problems and 'troublesome private events'. It had not been difficult for him to get access to drugs, but after his wife surprised him while

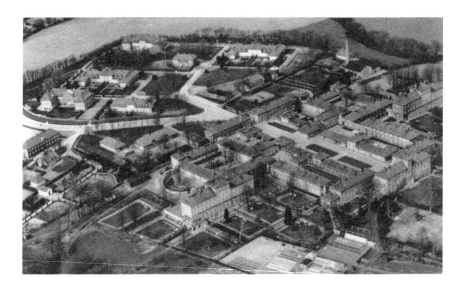

**Figure 8.2   The state mental hospital in Vordingborg from the 1940s.
             This institution, founded in 1858, was the second oldest of the
             Danish state mental hospitals.**
Photograph courtesy Medical Museion

injecting morphine, he could no longer conceal his habit and eventually had to accept treatment in a mental hospital. At the hospital in Vordingborg (Figure 8.2) he was not diagnosed with any psychiatric disorders other than drug abuse and a hospital psychiatrist noted the patient displayed no signs of 'the usual depravation of the morphinist'. During his stay at Vordingborg, he went through a withdrawal treatment where the dose of morphine was reduced by 20 per cent per day and terminated after a week. As part of the standard treatment at that time, he was requested to stay in the hospital for nine months. However, having decided to leave the institution after a shorter period of time, like many other patients receiving treatment for drug abuse, he relapsed into addiction.[3]

The addict physicians in Vordingborg were usually middle-aged when they had first used opiates, and most often claimed it was chronic diseases that had led them to addiction. Occupational stress and long working hours were also often cited as contributing factors, as well as financial trouble and marital problems.

Even though pain relief was given as the main reason for the use of morphine, some patients confessed that the euphoria of using morphine also played an important role. One physician had experienced a 'slight intoxication' when he started using morphine: 'My perception, ability to read, and memory abilities were

---

3   Case no 13,762, patient record males Statshospitalet i Vordingborg, Archive number HE-510, Landsarkivet for Sjælland (Statens Arkiver/The Danish National Archives).

considerably improved; my imagination came in motion, my energy increased, and it was always good and beautiful feelings that came up in me', he explained.[4] These pleasurable moments with morphine, however, were experienced in solitude, and like other drug users, this physician was not part of the drug subculture or a group of morphinists who had a mutual interest in drug-taking. Most such drug users obtained morphine on their own and kept it secret for as long as possible.

The National Health Service

The records of mental institutions such as the hospital in Vordingborg do not, however, contain information about all physicians with a drug problem. Many physicians did not receive drug-abuse treatment and managed to avoid mental hospital admission. Records of the National Health Service (NHS), however, provide further information about physicians taking drugs. The NHS kept records of physicians suspected of drug abuse. The names of 108 medical doctors were entered into the files of the NHS in the period leading up to the 1950s (the total number of physicians in Denmark was 4,952 in 1955). Of these 108 doctors, 15 were women. This is not, of course, a complete record of all physicians using morphine and other drugs. Many of the physicians admitted to the mental hospital in Vordingborg and other institutions, for instance, were not known to the NHS. However, these records do contain information about physicians who shunned treatment in psychiatric institutions. Approximately 40 per cent of the physicians listed by the NHS did not receive hospital treatment for drug abuse.

The NHS record can thus provide a more detailed picture of those physicians who used drugs. Most doctors began taking drugs when they were between 30 and 39 years old (45 per cent of the drug-taking physicians). There was also a large group, however, who began injecting morphine later in life, between 40 and 49 years old (31 per cent). Most were general practitioners (57 per cent) but physicians in higher positions were also among those registered by the NHS. Seven senior consultants were listed in the records.

Few of these physicians faced legal consequences, and the NHS does not appear to have been particularly interested in taking legal action against them. Some physicians had their rights to prescribe psychotropic drugs (such as morphine) revoked, but only three of the 108 physicians were denied the right to practice. Authorisation to prescribe was withdrawn in 37 cases, yet many of these doctors regained the right later on; and even though some physicians were stealing drugs from hospitals or forging prescriptions, they were rarely imprisoned or even fined (Nimb 1959, 46).

It was only in the late 1940s that the NHS accepted the need to support a stricter policy regarding drug use. This shift, however, had less to do with addicted

---

4   Case no 4,950, patient record males Statshospitalet i Vordingborg, Archive number HE-510, Landsarkivet for Sjælland (Statens Arkiver/The Danish National Archives).

physicians than with the new groups of drug abusers – groups considered a bigger societal problem than medical professionals' misuse of morphine.

Morphinist Surveys

Admissions statistics from the municipal hospital in Copenhagen, where Pontoppidan conducted his early morphinist studies, reveal that a change had occurred. In the early years of the twentieth century, female morphinists had begun to outnumber their male counterparts. During the period 1920–1932, for instance, women accounted for 55.6 per cent of morphinists admitted for treatment at the municipal hospital (Wimmer 1936, 89).

This predominance of female morphinists, however, remains somewhat ambiguous. Surveys from other hospitals, such as the Mental Hospital in Aarhus (Jutland) and the psychiatric clinic at Rigshospitalet (Copenhagen University Hospital), which opened in 1934, show a larger percentage of males – 53.4 and 61 per cent, respectively – in the first half of the twentieth century (see Table 8.3) (Helweg 1952; Strömgren 1944).

Among the morphinists registered by the NHS in the late 1940s and early 1950s, women accounted for 51.9 per cent of the total. The NHS during this period controlled the prescription process at all pharmacies, therefore the resultant database theoretically enabled them to identify new cases of abuse. Almost all drugs used by addicts in Denmark were believed to have been obtained by prescription, as drug-smuggling was not particularly common in this period. Police archives, however, show a different picture. Those users identified through police archives were found to have obtained their drugs largely by stealing from pharmacies, and such individuals were rarely known to the NHS; 68 per cent of the morphinists identified through police archives were male (see Table 8.3).

Table 8.3   Danish surveys on drug abuse, 1920–1954

	Cases	Men	Women
Municipal Hospital, 1920–32	106	44.3%	55.6%
Mental Hospital Aarhus, 1934–43	45	53.4%	46.6%
Rigshospitalet, 1945–49	87	61%	39%
National Health Service, 1949–51	227	48%	51.9%
Police Archives, 1949–56	216	68%	31.9%

Source: Wimmer 1936, 89; Strömgren 1944, 395; Helweg 1952, 507; Nimb 1959, 17, 21, 25

The Rise of Drug Control

Physicians still comprised a substantial percentage of the drug abuser population in the twentieth century. According to psychiatrist, Erik Strömgren, 'at least one third' of drug addicts in 1944 belonged to the medical profession (Strömgren 1944, 391). Large numbers of addicted physicians, however, were nothing new; Strömgren was only repeating the observations made by Pontoppidan 60 years prior. What was new was that, through an expansion of the health sector, morphine and other drugs – methadone in particular – were more widely available to the Danish population. From the late nineteenth century to the middle of the twentieth century, the number of medical doctors practising in Denmark had increased from 950 in 1890 to 3,995 in 1945; more than 40 per cent of those physicians were general practitioners (Jacobsen and Larsen 2007, 222; Valgårda 1992, 320). At the same time, wide-ranging health insurance programmes had made medical care considerably cheaper for those on low incomes. Doctors often paid little attention to the dangers of drug abuse in the twentieth century, and new drugs such as methadone were frequently dispensed to patients suffering from painful disorders, thereby increasing the risk of iatrogenic addiction.

Iatrogenic addiction, however, did not attract as much attention as the new phenomenon of 'group addiction'. During the Second World War, Denmark experienced a lawless period during which black market activities flourished. Groups of black market traders had also begun to sell drugs and 'eagerly and successfully sought to make converts to addiction' (Nimb 1959, 11). Whereas late nineteenth-century morphinists usually took their drugs in solitude, these new addicts, generally drawn from lower social classes, often gathered in bars and dives in the harbour areas of Copenhagen, where they shared and sold the drugs they had stolen from pharmacies or obtained by forging prescriptions.

Danish newspapers began to run stories about drug crimes committed by addicts in Copenhagen, and these articles led to the foundation of a state committee in 1950. Three years later, the committee issued a report on the misuse of psychotropic drugs recommending that legislative measures be taken to halt the increasing drug problem. In 1955, the Danish parliament passed the first national law intended to control narcotics. Stricter controls over prescriptions were introduced, together with a penal clause under which the commission of certain illegal acts could garner up to two years of imprisonment. It thus became punishable to import, sell or buy, distribute, manufacture, prepare or process prohibited or regulated drugs (Betænkning 1952, 24; Jepsen 2008, 155). The 1955 drug law led to an increase in police activities and in more control of individuals involved in drug abuse or illicit trafficking in psychotropic drugs. By 1958, the police registry contained information on more than 1,000 individuals (Nimb 1979, 28).

Different Responses to Drug Addiction

The shift in social class distribution among addicts prompted different methods of dealing with drug users. Drug users from lower social classes were often registered with the police or diagnosed as psychopaths. A fair share of these users were convicted and confined to the Psychopath Institution in Herstedvester (Stürup 1959). Conversely, psychiatrists only rarely diagnosed affluent drug abusers as psychopathic, and they were often processed by the NHS and the mental hospital system, rather than the police and penal system. Neither the NHS nor the mental hospital system, however, supported tough measures aimed at preventing morphinism. The NHS took few actions against morphinist doctors who might pose a risk to their patients, and doctors at mental hospitals did not encourage compulsory detention or treatment of drug abusers.

Contrary to studies emphasising the expansive aims of the medical profession, it appears that the medical community had a more ambivalent attitude towards drug abuse. The medical profession had little interest in drawing attention to the group of male and female addict physicians and was, for a long time, uninterested in advocating strict regulations or laws which would criminalise drug users. The regulations enacted in the 1950s had less to do with the interests of the medical profession and more to do with class, being largely motivated by the spread of drug addiction to people of lower socioeconomic status.

When compared to other countries, Danish drug abuse regulations were implemented rather late. In countries such as France, the UK, and Germany, stricter regulations had been introduced during or shortly following the First World War, largely due to the problem of addicted soldiers and reports about increasing use of opiates among civilians. Denmark's neutrality during the Great War might have delayed this type of reaction. Yet it is also important to point out that European countries tackled drug problems in diverse ways. As Howard Padwa has recently emphasised, variations in political culture and discourse shape how states respond to their drug problems, creating different ways of using law enforcement, prevention, and treatment measures (Padwa 2012, 5).

The claim advanced by American scholars, that the majority of morphinists were female, has not been confirmed by German, French or Danish sources. Bourgeois European women were not reported to be the largest group of morphinists in the late nineteenth century; male doctors were. Furthermore, hysteria was not the most common diagnosis associated with morphinism in Denmark. Only in two out of 25 female patient records from Vordingborg was hysteria associated with morphinism. The majority of female patients had begun to use morphine after receiving treatment for painful disorders. European physicians, however, were not only willing to prescribe morphine to female pain sufferers, they were even more eager to prescribe the drug for themselves.

There may well have been different patterns of addiction in Europe and the US, but it is also possible that the proportion of female morphinists has been overemphasised. American physicians do not appear to have been more reserved in their use of morphine than their European peers, and contemporary sources imply that addicted male physicians constituted a substantial percentage of American morphinists (Mattison 1883; Crothers 1899; see also Courtwright 2001, 41). As has been pointed out by Yvorell and Berridge, the notion of a majority of female morphinists often stemmed from sensationalist accounts in the press or from physicians who were not experts on drug abuse. Historical studies relying on these types of sources might provide a biased picture of gender distribution. Furthermore, precise American statistical data are lacking, and early surveys provide limited information on the number of female morphinists. Nevertheless, it is also possible that it was easier and less expensive for American women to use opiates on a regular basis, which may have resulted in higher numbers of female addicts. It remains difficult, however, to draw firm conclusions on this issue. Little comparative work, for instance examining differences in drug abuse between Europe and the US, has been conducted, and the issue of addiction among physicians has often been overlooked in writing the history of addiction.[5] It will be a task for future studies to determine the existence or absence of gender differences across borders.

The predominance of male morphinists can be associated with the characteristics of drug addiction in the late nineteenth century. The main cause of addiction in this period was administration of morphine by physicians. Drugs such as morphine were not sold on the black market and had to be obtained by prescription. Consequently, morphine was only available to small groups of people; such people had first experienced the effect of morphine in the course of medical treatment, or consisted of medical professionals who had self-medicated. In this period, male doctors – who had the greatest exposure to morphine – outnumbered all other demographic groups. Regular morphine use required not only easy access to morphine, a strong economic position was also essential. Well-educated people belonging to the middle and upper classes had the financial wherewithal to maintain their habit, and often had reason to prefer the use of morphine to that of alcohol; for male doctors, a morphine habit was easier to conceal than a heavy use of alcohol.

Similarly, morphine use could be less problematic for women than an alcohol habit, and morphinism was not described in the same negative terms as female alcoholism. Yet of the female morphinist patients admitted to Danish mental hospitals only very few thought of morphine as an intoxicant that produced euphoria. Most women had been introduced to the drug by doctors in the course of medical treatment. As often mentioned in the historiography of opiate abuse, medical practice during the late nineteenth century was one of the main reasons for female addiction. Indeed, women had a high risk of iatrogenic addiction in the late nineteenth century, but socio-economic factors restricted the number of female morphinists. Apart from nurses, physicians, and doctors' wives,

---

5 Few comparative studies have been published; see Gerritsen 2000. For a historiography of the topic, see Padwa 2012, 2–6.

most women did not have easy access to the drug or were not economically independent enough to sustain regular morphine use.

For men in elevated social positions, morphine appeared to be the solution to a range of problems and ailments. Like the female patients, most male morphinists stated that they had begun injecting morphine because of painful disorders and diseases. While this explanation was the least controversial, the sequence of events is often supported by both their medical history and the fact that many were middle-aged when they began using morphine. Compared with female morphinists, however, issues of working ability and drug use played a more important role in the accounts of male patients. Some men claimed that by using the drug, they were able to better pursue their work. As some patients asserted, regular and prolonged morphine use could be motivated by the apparent enhancement of mental faculties. There is no simple explanation, however, as to why various people began consuming morphine. Patient records and other sources do not reveal everything about addiction, and patients who were treated for drug abuse could not speak freely about their thoughts and feelings.

The number of addicted male physicians remained high throughout the late nineteenth century and into the middle of the twentieth century. With the expansion of the health sector during the early twentieth century, however, psychotropic drugs became more readily available to larger segments of the Danish population, and new groups of drug users emerged. In addition, few warnings about drug abuse were issued in this period, and addiction was not a heated topic in the press until the late 1940s. During the early twentieth century, more women began using drugs, often as a result of iatrogenic addiction. It was not until drug abuse was linked with black market activities and working class communities, however, that it came to be regarded as an important social problem.

An increased focus on crime and drug abuse had an impact on the use of illicit drugs among women, with lower rates of female drug abusers subsequently reported; by the 1960s and 1970s, the misuse of opiates was primarily associated with men (Dahl and Pedersen 2008, 22). This profile of the typical drug abuser has remained unchanged up to the present day. In the most recent Danish statistical survey on drug addiction, 78 per cent of addicts receiving treatment for drug abuse were male. However, other factors have changed. Modern-day patients have an entirely different social profile from their fellow drug users of the late nineteenth century. Drug abusers receiving treatment no longer have a middle or upper class background; the typical drug abuser of today tends to suffer from a lack of education, be unemployed, and homeless (Sundhedsstyrelsen 2013, 40).

References

Acker, C. J. (2002), *Creating the American Junkie: Addiction Research in the Classic Era of Narcotic Control* (Baltimore: Johns Hopkins University Press).

Ackerknecht, E. (1967), 'A plea for a "behaviorist" approach in writing the history of medicine', *Journal of the History of Medicine and Allied Sciences* 22:211–14.

Anonymous (1860), 'De subcutane Injectioner forsøgte i vore Hospitaler', *Hospitals-Tidende* 3:193–4.

Bachmann, C. and Coppel, A. (1989), *Le dragon domestique: deux siècles de relations étranges entre l'Occident et la drogue* (Paris: Albin Michel).

Beretninger om den kjøbenhavnske, den nørrejydske, Østifternes og den viborgske Sindssygeanstalt 1885 (1886) (Copenhagen).

Berridge, V. (1979), 'Morality and medical science: Concepts of narcotic addiction in Britain, 1820–1926', *Annals of Science* 36:67–85.

―――― (1999), *Opium and the People. Opiate Use and Drug Control Policy in Nineteenth and Early Twentieth Century England* (London: Free Association Books).

Betænkning om brug af euforiserede stoffer (1952) (Copenhagen: S. L. Møller).

Booth, M. (1999), *Opium: A History* (New York: St. Martin's Griffin).

Braslow, J. (1997), *Mental Ills and Bodily Cures. Psychiatric Treatment in the First Half of the Twentieth Century* (Berkeley: University of California Press).

Burkart, R. (1880), *Die chronische Morphium Vergiftung und deren Behandlung durch allmähliche Entziehung des Morphium* (Bonn: Kessinger).

―――― (1883), 'Zur Pathologie der chronischen Morphiumvergiftung', *Deutsches medizinische Wochenschrift* 9:33–6.

Calvet, L. (1876), *Essai sur le morphinisme aigu et chronique: Étude expérimentale et clinique sur l'action physiologique de la morphine* (Paris: Imp. V. Goupy).

Campbell, N. D. (2000), *Using Women: Gender, Drug Policy, and Social Justice* (New York: Routledge).

Chambard, E. (1890), *Les morphinomanes* (Paris: Rueff & Cie).

Collegium Sanitatis Regium Hafniense (1840), *Pharmacopoea Danica*, Editio 3 (Hafniæ: C. A. Reitzel).

Courtwright, D. (2001), *Dark Paradise: A History of Opiate Addiction in America* (Cambridge, MA: Harvard University Press).

Crothers, T. D. (1899), 'Morphinism among physicians', *Medical Record* 55:784–6.

Dahl, H. V. and Pedersen, M. U. (2008), *Kvinder og køn: stofbrug og behandling* (Aarhus: Center for Rusmiddelforskning).

Davenport-Hines, R. (2001), *The Pursuit of Oblivion: A Social History of Drugs* (London: Phoenix Press).

De Quincey, T. (1821–1822), *Confessions of an English Opium-Eater*. Available at: http://archive.org/search.php?query=title%3A%22Confessions%20of%20 an%20English%20Opium-Eater%22%20AND%20mediatype%3Atexts [accessed 11 February 2014].

Dormandy, T. (2012), *Opium: Reality's Dark Dream* (New Haven: Yale University Press).

Edwards, J. (1998), 'Case notes, case histories and the patient's experience of insanity at Gartnavel Royal Asylum, Glasgow in the nineteenth century', *Social History of Medicine* 11:255–81.

Erlenmeyer, A. (1883), *Die Morphiumsucht und ihre Behandlung* (Berlin: Heuser Verlag).

———— (1897), *Die Morphiumsucht un ihre Behandlung* (Berlin: Heuser Verlag).

Faust, E. S. (1900), *Ueber die Ursachen der Gewöhnung an Morphin* (Leipzig: J. B. Hirschfeld).

Fiedler, C. L. (1874), 'Ueber den Missbrauch subcutaner Morphium-Injectionen', *Deutsche Zeitschrift für praktischen Medicin* 27:231–9.

Foxcroft, L. (2007), *The Making of Addiction: The 'Use and Abuse' of Opium in Nineteenth-Century Britain* (Aldershot: Ashgate).

Gerritsen, J.-W. (2000), *The Control of Fuddle and Flash: A Sociological History of the Regulation of Alcohol and Opiates* (Leiden: Brill).

Gillis, J. (2006), 'The history of the patient history since 1850', *Bulletin of the History of Medicine* 80:490–512.

Helweg, H. (1952), 'Drug addiction', *Acta Medica Scandinavica* 142:507–13.

Hickman, T. A. (2004), 'Mania Americana': Narcotic addiction and modernity in the United States, 1870–1920', *The Journal of American History* 90:1269–94.

Hodgson, B. (2004), *Opium: A Portrait of the Heavenly Demon* (Oxford: Greystone Books).

Howard-Jones, N. (1947), 'A critical study of the origins and early development of hypodermic medication', *Journal of the History of Medicine and Allied Sciences* 2:201–49.

Jacob, W. (1925), 'Zur Statistik der Morphinismus in der Vor- und Nachkriegszeit', *Archiv für Psychiatrie* 76:87–96.

Jacobsen, K. and Larsen, K. (2007), *Ve og velfærd. Læger, sundhed og samfund gennem 200 år* (Copenhagen: Lindhardt og Ringhof).

Jennings, O. (1910), 'The frequency of morphinism', *The British Journal of Inebriety* 7:193–6.

Jepsen, J. (2008), 'Danish drug control policy 1945-2007' in Bagga B. et al. (eds) *Drug Policy: History, Theory and Consequences. Examples from Denmark and USA* (Aarhus: Aarhus University Press) 151–80.

Kandall, S. R. (1996), *Substance and Shadow. Women and Addiction in the United States* (Cambridge, MA: Harvard University Press).

Keire, M. L. (1998) 'Dope fiends and degenerates: the gendering of addiction in the early twentieth century', *Journal of Social History* 31:809–22.

Kohn, M. (1992), *Dope Girls. The Birth of the British Drug Underground* (London: Granta Books).

Kraepelin, E. (1896), *Psychiatrie. Ein Lehrbuch für Studierende und Ärzte* (Leipzig: Verlag von Johan Ambrosius Barth).

Krafft-Ebing, R. (1893), *Lehrbuch der Psychiatrie auf klinischer Grundlage für praktische Ärtze und Studirende*, 5. auflage (Stuttgart: Ferdinand Enke).

Laehr, H. (1872), 'Ueber Missbrauch mit Morphium-Injectionen', *Allgemeine Zeitschrift für Psychiatrie* 28:349–53.

Levinstein, E. (1878), *Morbid Craving for Morphine. A Monograph Founded on Personal Observations* (London: Smith, Elder & Co).

——— (1880), *La morphinomanie: monographie basée sur des observations personnelles* (Paris: G. Masson).

——— (1883), *Die Morphiumsucht. Eine Monographie nach eigenen Beobachtungen*, 2. Edition (Berlin: Verlag von August Hirschwald).

Lewy, J. (2008), 'The drug policy of the Third Reich', *Social History of Alcohol and Drugs* 22:144–67.

Maehle, A.-H. (1999), *Drugs on Trial: Experimental Pharmacology and Therapeutic Innovation in the Eighteenth Century* (Amsterdam: Rodopi).

Malcolm, M. T. (1999), 'Morphine withdrawal, treatments 1900-30', *History of Psychiatry* 10:13–26.

Mattison, J. B. (1883), 'Opium addiction among medical men', *Medical Record* 23:621–3.

Milligan, B. (2005), 'Morphine-addicted doctors, the English Opium-Eater, and embattled medical authority', *Victorian Literature and Culture* 33.541–53.

Nimb, M. (1959), *Some aspects of drug addiction in Denmark (1949–1958) with special reference to preventive measures and their results* (WHO/APD/118).

——— (1975), *Misbrug af euforiserende stoffer i Danmark i 1950'erne med efterundersøgelse i 1972* (Copenhagen: Villadsen & Christensen).

Noll, S. (1994) 'Patient records as historical stories: The case of Caswell Training School', *Bulletin of the History of Medicine* 68:411–28.

Norm, S., Kruse, P. R. and Kruse, E. (2006) 'Træk af injektionens historie', *Dansk Medicinhistorisk Årbog* 35:104–12.

Obersteiner, H. (1879–1880), 'Chronic morphinism', *Brain* 2:449–65.

——— (1882–1883), 'Further observations on chronic morphinism' *Brain* 5:324–31.

——— (1883), 'Der chronische Morphinismus', *Wiener Klinik* 9:1883, 61–84.

Padwa, H. (2012), *Social Poison. The Culture and Politics of Opiate Control in Britain and France, 1821–1926* (Baltimore: Johns Hopkins University Press).

Palmer, C. and Horowitz, M. (1982), *Shaman Women, Mainline Lady* (New York: William Morrow).

Parssinen, T. and Kerner, K. (1980), 'Development of the disease model of drug addiction in Britain, 1870–1926', *Medical History* 24:275–96.

Pichon, G. (1889), *Le morphinisme: impulsions délictueuses, troubles physiques et mentaux des morphinomanes, leur capacité et leur situation juridique: cause, déontologie et prophylaxie du vice morphinique* (Paris: Octave Doin).

Pontoppidan, K. (1883), *Den kroniske Morfinisme* (Copenhagen: Levin).

Retaillaud-Bajac, E. (2009), *Les paradis perdus: drogues et usagers de drogues dans la France de l'entre-deux-guerres* (Rennes: Presses Universitaires de Rennes).

Risse, G. and Warner, J. H. (1992), 'Reconstructing clinical activities: Patient records in medical history', *Social History of Medicine* 5:183–205.

Rodet, P. (1897), *Morphinomanie et morphinisme. Mœurs, symptómes, traitement, médicine légale* (Paris: Felix Alcan).

Schou, J. (1959), *Subcutan absorption af lægemidler* (Odense: Andelsbogtrykkeriet).

Schulsinger, F. et al. (eds), *The Department of Psychiatry. Kommunehospitalet Copenhagen 1875–1975* (Copenhagen: Munksgaard).

Seddon, T. (2008), 'Women, harm reduction and history: Gender perspectives on the emergence of the 'British System' of drug control', *International Journal of Drug Policy* 19:99–105.

Strömgren, E. (1944), 'Morfinismens klinik', *Maanedsskrift for Praktisk Lægegerning og Social Medicin* 22:385–411.

Stürup, G. K. (1959), *Forvaringsanstalten i Herstedvester: Beretning om arbejdet* (Copenhagen: Direktoratet for Fængselsvæsenet).

Sundhedsstyrelsen (1951), *Medicinalberetning for Kongeriget Danmark i året 1950* (Copenhagen: Hagerup).

——— (2013), *Narkotikasituationen i Danmark 2013* (Copenhagen: Sundhedsstyrelsen).

Vaczy Kragh, J. (2010), *Det hvide snit. Psykokirurgi og dansk psykiatri* (Odense: University Press of Southern Zealand).

Valgårda, S. (1992), *Sygehuse og sygehuspolitik i Danmark: Et bidrag til det specialiserede sygehusvæsens historie 1930–1987* (Copenhagen: Jurist-og Økonomforbundets Forlag).

Wimmer, A. (1936), *Speciel klinisk Psykiatri for Studerende og Læger* (Copenhagen: Munksgaard).

Yvorel, J. J. (1993), 'La morphinée: une femme dominée par son corps', *Communications* 56:105–13.

Zieger, S. (2005), 'How far am I responsible? Women and morphinomania in late-nineteenth-century Britain', *Victorian Studies* 48:59–81.

Chapter 9

'A gendered vice'? Gender Issues and Drug Abuse in France, 1960s–1990s

Alexandre Marchant

On March 1962, a special program on drug abuse was broadcast on ORTF, France's official television channel. Entitled *La Minute de Vérité*, the focus of the program was a lengthy interview with an elderly woman. She talked about her life as an opiate addict; an addiction she had developed during a stay in hospital, when, according to her recollection, she was administered morphine to combat her pain. Afterwards, she became addicted to pharmaceutical opiates (palfium and paregoric elixir), barbiturates obtained through complacent medical prescription or bought over the counter. Some details about the origin of her addiction were underlined by the staging of the interview; her weakness, her apathy, and her loneliness, as she was without a husband who might have taken care of her and saved her from addiction (INA 1962). In this gendered narrative, the woman was portrayed as a childish person lacking responsibility, a particular stereotype to be deconstructed, all the more so as she was presented as a 'typical' case of drug addiction.

This particular representation needs indeed to be deconstructed to reveal the social, cultural, historical or political logics that enabled this kind of narrative. In this chapter, I will therefore examine the role of gender perceptions in the making of the drug problem; that is, the type of links established between women and drug abuse. The two sides of drug abuse will be discussed, medical overconsumption and illicit drug-taking, the above example occurring at a time when the model of an iatrogenic origin for addiction predominated. As a constitutive element of social relationships based on a male/female dichotomy, these two categories have been analysed extensively for other cases (Scott 1988; Butler 1990). This chapter will address the issue of gendered identities as objects of discourses on drug abuse in France from the 1960s to the 1990s, and will also show the connection made with sexuality and motherhood in relation to drug abuse. Defined either as a pathological condition or a social plague, addiction became gendered in some narratives, allowing us to explore the political issues regarding the social roles of women and sexualised bodies within society.

These social and political narratives were constructed during the birth of drug abuse as a public health problem in France (1960s–1990s), as demonstrated by the law passed in 1970 which seriously strengthened the prohibition of illicit drug use, before the generalisation of harm reduction policies (programs of methadone or Subutex substitution and needle exchanges for heroin addicts, less repression for cannabis consumers) in the 1990s imposed a less catastrophist perception of the problem. Drug abuse as a social problem reached the dimensions of a public scandal when it raised the issue of the norms regulating society, and more particularly for the aim of this chapter, gender relations. Concerns about addiction expressed by a certain elite implicitly reflected, I would suggest, wishes to control social and symbolic relationships between women and men, so as to restore a 'normal' social order.

My research is based on printed sources – newspapers, magazines, and several novels – from the last third of the twentieth century in France, selected for their evocation and representation of women within the global issue of drugs. Since the pioneering work of Foucault (1976), it has been recognised that medical and political discourses can be utilised to support power strategies. I have therefore focused on discourses from a certain elite who intended to control, regulate, and condemn the use of drugs, as well as sexuality. Contextualising the production of depictions of women can reveal the implicit goals of this top-down discourse. For a wider landscape of discourses and practices, I also include material from the women themselves, through direct or indirect sources which allow consideration of these voices from the bottom.

The first part of this chapter is a historical reconstruction of the medical and social discourse regarding women drug addicts and their public images. I then analyse the changes affecting this gendered representation when (illicit) drugs abuse became a large social and political problem in the 1970s, and address the gendered representations of sexuality and body in the following years. Finally, I give prostitutes and addict-mothers a voice in my reconstruction of the turning point during the 1980s–1990s, when such women were most often the objects of narratives and perceptions originating from others.

The Genealogy of the Medical and Social Discourse Surrounding the Female Drug Abuser up to the 1960s

The way women were presented in the condemnation of drug abuse in the French TV program referred to above was the product of several heritages. Among the various contemporary narratives on women and drug abuse, medical discourse emphasised the idea of women's weakness predisposing them to drug abuse. Retracing the genealogy of this association, we can see nineteenth-century models in which addiction resulted from the 'natural' predisposition of women to hysteria as one origin of the construction of such a stereotype. Drug abuse was seen as a catalyst for impulses of a sexual type. In 1847, the physician François Magendie, Professor of Medicine at the Collège de France since 1831, explained in the Gazette Médicale de Paris, that the abuse by women of the anaesthetic ether was the result of 'hysteria crises' and 'uterine fury' (Yvorel, Dugarin and Nomine 1988). Toxic 'vice' was associated with defects usually attributed, in a quite misogynist period, to the so-called 'weak sex': debauchery, lust, sloth and a temptress attitude.

In the 1880s, a time when morphine had become a commonly prescribed painkiller, French medical literature was obsessed by the figure of the 'morphinée', a gendered pattern of the addicted hysteric woman from the upper classes of bourgeoisie and aristocracy, as described by the physician Edouard Levinstein in *La Morphinomanie* in 1880. Injecting herself with a hypodermic needle, a French invention by the physician Charles Pravaz in 1841, the 'morphinée' incarnated, to the eyes of the physicians who condemned her, the archetype of a woman dominated by her body and impulses. Unreasonable and forgetful of her duties as a wife, a mother and a housewife, her impulses were regarded as intolerable under the patriarchal norm of the bourgeois world in the nineteenth century. This is particularly surprising given that medical monographs in Europe at that time, as discussed in Jesper Vaczy Kragh's chapter in this volume, catalogued the predominance of male morphine addicts in the population, in contradiction with certain notions held by the physicians themselves. During the interwar period of the twentieth century, medical literature still focused on women's drug addiction as a product of the naturalised weakness of women. In 1929, the clinician Jules Ghelerter, similarly to other practitioners, described cases of divorced, abandoned and single women, who soothed the sorrow of being alone by consuming morphine and other opiates in his thesis about drug abuse (Retaillaud-Bajac 2009). In the 1950s, medical discourse abandoned the strong moralising dimension and began to explain addiction in terms of 'constitutive neurosis' (Delrieu 1988). But a link could still be made with women's 'predisposition' to weakness and hysteria. This legacy of discourses and models can explain the TV program of 1962. It was prepared with the help of the psychiatric staff at Saint Anne hospital in Paris, a renowned medical institution engaged in the progress of psychopharmacology at that time. New theories of addiction, however, were developed at the beginning of the 1970s, such as the approach of Claude Olievenstein. Founder of the Marmottan Clinic for addicts opened in Paris in 1971, Olievenstein considered addiction to be the encounter between 'a product, an individual and a socio-cultural circumstance' (Olievenstein 1970; 1984). If some genderised predispositions were still at work in the medical discourse of drug addiction, in terms of psychoanalytic concepts with links set between sexuality, transgression and abuse, they were reconstructed as the result of trauma, rather than in the biological terms of hormones and the moralist terms of women's weakness.

However, for a long time, some inherited features became stereotypes that went beyond medical sources, appearing in literature and popular culture. A song written in 1893 by Jean Lorrain, 'La Morphinée', echoed medical concerns. The song was written for the cabaret artist, Yvette Guilbert, and associated morphine taking with voluptuous pleasure, describing the injection leading to a sensation of 'fine pearl flowing into the bones' ('On dirait de la perle fine/coulant liquide dans les os', Yvorel 1993). Famous pictures such as 'Les morphinées' (1891) by Georges Moreau de Tours or 'La Morphinée' (1905) by Albert Matignon, depicted women, possibly as prostitutes and 'demi-mondaines', injecting themselves with morphine and, elongated in a languid pose, falling into ecstatic daydreams.

The sexual connotations were powerful. This stereotype persisted during the interwar period, alongside the negative image of the 'flapper', often a lesbian cocaine or opium consumer, as illustrated by Victor Marguerite in his famous novel, *La garçonne* (1922). Through selection and exaggeration, this cliché continued during the 1950s and 1960s, with addict women portrayed as prostitutes or lascivious girls in many tabloids, such as *Détective* or *Reportage*. Such representations, always made by men and often appearing in right-wing publications, make evident the fantasies of male journalists. The stereotype was also maintained within some popular literature: the journalist, Guy Champagne, in his best-selling confession, *J'étais un drogué* (Champagne 1967), narrated how he had fallen in love with a mysterious woman who, in her luxury apartment converted into an opium den, initiated him into opium smoking, then drove him to heroin. His story reactivated the image of a temptress woman in the depiction of a kind of modern 'morphinée'. The gendered imagery unveils male stereotypes regarding women's bodies.

This narrative was also reflected in newspapers, at a time when drug abuse was largely considered by the French public authorities in charge of the regulation of narcotics (namely the Direction of Pharmacy and Medication at the Health Ministry, or Joint Ministerial Commission on Narcotics) to result from the excessive availability of over-the-counter psychotropics or complacent prescriptions by physicians. By the 1960s, there was certainly an overconsumption in France of certain legal amphetamines with euphoriant and weight-loss properties, Preludine (phenmetrazin) in particular. In 1960, with the case of Miss Europe 1958, Johanna Ehrenstrasser of Austria, the phenmetrazin gained notoriety in the media. Ehrenstrasser, arrested in London for various thefts, claimed in her defence to have been under the influence of Preludine (Bachmann and Coppel 1989, 445). This amphetamine had indeed been considered a highly efficient product for the treatment of obesity since the mid 1950s. Even though available over the counter, the drug was also generously prescribed: clinical studies had indeed demonstrated very good results, both of significant weight loss and amelioration of mental state, among depressive patients (Roudier 1958). However, in the second half of the 1960s, the aforementioned administrations discovered an overconsumption among women of 10 to 20 times higher than the prescribed dosage. The Commission initially restricted the drug to medical prescription before prohibiting the drug entirely in 1969, having found a massive use of false prescriptions in pharmacies and crushed Preludine pills being injected in some extreme cases of addiction (Ministry of Health Archives 1969).

Meanwhile, the number of patients being prescribed anxiolytics was multiplying. Surveys by the French National Institute of Medical Research (INSERM) revealed that, from the 1960s, more than 60 per cent of French patients prescribed benzodiazepines or various antidepressants (Valium, Temesta, Tranxene or Prozac) were women (Reynaud, Chassaing and Coudert 1989). Valium pills could be perceived as 'mother's little helper', as in the famous 1966 song by the Rolling Stones, a criticism of the tranquillizer addiction of the middle class, the alienation felt by certain housewives and the hypocrisy of society (Pieters, Snelders and Geels 2007). This overconsumption also appeared in young people, as revealed by INSERM surveys of drugs consumption carried out in high schools in 1973 and 1980. For example, in a sample of 1110 boys under 20 years old, 9 per cent were found to take psychotropics, while in a sample of 960 girls, the figure was 20 per cent. About two thirds of the drugs consumed were legal and had been prescribed by general practitioners for 95 per cent of them. Among the drugs prescribed were tranquillizers such as Tranxene or Valium (21 per cent), hypnotics like Mogadon (20 per cent) and barbiturates (14 per cent) (Davidson and Choquet 1980). To explain this asymmetry between men and women, feminists in the 1970s would point to the weight of social norms placed upon women, rather than a supposed natural weakness (Coppel 2004).There may, however, be another explanation: Metzl (2003) has shown that the overprescription of anxiolytics in the US in the 1950s and 1960s was based on a vision of female disorders (anxiety, sexual frigidity and so on) based on a male representation of femaleness, the professional body being almost exclusively composed of men. The medical profession in France in the 1960s was also dominated by men: the committee of the National Order of Physicians, for instance, included a female doctor for the first time in 1967. As shown in the chapter by Jesper Vaczy Kragh, numerous cases of morphine addiction had already been directly caused by the medical prescription of opiates in the late nineteenth century. Overconsumption of pharmaceutical psychotropics was here inscribed in a power relationship between the male prescriber and the female patient. To conclude this historical contextualisation, the medical and social discourses concerning drug abusing women which focused on women's weakness, and the male construction of the subversive 'morphinée' or female addict during the 1960s–1970s, actually reveal the less powerful position of women in a society ruled by men.

The Renovated Representation of the Female Drug User and the 'Drug Epidemics' of the 1970s

Between 1968 and 1969, violations of drug law (use and trafficking of illicit drugs) experienced a dramatic surge of over 300 per cent, the number of arrests rising from 361 to 1,200 (then 1,861 in 1970, 2,592 in 1971, and 3,016 in 1972: Pelletier 1978). In the autumn of 1969, when around 80 articles on the 'drug phenomenon' were published in newspapers, the French parliament organised extraordinary hearings on the problem of drug abuse. The 1970 Act was passed one year later, with the Gaullist politicians in charge declaring a true war on drugs. 'Drug epidemics' became a metaphor used throughout the media for the consumption of LSD, marijuana and heroin by young people, symptomatic of a counter-culture, a beatnik and hippie movement (Bachmann and Coppel 1989). Within this new trend, women drug abusers were a very small minority, according to statistics based on the judiciary files of law enforcement agencies. In 1971, for example, women comprised 21 per cent of arrested drug users; in 1973, this had decreased to 18 per cent; and in the 1980s the figure fell to a yearly average of 12 per cent. Modern drug abuse, as captured by statistics but also as now conceived by physicians within the addiction sector, appeared to be essentially a male problem, associated with rebellion or transgressive behaviours (Pelletier 1978; Trautmann 1990).

Nevertheless, this was at odds with the particular way young women were portrayed in narratives about the rise of illicit drug use. This contrast between narratives and reality was not new: drug addiction at the end of the nineteenth century, although mostly a male trait as discussed in Jesper Vaczy Kragh's contribution, was still associated with the figure of a woman, as highlighted in this chapter. Addiction remained a largely male problem at the time of iatrogenic addiction, as it did at the time of recreational or politically oriented consumption. But addiction and overdose seemed more shocking when involving women rather than men. In France in the summer of 1969, a media frenzy was initiated by the heroin overdose of a teenage girl named Martine in a casino toilet in Bandol on the French Riviera. Several similar cases were remarked on in the press, predominantly affecting young people aged between 17 and 22 years old. Hundreds of articles were published about this new 'cancer spreading in the youth' from 1969 to 1973, the year the 'French Connection' (one of the most famous drug rings of that period: the clandestine production of heroin in the Marseilles area under the supervision of the local Corsican mafia) was dismantled, marking a pause in the frenzy (Picard 1973). Drug abuse was deemed a source of corruption and regarded as even more scandalous when affecting teenage girls. 'Drugs have killed Martine, only 17 years old', ran the headline of *Le Parisien Libéré* in August 1969: a title repeatedly reproduced was 'drugs have killed X, only 18/19 years old'; or 'on the sidewalk, several little girls, heroin addicts, none older than twenty', a terrible vision of the streets of Marseilles from a *Figaro* journalist in September 1969. In October 1972, *France Soir* published an article entitled 'The long calvary of a young female drug addict', which dwelt on her psychological degradation:

> Old at 24! Old at the age of freshness, of love, of enthusiasm, of *joie de vivre* in a word. Old and dying. Her destiny was meant to be cheerfulness and enthusiasm, and she died stupidly, heavily, in the darkness of a basement. (*France Soir* 1972)

All these articles, along with many others, were published with a photo of a young girl, eyes hidden by a black headband, a cliché often found in this series of sensationalist articles. Sensationalism met male imagery of addicted women and created a powerful representation of women's drug abuse. These images and rhetoric were particularly presented in titles addressing a conservative readership, such as the newspapers *Le Parisien libéré* and *France Soir*. In a resurgence of inherited gendered stereotypes, these commentaries emphasised the girls' weakness: they were often initiated into heroin addiction by young boys, or even injected by somebody else due to not having the strength to resist. But these portrayals were not limited to conservative publications: in November 1972, the weekly newspaper, *Le Nouvel Observateur*, a journal with a social-democratic readership, published a special issue entitled 'Why your children are taking drugs'. Its cover displayed a needle and a doll, representing young girls as consumers, revealing the passivity attributed by men to women's decision capacities regarding drug consumption. In this case, the intention of the journal was to maximise sales with a catchy cover on a fashionable topic, but the choice of such a pattern is fully gendered: it was not based on statistical reality but on a new stereotype then apparently fascinating the public.

The new cliché of the young female junkie can indeed be regarded as coherent with this gendered landscape. Numerous pictures in newspapers – a lot of them reconstructions – showed young anonymous girls injecting themselves. The association of young girls with heroin also appeared in the bestselling 'oeuvres de circonstance', such as *Satan qui vous aime beaucoup* by the journalists, Patrick Pesnot and Philippe Alfonsi (Alfonsi and Pesnot 1970). The authors described their exchanges with two young girls, one only 16-years-old, driven completely mad by their abuse of drugs; one of the girls apparently believed she was Satan. They ran away from home on multiple occasions, travelled to Iran and Turkey with drug traffickers, were involved in several pharmacy robberies to obtain classified narcotics, and ended up in the prison Les Baumettes in Marseilles. Another publishing success of these years was *L'herbe bleue, journal d'une jeune droguée* (anonymous 1972), actually a translation of the US book, *Go ask Alice* (1971). Although supposedly a genuine diary of a teenager, its authenticity was questionable: the real author very likely being the publisher, the therapist Beatrice Sparks, inventing a false testimony for moral edification (Di Folco 2006). It narrated the story of a 15-year-old girl, initiated into the use of LSD by friends, moving on to heroin, becoming a runaway, getting involved in thefts and prostitution and having various problems with the law, and finally dying from a heroin overdose. The preface was addressed to those parents who needed to monitor their children under the influence of pop culture and its permissiveness. The publication of these books where girls' testimonies were framed or reconstructed, however, also coincided with the release of autobiographical novels by young women returning from the Eastern 'hippie trail'. A good example is *H* from the French-speaking Belgian, Brigitte Axel, published in France in 1970. It narrated her experiences of many drugs, her trip to India and her 'bad trip' on LSD: discovered in the streets of Kathmandu naked and raving, she underwent emergency repatriation to Europe. These three examples had different motivations (a work of investigative journalism, a right-wing source adopting the tone of scandal, and a testimony from a former hippie who adopted leftist and counter-cultural ideas) but they converged in the same representational *cliché* of the young female junkie. The young junkie girl was presented as a childish person, irresponsible, making the wrong choices, forgetting any moral barriers, and sometimes licentious. She is the modern avatar of the 'morphinée', with added subversiveness and a nomadic dimension, incarnating a conception of liberty not in accordance with the traditional role assigned to women by society. Right-wing voices denounced both the moral and sexual liberty of the female drug addict. During the parliamentary sessions in which the 1970 Act was prepared, two particular 1969 films – *More*, by Barbet Schroeder, and *Les Chemins de Katmandou*, by André Cayatte (based on a scenario by René Barjavel who also wrote a novel on that topic with the same title) – were cited as bad examples to youth, given their portrayals of debauchery and idleness. The two films did feature single women – a hippie in Cayatte's movie – experiencing drugs and sexual liberty. Drug-taking became a motivation for Gaullist politicians, still traumatised by the May 1968 student riots, to stigmatise counter-cultural ideas and youth protests (Assemblée Nationale 1969).

At this time, however, a transformation of the roles and places of women within society was occurring. Two important laws were approved: the Neuwirth Act of 1967 which gave women the right to contraception, and the Veil Act of 1975 which authorised abortion under certain conditions. Nevertheless, beyond this legal emancipation, a strong feminist movement was emerging that wanted to go further, such as the *Mouvement de Libération de la Femme* in 1970, which denounced a 'phallocentric' culture (Duchen 1986, ch. 5). If this latter movement has produced few thoughts about illicit drugs, the hippie movement did depict examples of emancipated women, as in the novel, *L'Antivoyage*, by Muriel Cerf, in which she poetically related her pilgrimage to Mumbai, Kathmandu and Bangkok, and her experiences of various drugs and sexual initiations (Cerf 1974). This novel, of high stylistic quality, was even praised by the Minister of Culture, André Malraux: the text was indeed rather different than other novels narrating only hippie experiences, being not only the testimony of a runaway but a literary ode to liberty. Moreover, pop culture also featured a number of emancipated female icons: two singer-actresses, Zouzou (Danièle Ciarlet) and Dani (Danièle Graule), incarnated this in their widely rumoured recreational drug use that would later become heroin and cocaine addiction and repeatedly put them in jail in the 1980s and 1990s (Dani 1987; Zouzou 2003). As a voluntary action upon their own body, drug-taking was associated with the emancipation of women, although the elderly and supporters of the traditional patriarchal order still tended to interpret women's drugs consumption as debauchery. The drug debate was one between cultural representations of women, and grafted onto the changing power relationships between women and men within society.

The Evolution of Narratives on Drug-Taking and Sexuality

Allowing a certain representation of the body, narratives on drug abuse also engaged with issues surrounding sexual identities and practices. They revealed moments of confrontation between, on the one hand, a certain elite, that is Gaullist and post-Gaullist politicians or those writers and journalists shocked by the sexual liberation rhetoric of May 1968 and its legacy, and on the other hand, some socio-cultural minorities attempting to resist symbolic attempts at normalisation.

The 'drug epidemic' was indeed interpreted by some conservative intellectuals, such as Jean Cau or Pierre Gaxotte, as a sign of both spiritual and sexual decadence. In 1966, Cau described in the weekly newspaper, *Paris Match*, some 'drug parties' he attended within the artistic bohemia of Saint Germain des Prés, Paris, during which the debauchery of young people under the influence of LSD shocked him. In several texts published during this time, he warned parents about the dangers of physical and moral corruption their children faced (Cau 1969b). The satirical newspaper *The Crapouillot* produced a special issue on LSD, directed by Cau and entitled 'An atomic bomb in the head', reporting on the same drug party, significantly depicted on the cover with a disturbing photo of a wide-eyed young girl, face contorted and probably under the influence of hallucinogens. Once again, using a representation of a young girl stained by drugs appeared to be a winning marketing strategy (Cau 1966; 1969a). During the 1970s, many newspaper articles and TV documentaries condemned the use of LSD, cannabis and heroin in French orgies and the wider hippie communities of Europe. In a striking example in 1970, a writer in the newspaper *Ici Paris* was particularly virulent about the behaviour of hippies at the international Isle of Wight festival:

> Naked, covered with parasites, drug addicts: they make love in public ... They come, butts in the air, to the place of concert, no one is shocked. I stepped over a couple making love on the floor, in the mud ... A girl was doing her personal hygiene ... In a few minutes, drugs will make them unconscious wrecks ... hippies reduced to animals diggings burrows with their own hands. (*Ici Paris* 1970)

Another journal, *Le Parisien libéré*, in April 1973, made similar observations about the debauchery of young drug users:

> Hirsute, dirty and ragged, the hippies have broken into the world, carrying the 'message' enunciated by philosophers of renunciation and apostles of forfeiture ... The evil is extended with the benevolent protection of the admirers of the 'society of tolerance' that, 25 years after the closing of houses with the same name, will hasten our downfall and our enslavement. (*Le Parisien libéré* 1973)

The reference made to the 1946 closure of French 'tolerance houses' – legal brothels – makes a direct link between drug-taking and prostitution, between the liberation of sexuality and the return of an unacceptable form of moral decadency (Picard 1973).

In the frame of a conservative counter-reaction, therefore, the alleged corruption of body and mind by drugs legitimated discourses advocating a return to 'traditional' sexual social roles, as seen in the books of the journalist, Suzanne

Labin, *Hippies, sexe, drogue* in 1970, and *Le Monde des drogués* in 1975. This reporter attacked the hippie movement, labelling it a threat to the future of Western civilisation. The 'unbridled eroticism or pornography spreading freely in columns of newspapers and suggestive small ads' that showed young addicts going into homo- or bi-sexual prostitution, was, according to Labin, a degradation induced by the necessity to obtain easy money for drugs (Labin 1970; 1975). Appreciated by a conservative readership for her commitment to anti-communism, Labin was an interlocutor for many US attorneys and put forward by her editor as a witness for the US Senate commission on drug abuse in 1972. Popular literature about criminality, such as *Paris sur drogue* (1978), a novel supposedly based in fact by the former chief of the Paris Vice Squad and Narcotics Brigade, Roger Le Taillanter, shared these concerns. This novel had a gallery of stereotypical characters: Mahmoud the dealer, necessarily black and actively homosexual, manipulated and raped his punter, a young heroin-dependent white man unable to defend himself; a female Afro-American jazz artist had initiated the latter into smoking marijuana and taking heroin. All these characters were part of a typical description of the 'hell of drugs', reinforced within a racist and sexist discourse (Le Taillanter 1978).

It was within this environment that the vote and enforcement of the prohibitionist law of 1970 originated. Confronted by leftist student groups and young activists considered by the Minister of the Interior, Raymond Marcellin (1968–1974), to be a real threat, many politicians were determined to fight back against what they saw as both a political revolt and a dissolution of morality. One of the most surprising arguments heard during the parliamentary debates in October 1969 came from the Gaullist Pierre Mazeaud:

> We can notice in this country a resurgence of syphilis. According to several physicians, the sexual liberty of the young drug addicts is one of the direct causes. Besides, narcotic use in its final depressive phase weakens sexual function. It is therefore easy to understand that multiple partner orgies are multiplying to support with a pornographic placebo some deficient physical capacities. (Assemblée Nationale 1969, 2395)

Alain Peyrefitte, the Gaullist Member of Parliament who supervised the exceptional hearings of autumn 1969, published their contents a few months later in a book with a preface that directly associated sickness and moral degradation with excessive freedom:

> The drug phenomenon is one element of a more serious and extended sickness, that of the general alteration of individual and collective behaviours, that is, the degradation of morals in our developed society. This moral degradation takes so many forms: delinquent communities, outbreaks of violence, alcoholism, prostitution, extension of male and female homosexuality and the invasion of pornography … Everything is connected, and drug abuse is one aspect of

> the upsurge we are confronted with ... Excessive freedom is the cause of this
> degradation which does not seem to exist with this intensity, at least regarding
> drugs and pornography, in the socialist [communist] countries strongly controlled
> by the collective superego, denunciations, and police ... (Peyrefitte 1970, 10)

Such words call for more control and legislation on manners. The model of a
'tolerant society', set against the background of a cultural conflict between
generations, was the focus. Drug-taking was inserted into a political discourse
against the May 1968 protestors, who had claimed the right to individual happiness
while rejecting a consumerist society. Far-Left activists also rejected the moral and
social attitudes contained in such slogans as 'enjoy without restraint!' or 'making
love is making revolution' (Zancarini-Fournel 2008).

On the other side, for those who were stigmatised by a bourgeoisie elite, the
reversal of sexual norms was the basis of a particular subculture that overthrew codes
of a sexuality deemed 'bourgeois' or 'puritanical'. The monthly journal *Actuel*,
edited by Jean-François Bizot, or booklets published by the Parisian bohemia of
artists and poets, like *Le Dossier LSD* (Mandala 1967), introduced the reflections of
US writer Timothy Leary, including his description of hallucinogens as 'the most
powerful aphrodisiac substances man has ever imagined' (Leary 1979). Regarding
alternative sexual practices or identities, radical homosexual movements which
emerged at that time, such as the *Front Homosexuel d'Action Révolutionnaire*
(FHAR) founded in 1971, have clearly seen in the character of the drug addict
another victim of the 'phallocratic' order and a brother in the experience of
repression (FHAR 1971), but drug-taking was not the object of deep theorisations.
The hippie movement, however, went further, claiming sexual liberation could be
achieved through multiple sexual practices, including the sensitive experience of
drugs, an essential adjuvant for sexual ecstasy (Balland and Bernard c1970). Such
practices, supposedly challenging the traditional social order, acquired political
dimensions. But in these narratives, emancipation did not appear always to be
favourable to women: in the aforementioned references, written by men, the vision
of woman is that merely of a sexual partner, interchangeable with others.

This dimension would remain in the literature produced by drug addicts
a decade later, when counter-cultural references had receded. What was said
regarding the 'moral crusade' against sexuality was related to a specific moment
of French socio-cultural history: the sexual revolution of the 1960s and 1970s.
In the 1980s, tensions surrounding sexual emancipation would slowly disappear,
and condemnations by right-wing actors of unbridled sexuality coupled with illicit
drug-taking would focus on heroin users and male homosexuality at the time of
the AIDS epidemic. On the other hand, however, women were not advantaged
by the iconography in the 'underground' publications issued by injecting heroin
users, such as the fanzine *Viper*, an ephemeral strip cartoon magazine published
by Gérard Santi from 1981 until 1984, when it was banned for promoting illicit
drug use. Pictures had clear pornographic dimensions, with fictional characters
aimed at a largely male readership of heroin injectors: 'Bloodi', the most popular

character created by Pierre Ouin, was a heroin addict punk with an unbridled sexuality, loving prostitutes and easy women full of venereal diseases. The latter character would reappear in the current drug users' association journal, ASUD, established in 1992. The representation of women in *Viper* tended to be rather negative; portrayed as merely partners or objects for the satisfaction of a male sexual compulsion. Divisions were thus far from simplistic and sexism can be found in the politically subversive material produced by addicts groups promoting the liberation of sexuality from traditional norms (*Viper* 1981–1984).

Paradoxical Figures of Voiceless Women

As shown, women have been the objects of narratives far more often than the producers of visible narratives themselves. This invisibility was particularly apparent at the turn of the 1980s and 1990s in the way some public health institutions considered the special cases of precariously addicted women. In the 1980s and 1990s, prostitution was seen as an important element of the picture of the 'hell of drugs' and a public health problem due to the AIDS epidemic. The representation of links between prostitution and drugs – including the female drug abuser – was reactivated by the popular success of an autobiographical German novel by Christiane Felscherinow, adapted into a movie, *Wir Kinder von Banhof Zoo*. In France, the film, provocatively titled *Moi, Christiane F., 13 ans, droguée, prostituée*, was designated 'the movie of a generation' by the newspaper *Le Monde* (Felscherinow 1978; Edel 1981). In Paris, the main prostitution areas – the historical scene of Rue Saint Denis in the 2nd district, Pigalle in the 18th district, Place de Stalingrad and city gate areas like Porte de Vincennes and Bois de Boulogne – were well known in the 1980s by users, dealers and the police, as places where heroin, and later crack, could be bought. In 1993, a report from the Research Institute on the Epidemiology of Pharmacodependence (IREP) by Dr François-Rodolphe Ingold, summarising field research conducted between 1989 and 1993, revealed massive use of cannabis, heroin, cocaine and crack coupled with Temgesic, Tranxen, Rohypnol and Valium among prostitutes. Moreover, of 294 women interviewed, 114 were HIV-positive (Ministry of Health Archives 1993). But this kind of epidemiological study, stimulated by the necessity of fighting AIDS, also imposed a new reading of the phenomenon through a sociological model, breaking down negative stereotypes. These studies introduced 'the interface of prostitution and drug abuse' as 'a functional one'. Rain, cold, boredom, prolonged standing, and confrontation with unknown clients were situations made more bearable by stimulants or sedatives. This new, emerging discourse about prostitution therefore imposed the image of prostitutes as victims. In the 1970s, the young female junkie could come from any social background, mostly in the examples given, bourgeois or middle class backgrounds, influenced by beatnik or hippie cultures. What the AIDS epidemic revealed in the 1980s was, on the contrary, the circumscription of narratives about addict women to the most socially weak ones. Class issues crossed gender issues, reflecting a 1980s trend: the spread of drug addiction to people of lower socioeconomic status and consequently the 'proletarianisation' of representations of addiction (Duprez and Kokoreff 2000).

These images still marginalised women in a discourse pretending to characterise them but not originating from them. Narratives about drug abuse and the associated depictions of women reveal a relationship of social domination. When the opportunity to speak was afforded to this voiceless group, collected discourses shattered any imposed model. Such an opportunity occurred in 1989 in research carried out in Paris by the sociologist, Anne Coppel. With the aim of collecting narratives from prostitutes themselves, Coppel collected 50,000 letters from Parisian prostitutes between January and June in 1990. These reveal a plurality of paths, centered on problems such as children, housing and, for foreigners, residence permits. Empowered, they talked in a different way about drug-taking and raised other particular representations of bodies, sexual practices and gender identities. There was no consensus found on the status of prostitution (freely chosen or imposed) and its link to AIDS. The studies did, however, put forward new claims, such as social security for prostitutes, an end to police harassment and the need for hygienic places to work. For the first time, prostitutes entered the public debate about themselves, AIDS and drug abuse, and began to exist as real subjects with voices. 'We have rights, the same rights as other women', 'We are hunted like animals', 'We cannot live as criminals' were some of the statements in a collective letter by Ghanaian prostitutes, a group particularly isolated due to the language barrier (Coppel 2002, ch. 2 and 3; 2009). In response to their claims the 'Women's Friends' Bus' was implemented in November 1990, a service which still operates. The bus offers shelter for emergency situations, and distributes drinks, condoms and health messages about sex and drugs. It was a harm-reduction policy instrument, and contributed to the abolition of the offence of passive solicitation, removed from the Criminal Code in 1994 (however restored in 2003 by a new law on prostitution and safety, before being abrogated again by another law in 2013). This unique experience demonstrated the extreme difficulty that collectives of women had being heard, their bodies and sexual behaviours being subject to the discourses of doctors, researchers, and public authorities – all usually male – and public opinion, in the making of a policy that directly concerned them.

There is also another surprising blind spot regarding women addicts, which relates to those experiencing pregnancy and motherhood. Sociological works based on these women's own perceptions have only recently been published. Before this, being voiceless objects of medical studies focusing on physiological symptoms, they appeared as a devalued minority, as the aforementioned prostitutes. Their lifestyle has for a long time been blamed for diseases affecting newborns, such as the 'newborn withdrawal syndromes' (NWS) in the case of mothers addicted to opiates or crack. They were described as 'monsters', having lost their maternal instinct or being indifferent to the destiny of their child (Simmat-Durand 2009). To exist as political subjects with specific demands, particularly regarding their therapeutic care, they required intervention from associative actors engaged in street-level care, such as the activist Anna Fradet. The latter created in 1993 the first 'sleep-in' for hard drug addicts in Paris, a centre offering collective accommodation regardless of social conditions and not requiring abstinence. She managed to break the logic of 'therapeutic distance', imposed by the medical profession, that did not fit the needs of extremely marginalised populations such as crack addicted, pregnant and often homeless women (Fradet 2004). Similarly, in the context of the AIDS epidemic, some progressive physicians have also been relays for their claims. Dr Aimé Charles-Nicolas, director of the post-cure centre Pierre Nicole in Paris, opened the first service welcoming mothers and children in 1987, with an experimental unit of four mother-child beds. From that moment, addict mothers acquired a life, a discourse and a body that needed to be cared for (Coppel 2004). This case also points out a paradox of the AIDS epidemic: affecting in so cruel a way the most stigmatised fringes of the population (drug addicts, single and poor mothers, homosexuals, uprooted immigrants, prostitutes and individuals crossing some or all of these categories), it forced the public, physicians and public authorities to 'recognise' and give voice to groups previously invisibilised and silenced, unable to take part in the debates that directly concerned them.

These issues lead us to reintroduce the relationship between medical authorities and addict women, as discussed at the beginning of this chapter. At that particular moment a blockage was revealed that would only be gradually removed from the end of the 1990s. The new specialised medical sector on addiction that appeared in the wake of the 1970 Act, on the basis of the psycho-social approaches of Olievenstein, was indeed highly insensitive to gender differences among the public, the latter being essentially a masculine population: care was thus constructed on a masculine addiction pattern. Later, physicians and paramedics involved in harm-reduction policies, such as needle exchange programs, were concerned about equality of treatment, without gender distinctions. Nevertheless, as they did not find a shelter that met their expectations, many women avoided the existing health care system. In the late 1990s, for instance, less than 10 per cent of the clientele of a needle exchange program in La Goutte d'Or, a neighbourhood of Paris with a huge drug scene, were women. This marginal presence was due to the fear these women had that their children could be removed by social services (a situation affecting 40 per cent of addicted mothers according to INSERM surveys), and also the status of inferiority that can affect women in the Maghreb and African communities, a large proportion of this district's population (Pachoud 1997). Specialised care centers for drug addicts – the CSST – were also finding only a quarter of their waiting lines were women. Sociological and INSERM surveys about this issue, starting in the mid 1990s and continuing up to today, reveal that, in terms of treatment, women prefer going to general practitioners for synthetic opiate prescriptions or kicking the habit alone without treatment or social support (Coppel 2004 and 2007). As recently as 2003, half of addicted women would never talk to their attending physicians when pregnant, fearing shame or consequences for their childcare. Moreover, these surveys have revealed that 40 per cent of addicted women have in the past suffered from psychological abuse, 40 per cent from physical abuse, and 20 per cent from sexual abuse within their own families. Forty-three per cent of them discussed these problems for the first time when surveyed by the INSERM. Women have such a specific addiction profile, however, that for a long time the problems particular to them were not taken into account by socio-medical services. Nevertheless, when structures addressing women have been established, women become visible. A good example is the 'boutique for women', a needle exchange program opened in 1996 in the 18th district of Paris, at the boundary of three important drug zones (Place de Stalingrad, Porte de la Chapelle and the Goutte d'Or neighbourhood) following the discovery that women seemed to avoid the existing mixed centre due to the presence of men, many of them pimps or dealers. In only a few months, tens of women attended, even though 80 per cent of them still belonged to the particularly precarious category of prostitutes (Desplanques 2003). Voiceless women addicts regularly find themselves at a disadvantage as regards the socio-medical system. Although former medical stereotypes may have disappeared since the 1970s, women still regularly suffer from a lack of specialised shelters, and are therefore placed in a position of relative inferiority to the healthcare system.

In conclusion, this contribution, opening with the striking image from a famous TV program of the 1960s, has aimed to discuss the representation of drug abuse as a 'feminine vice'. Former medical and social narratives frequently depicted woman as a naturally weak prey for substance abuse. Although the medical approach changed during the social dispute surrounding the 'new social plague' of drug abuse at the turning point of the 1960s–1970s, some stereotypes remained and biased perception of the problem in some media outlets. Debates on drug abuse were also the pretext of a new portrayal of the body of woman, liberation or decadency, depending on the view and cultural background of agents. Narratives on the links between drugs and sexuality revealed a moral confrontation about the standards of 'good' sexuality or bodily integrity, biased or sexist representations of women not necessarily being simply partitioned by dichotomies such as Left or Right, conservative or progressive, established authority or underground movement. In many cases, however, narratives on drugs, women and sexuality reveal relationships of domination, with certain stigmatised groups, such as prostitute addicts and addict-mothers, only having a voice at rare moments in the debates concerning them.

As a final remark, I need to emphasise that the materials selected here do not reflect the view of French society in its totality, which obviously cannot be reduced to a single position. Although the politicians in charge, whether from Right or Left, have never approved of illicit drug abuse, many progressive intellectuals such as Michel Foucault, fascinated by mind-altering drug experiences, have advocated drug use, while the writers and philosophers who signed 'L'Appel du 18 joint' in *Liberation* in 1976, a petition for the decriminalisation of marijuana (signed by Gilles Deleuze, Félix Guattari, Edgar Morin, Philippe Sollers and François Châtelet), were also in favour of the associated sexual emancipation. Some situations I have dealt with, however, reveal virulent reactions, 'moral crusades' against the massification of recreational psychotropics use among the young: 'moral entrepreneurs' attempted to restore, what were in their opinions, traditional norms (Becker 1973, ch. 6). Taking into account the voices of stigmatised groups of women, they also reveal situated cultural or institutional mechanisms that, in the field of the political or medical treatment of addiction, reproduced the inherited inequalities between women and men.

Acknowledgements

I would like to thank María Jesús Santesmases and Teresa Ortiz-Gomez sincerely for their patient re-readings of this chapter, and their many suggestions that helped to significantly improve my initial contribution.

References

Alfonsi, P. and Pesnot, P. (1970), *Satan qui vous aime beaucoup* (Paris: Robert Laffont).
Anonymous (1972), *L'Herbe bleue; journal intime d'une jeune droguée* (Paris: Pocket).
Assemblée Nationale, Session Records (1969), *Séance extraordinaire du 24 Octobre 1969* [record] (Paris: Assemblée Nationale Archives).
Axel, B. (1970), *H.* (Paris: Flammarion).
Bachmann, C. and Coppel, A. (1989), *Le dragon domestique; Deux siècles de relations étranges entre l'Occident et la drogue* (Paris: Albin Michel).
Bailly, J.-C.and Guimard, J.-P. (1969), *Essai sur l'expérience hallucinogène* (Paris: Belfond).
Balland, A. and Bernard, M. (c1970), *More Love* (Paris: Editions André Balland).
Becker, H. (1973), *Outsiders: Studies in the Sociology of Deviance* (New York: the Free Press).
Butler, J. (1990), *Gender Troubles: Feminism and the Subversion of Identity* (London: Routledge).
Cau, J. (1966), 'Une bombe atomique dans la tête', *Le Crapouillot*, n°71.
———— (1969a), 'J'accuse', *Paris Match*, 15 October, pp. 97–101.
———— (1969b), 'La Drogue c'est la peste', *Elle*, n° 1245, 27 November.
Cerf, M. (1974), *L'Antivoyage* (Arles: Actes Sud).
Champagne, G. (1967), *J'étais un drogué* (Paris: Editions du Seuil).
Coppel, A. (2002), *Peut-on civiliser les drogues? De la guerre à la drogue à la réduction des risques* (Paris: La Découverte).
———— (2004), 'Figures de femmes', *Le courrier des addictions*, 6/2, pp. 54–8.
———— (2007), 'Usage de drogues et femmes: le déni français', *Le courrier des addictions*, 9/1, pp. 3–4.

———— (2009), 'Ecrire pour exister [article, extracts of letters]', *Vacarme*, n°46, pp. 29–34.

Dani (1987), *Drogue, la galère* (Paris: Carrère).

Davidson, F. and Choquet, M. (1980), *Les lycéens et les drogues licites et illicites* (Paris: INSERM).

Delrieu, A. (1988), *L'inconsistance de la toxicomanie: contribution à l'histoire des discours et des pratiques médicales*, *Analytica*, volume 53 (Paris: Navarrin).

Desplanques, L. (2003),'Femmes et addiction', *Swaps* n. 29.

Di Folco, P. (2006), *Les grandes impostures littéraires* (Paris: Ecritures).

Duchen, C. (1986), *Feminism in France, from May 68 to Mitterrand* (London: Routledge).

Duprez, D. and Kokoreff, M. (2000), *Les Mondes de la drogue. Usages et trafics dans les quartiers* (Paris: Odile Jacob).

Edel, U. (Director) (1981), *Christiane F. – Wir Kinder vom Bahnhof Zoo* [film]. Germany.

Felscherinow, C. V. (1978), *Wir Kinder vom Bahnhof Zoo* (Hamburg: Gruner und Jahr).

FHAR (1971), *Rapport contre la normalité* (Paris: Champ libre).

Foucault, M. (1976), *Histoire de la sexualité, 1: la volonté de savoir* (Paris: Gallimard).

Fradet, A. (2004), *Chez moi, on ne crache pas par terre* (Paris: L'Esprit frappeur).

France Soir (1972), 'Tant mieux si cette histoire écoeure', 27 October.

Ici Paris (1970), 'Les hipies: ils vivent comme des bêtes', n°1313.

INA Archives, ORTF (1962), *La Minute de Vérité (09/03/1962) "La Drogue"* [audiovisual file]. Available at: http://www.ina.fr/economie-et-societe/vie-sociale/video/CAF93014165/la-minute-de-verite-la-drogue.fr.html [accessed 26 March 2013. Only 1 minute of access is free].

Labin, S. (1970), *Hippies, drogue et sexe* (Paris: La Table Ronde).

———— (1975), *Le Monde des drogués* (Paris: Edition-France Empire).

Le Taillanter, R. (1978), *Paris sur drogue* (Paris: Julliard).

Leary, T. (1979), *La Politique de l'extase* (*Politics of ecstasy*, 1968) (Paris: Fayard).

Mandala (1967), *Le Dossier LSD* (Paris: 1967).

Metzl, J. (2003), *Prozac on the Couch: Prescribing Gender in the Era of Wonder Drugs* (Durham: Duke University Press).

Ministry of Health, Direction of Pharmacy and Medication (1969), *Problèmes des stupéfiants* [note to the Minister Cabinet]. Fontainebleau: Center for Contemporary Archives.

Ministry of Health, Direction of Social Action (1993), *Le travail sexuel, la consommation des drogues et le HIV: investigation ethnographique de la prostitution à Paris, 1989–1993* [IREP report] 19980329/65. Fontainebleau: Center for Contemporary Archives.

Olievenstein, C. (1970), *La Drogue: drogués et toxicomanes* (Paris: Editions Universitaires).

———— (1984), *Destin du toxicomane* (Paris: Fayard).

Pachoud, S. (1997), 'Femmes et drogues: quelle approche spécifique?', *Swaps* n. 6.

Le Parisien libéré (1973), 'Une catastrophe nationale ... On meurt de la drogue à 17 ans', 7 April 1973.

Pelletier, M. (ed.) (1978), *Rapport de la mission d'études sur l'ensemble des problèmes de la drogue* [report] (Paris: La Documentation Française).

Peyrefitte, A. (1970), *La Drogue: ce qu'ont vu, ce que proposent médecins, juges, policiers, ministres* (Paris: Plon).

Picard, G. (1973), *La drogue dans certains quotidiens et périodiques français* (Paris: UNESCO publications).

Pieters, T., Snelders, S. and Geels, F. (2007), 'Cultural Enthusiasm, Resistance and the Societal Embedding of New Technologies: Psychotropic Drugs in the 20th Century', *Technology Analysis and Strategic Management* 19(2):145–65.

Retaillaud-Bajac, E. (2009), *Les paradis perdues; drogues et usages de drogues dans la France de l'entre-deux-guerres* (Rennes: PUR).

Reynaud, M., Chassaing, J.-L.and Coudert, A.-J. (1989), *Les toxicomanies médicamenteuses* (Paris: PUF).

Roudier, C. (1958), *Etude d'un modérateur de l'appétit (A 66 ou Préludine) dans le traitement des obésités* [Thesis in medicine] Université de Toulouse.

Scott, J. (1988), *Gender and the politics of history* (New York: Columbia University Press).

Simmat-Durand, L. (ed.) (2009), *Grossess avec drogues: entre médecine et sciences sociales* (Paris: L'Harmattan).

Trautmann, C. (ed.) (1990), *Lutte contre la toxicomanie et le trafic de stupéfiants* [report] (Paris:La Documentation Française).

Viper (1981–1984), (Ecommoy: Sinsémilla Editions). Private Archives Jimmy Kempfer, Paris.

Yvorel, J.-J. (1993), 'La morphinée: une femme dominée par son corps', *Communications* 56:105–13.

Yvorel, J.-J., Dugarin, J., Nomine, P. (eds) (1988), *Consommation des drogues, représentations sociales et attitudes du pouvoir en France 1800–1988* (Reims: Institut de Recherches spécialisées).

Zancarini-Fournel, M. (2008), *Le Moment 68. Une histoire mouvementée* (Paris: Le Seuil).

Zouzou, (2003), *Jusqu'à l'aube* (Paris: Flammarion).

Chapter 10

Learning to be a Girl: Gender, Risks and Legal Drugs Amongst Spanish Teenagers[1]

Nuria Romo-Avilés, Carmen Meneses-Falcón, Eugenia Gil-García

Gendered Risky Behaviour

Risk is inherent in life and part of our everyday experience; it cannot be avoided and we have to live with it. Risk helps adolescents acquire maturing experiences, become aware of their limitations and gain knowledge about themselves (France 2000; Lupton and Tulloch 2002; Meneses, Gil and Romo 2010). Risk behaviours are not uniform, and gender, ethnicity and social class are essential factors for understanding the perception of risk and responses to it (Bimbela and Cruz 1997; Romo 2005). Risk behaviours relating to drug use, vehicle driving or unprotected sexual relationships are usually associated with, and determined by, transversal categories such as gender (Best et al. 2001). Thus, according to the so-called 'white male' effect, the perception and assessment of risk by white men differs from that of women and of other ethnic groups (Finucane et al. 2000), or to frame it in another way, risk perception differs between people with higher and lower socioeconomic power or status (Kawachi and Kennedy 1997; Mackenbach 2006). The differential socialisation and education of boys and girls means that this situation, observed in adulthood, can also be discerned in adolescence.

The usual approach in studies of adolescence and risk is to consider risk as associated with danger or injury and with circumstances and behaviours to be prevented and avoided (Douglas and Wildavsky 1983). However, this association between risk and injury does not usually match the assessment made by adolescents themselves, for whom risk can be positive (Coleman and Hagell 2007). Our analysis of risk behaviour associated with the use of legal drugs by Spanish adolescents adopts a similar perspective to that of the adolescents themselves. By not directly associating risk with harm, we can gain a more comprehensive view of their behaviours.

However, adolescents are not a homogeneous group. A gender perspective is useful for the observation of differences in risk behaviours between adolescent

1   This work is part of the National R+D+i Project, 'Adolescence and Risk: a comparative study in three Autonomous Communities', subsidised by the Ministry of Education and Science, Reference: SEJ2005-03839, the general aim of which is to study risk behaviours in adolescents.

females and males, and is indispensable when the objective is to understand the reasons for their risk behaviours and their meanings.

Within this gender analysis, the dominant representations associated with masculinity and femininity are determinant of the culture and social lifestyles of male and female adolescents. For instance, the dominant constructions of masculinity lead to the consideration of passivity as a quality of 'appropriate femininity', which in turn leads females to adopt unsafe sexual strategies (Ryan and Edward 2000). In contrast, males usually interpret masculinity as a legitimisation of social patterns that include exposing their girlfriends to risk (WHO 2012).

Behaviours that pose health risks are not part of the conventional construction of feminine identity. However, cultural trends towards equality entail, for some female adolescents, the adoption of risk behaviours previously considered to be typically male. In fact, intergenerational research indicates there has been an increase in risk behaviours among adolescent females when compared to their mothers' generation, with a reduction in the conventional gender gap with regard to risk taking (Abbott-Chapman, Denholn and Wyld 2007).

Therefore, if the reasons leading individuals to adopt risk behaviours are to be fully understood, investigations need to take account of social relationships, situations and interactions, and move beyond theoretical psychological perspectives that consider actions as resulting from a rational assessment of the costs and benefits (Rhodes 2009).

Use of Legal Drugs by Females

The view of the consumption of certain psychoactive drugs as a social problem is part of a historical process that began in the late nineteenth century, with the introduction of state interventionist policies. In 1914, the Harrison Narcotic Law was enacted in the US to ban the use of narcotics without medical prescription, leading to the subsequent criminalisation of certain psychoactive substances in that country and around the world (Markez Alonso 2010; see also chapters by Kragh and Marchant in this volume). Since that time, drugs have remained bound in the Western collective imaginary to drug dependency, described by Oriol Romaní (1999) as a complex phenomenon characterised by the more or less compulsive consumption of one or more drugs, or by the organisation of an individual's daily life around this habit. Differentiation between legal and illegal drugs has become the main way of explaining differences between psychoactive substances, with little attention paid to other characteristics, such as the damage their consumption might inflict on the health of populations.

Thus, perception of the risks derived from the use or abuse of a psychoactive substance became determined by its legal or illegal status and by the attempts of governments to control its consumption. International classifications that guide the penalisation of psychoactive substances offer no clear correlation between their effects and their possible damage to health. The legality of a substance is determined by the way in which it is used rather than by its health effects. For instance, despite the severe individual and public health problems caused by tobacco and alcohol, these substances remain legal.

In the same way that risk behaviour is considered nowadays a part of masculine culture, so is drug dependency. The androcentric positions that have dominated relevant literature have masked the social construction of the legal or illegal character of psychoactive substances that took place throughout the nineteenth and twentieth centuries. Despite the fact that the construction of the 'drugs problem' was initially associated with illegality and masculinity, women have generally consumed socially accepted drugs and medicines (Aldrich 1994; Kandall 2010; and Kragh's chapter in this volume), explaining in part the tendency for females to be ignored in public policymaking on drug dependency. Hence, a feminist and gender perspective is necessary to develop a better understanding of drug consumption cultures (Measham 2002). This approach also allows the risk behaviours of women and men and their possible health repercussions to be analysed from a public health perspective.

Since the 1990s, young females appear to have overtaken young males in the consumption of legal drugs (tobacco, alcohol and non-prescribed tranquillizers) in Spain. According to the most recent school survey by the Spanish Drug Observatory in 2010, a higher proportion of females than males aged between the ages of 14 and 18 consumed alcohol and tobacco. In addition, non-prescribed tranquillizers were used by 3 per cent of females in this age group, compared to only 1.8 per cent of males. In contrast, there was no gender difference in cannabis consumption, the most prevalent illegal drug among Spanish adolescents (DGPNSD 2011).

The consumption pattern for non-prescribed tranquillizers appears to be related to new modes of female drug consumption in Spain. These are legal substances when medically prescribed but are considered illegal when their use is not under the control of a healthcare professional. The consumption of psychoactive drugs has undergone a transformation since the 1950s, becoming widespread among individuals with no psychological disease, especially females (Romo et al. 2003; Gil et al. 2004; Arrizaga 2007). Health surveys conducted in Spain have reported that around 10 per cent of the female population had consumed a tranquillizer without medical prescription in the previous month (Hidalgo, Garrido and Hernández 2000).

Some adolescent females are treated with psychoactive drugs by their physician. Others start to use them without a medical prescription, however, often obtaining them from family members or friends for whom they have been prescribed (Romo et al. 2003). These self-prescribers have been described as generally healthy individuals who simultaneously begin to consume other legal and illegal drugs; in both cases (medical and self-prescription), the girls perceive the risk associated with psychoactive drugs to be low (Meneses 2002; Romo and Gil 2006).

The aim of this chapter is to analyse the relationship of young Spanish females with risk behaviours associated with the use of legal drugs (tobacco, alcohol and non-prescribed tranquillizers) and compare these behaviours with those of young Spanish males, taking into consideration their ethnic origin, social class, and sexuality.

Observing the New Forms of Articulating Risk Among Adolescent Women from an Intersectionality Perspective

Gender analysis reports and explains differences and inequalities between males and females in health and drug consumption. However, neither females nor males constitute a homogeneous group and there are other forms of inequality (McCall 2005; Simien 2007; Shields 2008; Bowleg 2012). Intersectionality offers a theoretical and methodological framework for explaining inter-gender and intra-gender inequalities (Mahalingam, Balan and Haritatos 2008; Nash 2008; Shields 2008). Social class, ethnicity/race, sexual orientation, age and religion, all contribute to experiences of oppression, inequality or privilege, and their consideration as analytical categories alongside gender can assist in elucidating the organisation of risk behaviours around drug consumption. Thus, in her paper on gender construction in psychoactive drug consumption patterns, "'Doing gender" – "doing drugs"', Fiona Measham (2002) underscored the relationship between their utilisation and gender identity.

Health promotion policies have been guided by the assumption that more risks are taken by young males than females, but it is possible that the behaviour of girls has been masked within some risk behaviour models. It is important to investigate gender differences in these behaviours and interactions between male and female adolescents.

Methodology: Samples and Procedures

This study adopted a mixed qualitative and quantitative approach, employing both discussion groups and a questionnaire. The subject group was a representative sample of secondary school students in the autonomous communities of Madrid and Andalusia, during the academic year 2007–2008. Discussion groups were used to obtain the meanings participants associated with these behaviours. The results also served to support the design of the questionnaire, and the analysis of responses (Meneses et al. 2009).

Two groups of adolescents aged between 13 and 17 were established in the Andalusia region and four groups in the Madrid region. Firstly, two discussion groups were held to validate the procedure to be followed with the six groups that formed part of the main study. A total of 58 adolescents participated in the six discussion groups. Gender acted in two of the groups as a homogeneity criterion (males alone and females alone) and in the other four groups as a heterogeneity criterion (mixed males and females). Age was a homogeneity criterion, given that fewer risks are perceived and assumed during the early years (first and second) than in the latter years (third and fourth) of secondary school. All groups included at least one student not born in Spain. The moderators were close in age to the participants to avoid any bias that might result from age difference. The only exception to this was the group for female adolescents alone, which was moderated by the principal investigator and, in this all-female setting, achieved a positive atmosphere of dialogue and participation. Written consent from parents or guardians was mandatory for the adolescents to participate. All discussions, including those in the Basque country, were conducted in Spanish. The adolescents were given a guarantee of strict confidentiality and anonymity, and assured the information would be used for social research purposes only. They also received a small gift in appreciation of their participation.

The discussion groups followed a standardised protocol. The aim was to elucidate the meaning of risk for the participants and their perception and assessment of risk behaviours, either their own or those of their peers. In general, it proved unnecessary for moderators to introduce the behaviours in question (drug consumption, sexual relationships, violence, and road insecurity), because debates on these points tended to emerge spontaneously in the course of discussion.

A questionnaire designed by the research team was used to gather data for quantitative analysis. This questionnaire included 57 questions on socio-demographic characteristics, risk behaviours and situations relating to drug use, violence, sexual relationships, road safety and eating disorders. The time period referred to was the previous year, with the exceptions of cigarette consumption (current daily number of cigarettes) and physical exercise (current weekly frequency). Two discussion groups were conducted to adapt the instrument to the language and perspectives of the adolescents. In a pilot test, the draft questionnaire was tested in two educational centres in a town of around 15,000 inhabitants in the Madrid region that was not involved in the main study.

The study populations for the questionnaires in Andalusia (n=1907) and Madrid (n=1720) were representative of the secondary school populations of these regions. The sample size was estimated by multistage simple random sampling for a sample error of 2.5, population variance of 50 per cent and 95 per cent confidence interval, yielding a minimum of 1,600 questionnaires for each region. The educational centres were selected to represent the types of secondary school in each region, including state schools, state-subsidised private schools (religious and non-religious) and private schools. Classes from years one, two, three and four were randomly selected at each centre. It was necessary to involve more centres in Andalusia than in Madrid to recruit the requisite number of participants.

The final study sample comprised 3,627 secondary school students from 17 centres (60 classes) in Madrid and 23 centres (83 classes) in Andalusia. Questionnaires were administered to the different groups during the same academic year (2007–2008). Participation was always voluntary, and the confidentiality of responses was explicitly guaranteed; 49.1 per cent of participants were male and 50.9 per cent female; 25.8 per cent of participants were in the first year, 24.5 per cent in the second, 25.7 per cent in the third, and 24 per cent in the fourth. The mean age was 14.8 years (standard deviation [SD] = 1.3, ranging between 12 and 19). With regard to school type, 38.6 per cent studied at a state school, 52.8 per cent at a state-subsidised private religious school, 2.7 per cent at a state-subsidised private (non-religious) school and 5.9 per cent at a private school. Place of birth was reported as Spain by 92.6 per cent, Latin-America by 5.1 per cent, Eastern Europe by 1.5 per cent and Africa by 0.8 per cent.

The ethnicity of the participants was self-determined from a list of different ethnic groups (White, Gypsy, Black, Asian, and so on) drawn up by the adolescents themselves and using their own designations. Because a large majority of the participants recruited at the centres defined themselves as 'white', all other ethnicities were grouped as 'other ethnic groups', the scant representation of which prevented the analysis of differences among them.

The questionnaires were self-administered in the classroom, in the presence of one of the research team. The adolescents took an average of around 40 minutes to complete the task.

SPSS 17 (SPSS, IBM, Chicago, IL) was used for the statistical analyses. Qualitative and categorical data were expressed as frequencies and percentages, and quantitative data as measures of central tendency and dispersion. The chi-square test was used for contingency analyses of relationships among variables and the Student's t-test was used to compare means. $P<0.05$ was considered significant. Multivariate analysis of risk behaviours was not possible due to inadequate sample sizes, given the small number of female consumers of tranquillizers.

Regarding the perception of family economic level, 78.2 per cent reported a good economic level, 20.2 per cent barely made it to the end of the month, and 1.6 per cent described many economic problems. According to parents' profession, participants were classified as having a high socioeconomic position (29.9 per cent), medium position (35.6 per cent), or low socioeconomic position (23.1 per cent); 11.5 per cent could not be classified due to the lack of relevant data.

Drug Use and Accessibility to Drugs

In this survey of female and male secondary school students, the majority of drugs consumed were legal. The consumption of these drugs (tobacco, alcohol, and non-prescribed tranquillizers) was more frequent among females than among males. Table 10.1 shows that the consumption of legal drugs was more frequent among females in both lifetime-prevalence and 12-month-prevalence.

Table 10.1   Drugs consumed by female and male adolescents in Andalusia and Madrid, 2007–2008

Drug Use	Females %	Males %	χ^2	P
At some time in their life				
Alcohol	67.0	63.0	6.187	.013
Tobacco	46.2	34.8	46.123	.000
Cannabis	9.5	11.6	3.894	.048
Non-prescribed tranquillizers	8.8	5.6	12.892	.000
Analgesics	12.3	7.5	21.703	.000
Ecstasy	0.7	0.7	0.004	.949
Inhalants	1.5	1.8	0.560	.454
Heroin	0.6	0.5	0.336	.562
Cocaine	1.6	1.8	0.221	.638
Previous year				
Alcohol	58.3	52.1	12.940	.000
Tobacco	35.7	24.4	50.806	.000
Cannabis	7.2	9.0	3.866	.049
Non-prescribed tranquillizers	5.0	3.0	9.255	.002
Analgesics	9.6	5.1	24.686	.000
Ecstasy	0.2	0.5	2.560	.110
Inhalants	0.8	0.8	0.001	.970
Heroin	0.2	0.3	0.171	.679
Cocaine	0.9	1.0	0.108	.743

These results are consistent with other studies conducted within Spanish populations (Inglés et al. 2007; Romo 2011). Initiation into illegal drug use is uncommon at these ages, with cannabis being more frequently consumed for the first time at later stages of adolescence. In the discussion groups, both female and male adolescents evidenced a low perception of the risks associated with legal drug consumption, regarding risk as omnipresent and seeing no reason why it would affect them in particular:

> 'People of our age may face many types of risks. On the street, at school, everywhere. I think it's the same ... well, not the same because we're not the same age as the adults, we are maybe more ... sensitive, we're more easily misled and all that but ... I think it's practically the same for us as for adults. Risk is everywhere.'
>
> (Mixed group: males and females)

Alcohol is the stellar substance. It stood out in discussions and in the high prevalence of its consumption among both males and females; results in line with the reports of other researchers in Spain (Moral, Sirvent and Rodríguez 2005; Gómez 2006). Alcohol was consumed by a higher proportion of females than males, but males consumed greater amounts than females:

> 'Alcohol ... almost everyone drinks it and for older people or whatever ... it
> is like they were drinking a coca-cola among friends and such: drink and drink
> and drink and they binge drink to get drunk and it's no big deal.'
> 'Alcohol consumption has become very generalised. The starting age has
> dropped a lot ... to 14, 13 ...'
>
> (Mixed group: males and females)

The widespread consumption of legal 'drugs', such as alcohol, and of officially prohibited substances considered 'legal' by young people, like cannabis, leads to the normalisation of these substances and facilitates access to them:

> 'Because so many people smoke joints, it's like you're less afraid to try it'
> 'With pills ... it's like more .. risky. You see people smoking joints and nothing
> happens to them so you know it won't happen to you either ...'
> 'It's like, it's more natural, isn't it?'
> 'If nothing happens to him, there's no reason why it would happen to you.'
> 'So, because everyone smokes joints, you're less afraid to try them aren't you?'
>
> (Mixed group: males and females)

Male and female adolescents categorised substances according to the potential danger they posed to health. Although some substances were considered 'natural', because they were used by everybody and therefore normalised, others were perceived as more dangerous or risky. This also related to the possibilities and difficulties of obtaining the substances. The legal or illegal status of the substances affected the perceptions associated with their consumption.

Table 10.2 shows that these adolescents considered it easy to gain access to legal substances, with no significant gender differentiation.

In the discussion groups, both males and females agreed they had no problems in gaining access to substances. When they could not buy them in public places because of their age, they would find other ways of obtaining them without difficulty:

> 'Well the truth is that ... regardless, it's prohibited to buy it under a certain age
> but in some bars they don't stop you, what do I know, at first glance maybe they
> can't tell that we're only 13 or 14 years old or whatever, you know? But if they
> don't say anything to you, you buy it.'
>
> (Mixed group: males and females)

Table 10.2   Perception of female and male adolescents of the accessibility of substances

Easy access to substances	Females % (n)	Males % (n)	$\chi2$	P
Tobacco	78.0 (1395)	76.6 (1271)	3.725	.054
Beer	78.0 (1386)	78.6 (1321)	0.234	.629
Wine	72.3 (1281)	75.5 (1269)	4.573	.032
Cocktails	58.4 (1024)	59.8 (991)	0.651	.420
Cannabis	26.5 (469)	32.9 (549)	16.771	.000
Ecstasy	13.3 (235)	15.4 (257)	3.066	.080
Inhalants	15.6 (274)	20.5 (341)	13.747	.000
Heroin	8.4 (149)	12.3 (205)	13.773	.000
Cocaine	12.5 (221)	15.2 (254)	5.326	.021

'If you have 18-year-old friends they can easily buy it for you.'

'And do they buy it for you?'

'Yes, but they always tell you that when someone asks you: Who bought it? Not to say it was them.'

'Of course, or ... we go to another place. For example, in the 24-hour store here (a store that's open 24 hours) if you buy alcohol, which they sometimes sell us, they give us white bags so you can't ...'

'So the label can't be seen ...'

'Or an older person comes up to you: look, I'll buy it for you but if they ask who sold it to you or who bought it for you, don't say it was me. Or, it's like with joints, if you score off a Moroccan and the police catch you ... they'll go after him. So you say you just found it, or someone you don't know gave it to you, or something.'

(Mixed group: males and females)

These extracts from the discourses of male and female adolescents highlight the strategies they use for obtaining legal psychoactive substances that are prohibited to them due to their age. The ability to gain access to these substances is most frequently attributed to the permissiveness of sales or bar staff and to the assistance of over 18-year-olds. Older teens provide this service because they had recently been in the same situation and had found someone to help them. This offers insight into how and why young people help each other. On other occasions, this service is provided in exchange for something, usually alcohol.

Female Drug Use and Other Risky Behaviours

Our study revealed a higher frequency of legal drug consumption among the female than male adolescents, consistent with the findings of other national studies. We focused on the questionnaire results for female adolescents, who represented almost 50 per cent (n=1827) of the study population.

Out of the 1827 females in the study, 87 (5 per cent) had consumed tranquillizers without a medical prescription in the previous 12 months; they showed no significant differences with the other females as a function of region (Madrid vs Andalusia ($p=0.451$), school year ($p=0.102$) or nation of birth (0.533). Among these 87 female adolescents, 85 per cent also consumed alcohol and 59 per cent smoked tobacco. In other words, other legal substances were usually consumed by the users of mood-altering drugs. According to statements made in one of the all-female discussion groups, alcohol played a key role in the structuring of relationships in leisure time and space:

> 'Okay, okay, I'll say it. For example, let's say, since we're on the subject of alcohol, if you go to a botellón [outdoor gathering of young people to consume alcohol bought from shops], it's obvious that you're going to drink, you're not going to stick to a glass of water.'
>
> (All-female group)

The only significant differences between the females who had and had not consumed non-prescribed tranquillizers during the previous year were in type of family, perception of the domestic economic situation, and age (see Table 10.3). Thus, non-prescribed tranquillizer consumption was more frequent among those not living with a parent, in comparison to those living with one or two parents, and among those perceiving many financial problems at home. The mean age of females who had taken tranquillizers was around one year older (around 15 years old) than that of females who had not.

Parents were continually referred to in the females' discourse, but were perceived as being unable to act:

> 'I think parents can't do anything to help us avoid the risk, because if you want to do it, you're going to do it, whether they help you or not. I don't know how to explain it.'
>
> (All-female group)

Many believed that their mothers had lived through the same situation and should therefore understand; they did not expect their mothers to stop them.

Table 10.3 **Socio-demographic characteristics of female adolescents as a function of their use of tranquillizers without medical prescription (n=87)**

	Use previous year (%)	No use previous year (%)	χ2	P
Region				
Andalucía	55.2	51.0	0.567	.451
Madrid	44.8	49.0		
Secondary school year				
1st	12.6	23.9		
2nd	25.3	24.4	6.207	.102
3rd	31.0	25.3		
4th	31.0	26.4		
Born in Spain				
Yes	90.8	92.6	0.388	.533
No	9.2	7.4		
Type of family				
Live with father alone	-	1.2		
Live with mother alone	17.2	11.6		
Live with both parents	75.9	82.0	11.107	.025
Live with step-family	2.3	4.1		
Other	4.6	1.2		
Social Class				
High	34.1	31.1		
Medium	36.6	41.1	0.751	.687
Low	29.3	27.5		
Perception of domestic financial situation				
Quite good	67.4	76.9		
Barely make it to the end of the month	26.7	21.5	10.523	.005
Many financial problems	5.8	1.5		
Ethnicity				
White Caucasian	85.7	83.0	0.421	.517
Other ethnic groups	14.3	17.0		
Mean age	15.2	14.8 years	-2.995*	.003

* Student's t test

Table 10.3 shows that the consumption of tranquillizers was not related to social class, ethnicity (self-identified) or nation of birth and was only significantly associated with type of family and subjective economic perception. Data suggests that there were significant links with living in female-headed households, barely making it to the end of the month, and experiencing financial problems. But we cannot know to what extent those variables are related. Although our series is representative, the sample size of females taking tranquillizers may be inadequate to detect differences relating to social class or ethnicity. These differences may be explained by various circumstances detectable through qualitative research.

Legal Drug Use and Risk

The female adolescents who had consumed non-prescribed tranquillizers in the previous year also reported other risky behaviours. In comparison to the other females, a higher proportion reported: riding on a scooter (term used in this chapter to cover all types of motor bicycle or moped) after consuming alcohol; losing consciousness after taking a drug; becoming inebriated; taking medicines or drugs with alcohol; consuming cannabis or some other illegal drug; riding on a scooter after the consumption of cannabis or other substance; and smoking cigarettes (see Table 10.4).

Table 10.4   Risk behaviours with drug use among the sample of females, based on the use of tranquillizers without medical prescription in the previous year

	Use previous year %	No use previous year %	$\chi 2$	P
Drink alcohol at a botellón and ride on a scooter afterwards	39.3	21.7	14.076	.000
Take too much of a drug and lose consciousness	8.3	3.4	5.97	.020
Get drunk	54.8	29.6	23.796	.000
Take medicines with alcohol	14.3	4.7	14.765	.000
Smoke cannabis	18.8	11.4	4.305	.038
Use illegal drugs other than cannabis	10.8	1.2	45.729	.000
Ride on a scooter when you have smoked cannabis or taken other drugs	8.3	3.1	6.872	.009
Sell cannabis and other drugs	4.8	1.3	6.685	.010
Smoke cigarettes	29.4	16.5	9.437	.002

Drug Use, Risk and Sexuality

A significant relationship was observed between the consumption by females of non-prescribed tranquillizers in the previous year and risky behaviour in sexual relationships (Table 10.5).

Table 10.5   Risk behaviours of female adolescents in sexual relationships as a function of their use of non-prescribed tranquillizers in the previous year

	Use in previous year %	Non-use in previous year %	$\chi 2$	P
Intercourse	31.0	18.8	7.480	.006
Use of condoms	92.3	89.6	0.192	.661
Having sex when asked to by boyfriend despite not wanting it	9.6	4.1	5.934	.015
Becoming pregnant	2.4	0.9	1.657	.198
Having sex after drinking	15.7	4.4	21.561	.000
Attempt at non-consensual sexual relations	20.7	11.6	6.451	.011

Females who consumed non-prescribed tranquillizers more frequently reported engaging in sexual relations with penetration and without protection, in comparison to those who did not. Although we cannot determine the extent to which they were victims or active agents in their sexual behaviours, they were also more likely to have sex when requested to by their boyfriends, either against their wishes or after drinking alcohol, and to have experienced attempted sexual abuse. These data provide evidence that adolescent females who use non-prescribed tranquillizers are more sexually active than non-users and yet are more vulnerable in their sexual relationships and more likely to be exposed to involuntary risks.

Risks associated with sexuality tended to emerge spontaneously in the all-female discussion groups. Pregnancy remained one of the main perceived risks, especially for females, although this situation may be changing, given that the risk can be controlled by new drugs, such as the morning-after pill. However, the same is not true for the risk of sexually-transmitted diseases:

> 'I think sex is what worries you most.'
> 'In terms of diseases, because you can take morning-after pill to stop yourself getting pregnant, and well, just carry on.'

> (All-female group)

Although condoms were known to be a good safety measure, the risk of condom failure was raised in some of the discussion groups:

> 'It could split and then you catch something ...'
> 'Even if you buy them in a chemists or wherever (talking at same time), even if you buy them in a chemists they can still split. There isn't, no ... I think there isn't any like that or ...'
> 'It's not 100 percent probability against, it's 99 and ...'

(All-female group)

Drug Use and Other Risk Behaviours

In previous studies by our group, incidents of unsafe behaviour on the road (Meneses, Gil and Romo 2010) and violent behaviour (Gil and Romo 2008; Meneses et al. 2009) were more frequent in young males than females. In the present study, female adolescents who had used non-prescribed tranquillizers reported fights and traffic violations in the previous year more frequently, and a greater liking for risk in comparison to those who had not (Table 10.6). The performance of these risky behaviours appears to reflect a different way of being a girl.

Table 10.6   Other risk behaviours by female adolescents as a function of their use of non-prescribed tranquillizers in the previous year

	Use in previous year %	Non-use in previous year %	χ^2	P
Fight in the previous year	26.7	14.9	8.845	.003
Fight after drinking	19.0	4.0	40.093	.000
High-speed racing				
Never	31.0	49.4	26.187	.000
At some time	32.2	34.4		
Often	36.8	16.2		
I like risks				
Never	18.4	34.8	13.317	.001
At some time	39.1	37.8		
Often	42.5	27.4		
Competing with others on the road				
Never	73.6	87.9	16.114	.000
At some time	18.4	9.2		
Often	8.0	2.9		

It was generally stated within discussion groups, that girls do not usually fight as often or with the same intensity as boys. Conflictive interaction between girls was mostly associated with verbal violence, with physical violence usually arising under the effects of alcohol and other drugs:

> 'Let's see, what I think is it's not only this about going into a coma or whatever, but rather alcohol, most of the fights, or whatever, perhaps at some parties it is because people go into a 'fog', they don't know what they're doing, … it's not necessary to join in everything, but because of the alcohol, the situation, it's no longer that you can just fall into a coma, or whatever if you don't control yourself, because you may control yourself and get into a fight, and that's when you lose control.'

> (All-female group)

Road safety risks also appear to be a gender issue, with fewer girls having scooters or feeling drawn to them:

> 'I think it's because they do more stupid things with a scooter, for example, you give a girl a scooter and she doesn't think: Hey, I'm going to do wheelies until I crack my head!'

> (All-female group)

Hence, the girls who adopt this type of behaviour, whether or not combined with other risk behaviours, appear to be in a distinct dimension with different meanings. Explanations may include rebelliousness, participation in the male world, or experimentation and learning in areas previously forbidden to women. It should not be forgotten that risk is inevitable and necessary for learning and discovering our limits and for forming our own identity (Lupton and Tulloch 2002).

Thinking About New Ways of Learning to be a Girl

Our investigation reveals a trend towards an increase in drug use and risk behaviours by young females in two Spanish regions. Both elements appear to be intertwined with gender.

The use of non-prescribed tranquillizers was associated with the consumption of other legal drugs, such as tobacco and alcohol. The same girls also adopted some risk behaviours considered masculine, including reckless driving, violence and risky sexual practices. These are particular ways of becoming an adult that should not serve to stigmatise this group but rather to strengthen it in a preventive approach. These forms of consumption, very distinct from conventional feminine passivity, require adapted public health interventions that include a gender perspective.

This study contributes evidence for a new 'female drug consumption model' organised around legality. Consumption may be a way of standing out and rebelling against what is expected of them, presenting behaviour that could be considered more masculine, but is at the same time distinctly female in terms of the choice of substance. This relatively small group of girls demonstrated a different way of constructing their identity, adopting an approach to learning and an experimentation strategy that might either make them more vulnerable, or endow them with greater knowledge and maturity. This represents one way for today's female teenagers to draw level with their male peers in terms of knowledge and discovery of their limits, self-control, and living with everyday and exceptional risks. Our study appears to unmask a group of female adolescents who engage in the most risky behaviours and are close to illegality in a similar way to males and in interaction with them. The risks faced by this group may be transient or become deep-rooted, but both can have negative repercussions on their health, requiring adequate preventive measures.

Wider studies with different methodologies are required to verify whether the present results are reproducible in other socio-cultural settings. Qualitative research is also warranted to explore some of our conclusions and enhance our understanding of these findings.

Previous studies indicating a trend towards an increased use of alcohol, tobacco and drugs by young females have questioned whether preventive policies are yielding adequate results for females. Two issues are at the core of this question: the gender-specific context of risk for substance use, and the implication of this context for prevention strategies (Amaro et al. 2001; Meneses et al. 2009). It is essential to address the health and development needs of adolescents if they are to make a healthy transition into adulthood. Societies must tackle the factors that promote potentially hazardous habits in relation to sex, tobacco and alcohol use, and must provide adolescents with the support they need to avoid these behaviours. In many high-income countries, adolescent females are increasingly using alcohol and tobacco, and obesity is on the rise. Supporting adolescents to establish healthy habits can yield major health benefits later in life, including a reduction in the risk of mortality or disability due to cardiovascular disease, stroke or cancer (WHO 2012). It may be that we should address the context of inequality in which these substances are consumed rather than working on specific groups (Frieden 2010). In agreement with Ettorre (2004 and 2007), we suggest that the inclusion of a gender perspective in the field of drug dependency would allow the creation of harm-reducing policies that cannot be successful without the full consideration of gender differences.

References

Abbott-Chapman, J. A., Denholm, C. J. and Wyld, C. (2007), 'Gender differences in adolescent risk taking: Are they diminishing? An Australian intergenerational study', *Youth and Society* 40:1, 131–54.

Aldrich, M. R. (1994), 'Historical notes on women addicts', *Journal of Psychoactive Drugs* 26:1, 61–4.

Amaro, H., Blake, S. M., Schwartz, P. M. and Flinchbaugh, L. J. (2001), 'Developing theory-based substance abuse prevention programs for young adolescent girls', *Journal of Early Adolescence* 21:3, 256–93.

Arrizaga, C. (2007), *La Medicalización de la Vida Cotidiana. El Consumo Indebido de Psicotrópicos en Adultos* (Buenos Aires: Observatorio Argentino de Drogas, SEDRONAR).

Best, D., Rawaf, S., Rowley, J., Floyd, K., Manning, V. and Strang, J. (2001), 'Ethnic and gender differences in drinking and smoking among London adolescents', *Ethnicity and Health* 6:1, 51–7.

Bimbela, J. L. and Cruz, M. T. (1997), *Sida y Jóvenes. La Prevención de la Transmisión Sexual del VIH* (Granada: Escuela Andaluza de Salud Pública).

Bowleg, L. (2012), 'The problem with the phrase women and minorities: intersectionality an important theoretical framework for public health', *American Journal of Public Health* 102:7, 1267–73.

Coleman, J. and Hagell, A. (2007), *Adolescence, Risk and Resilience. Against the Odds* (West Sussex: John Wiley & Sons, Ltd).

DGPNSD (2011) Encuesta Estatal Sobre Uso de Drogas en Enseñanzas Secundarias (ESTUDES). Ministerio de Sanidad, Política Social e Igualdad. [Online: Delegación del Gobierno para el Plan Nacional sobre Drogas] Available at: http://www.pnsd.es [accessed 10 December 2012].

Douglas, M. and Wildavsky, A. B. (1983), *Risk and Culture: An essay on the Selection of Technical and Environmental Dangers* (Berkeley: University of California Press).

Ettorre, E. (2004), 'Revisioning women and drug use: gender sensitivity, gendered bodies and reducing harm', *International Journal of Drugs Policy* 15:5–6, 327–50.

——— (2007), *Revisioning Women and Drug Use: Gender, Power and the Body* (Basingstoke: Palgrave).

Finucane, M. L., Slovic, P., Mertz, C. K., Flynn, J. and Satterfield, T. A. (2000), 'Gender, race, and perceived risk: the "white male" effect', *Health, Risk and Society* 2:2, 159–72.

France, A. (2000), 'Towards a sociological understanding of youth and their risk-taking', *Journal of Youth Studies* 3:3, 317–31.

Frieden, T. R. (2010), 'A framework for public health action: The health impact pyramid', *American Journal of Public Health* 100:4, 590–95.

Gil, E. and Romo, N. (2008), 'Conductas de riesgo en adolescentes urbanos andaluces', *Miscelánea Comillas* 66:129, 493–509.

Gil, E., Romo, N., Poo, M., Meneses, C., Markez, I. and Vega, A. (2004), 'Género y psicofármacos. La opinión de los prescriptores a través de una investigación cualitativa', *Atención Primaria* 5:8, 402–8.

Gómez, J. (2006), 'El alcoholismo femenino, una verdad oculta', *Trastornos adictivos: Órgano Oficial de la Sociedad española de Toxicomanías* 8:4, 251–60.

Hidalgo, I., Garrido, G. and Hernández, M. (2000), 'Health status and risk behavior of adolescents in the north of Madrid (Spain)', *Journal of Adolescent Health* 27:5, 351–60.

Inglés, C. J., Delgado, B., Bautista, R., Torregrosa, M. S., Espada, J. P., García, J. M., Hidalgo, M. D. and García, L. J. (2007), 'Factores psicosociales relacionados con el consumo de alcohol y tabaco en adolescentes españoles', *International Journal of Clinical and Health Psychology* 7:2, 403–20.

Kandall, S. R. (2010), 'Women and drug addiction: a historical perspective', *Journal of Addictive Diseases* 29:2, 117–26.

Kawachi, I. and Kennedy, B. P. (1997), 'The relationship of income inequality to mortality: Does the choice of indicator matter?', *Social Science and Medicine* 45:7, 1121–7.

Lupton, D. and Tulloch, J. (2002), 'Risk is part of your life. Risk epistemologies among a group of Australians', *Sociology* 36:2, 317–34.

Mackenbach, J. P. (2006), 'Socio-economic inequalities in health in Western Europe: from description to explanation to intervention' in Siegrist, J. and Marmot, M. (eds) *Social Inequalities in Health. New Evidence and Policy Implications* (Oxford and New York: Oxford University Press) pp. 223–50.

Mahalingam, R., Balan, S. and Haritatos, J. (2008), 'Engendering immigrant psychology: an intersectionality perspective', *Sex Roles* 59:326–36.

Markez Alonso, I. (2010), 'Dependencias: de la coerción a la reducción de daños', *Crítica* 60:967, 33–8.

McCall, L. (2005), 'The complexity of intersectionality', *Signs: Journal of Woman in Culture and Society* 30:3, 1771–800.

Measham, F. (2002), '"Doing gender" – "doing drugs": conceptualising the gendering of drugs cultures', *Contemporary Drug Problems* 29:2, 335–73.

Meneses, C. (2002), 'De la morfina a la heroína: el consumo de drogas en las mujeres', *Miscelánea Comillas* 60:116, 217–43.

Meneses, C., Gil, E., and Romo, N. (2010), 'Adolescentes, situaciones de riesgo y seguridad vial', *Atención Primaria* 42:9, 452–62.

Meneses, C., Romo, N., Uroz, J., Gil, E., Markez, I., Jiménez, S. and Vega, A. (2009), 'Adolescencia, consumo de drogas y comportamientos de riesgo: diferencias por sexo, etnicidad y áreas geográficas en España', *Trastornos Adictivos* 11:1, 51–63.

Moral, M. V., Sirvent, C. and Rodríguez, F. J. (2005), 'Motivadores del consumo de alcohol en adolescentes: análisis de diferencias inter-género y propuesta de un continuum etiológico', *Adicciones: Revista de Socidrogalcohol* 17:2, 105–20.

Nash, J. C. (2008), 'Re-thinking intersectionality', *Feminist Review* 89, 1–15.

Rhodes, T. (2009), 'Risk environments and drug harms: A social science for harm reduction approach', *International Journal of Drug Policy* 20, 193–201.

Romaní, O. (1999), *Las Drogas: Sueños y Razones* (Madrid: Ariel).

Romo, N. (2005), 'Género y uso de drogas: la invisibilidad de las mujeres', *Monografías Humanitas* 5, 65–83.

———— (2011), 'Cannabis, juventud y género: nuevos patrones de consumo, nuevos modelos de intervención', *Trastornos Adictivos: Órgano Oficial de la Sociedad Española de Toxicomanías* 13:3, 91–3.

Romo, N. and Gil, E. (2006), 'Género y uso de drogas. De la ilegalidad a la legalidad para enfrentar el malestar', *Trastornos Adictivos* 6:4, 243–50.

Romo, N., Vega A., Meneses, C., Gil, E., Márquez, I. and Poo, M. (2003), 'Sobre el malestar y la prescripción: un estudio sobre los usos de psicofármacos por las mujeres', *Revista Española de Drogodependencias* 28:4, 372–80.

Ryan, R. M. and Edward, L. (2000), 'Intrinsic and extrinsic motivations: Classic definitions and new directions', *Contemporary Educational Psychology* 25:1, 54–67.

Shields, S. A. (2008), 'Gender: An intersectionality perspective', *Sex Roles* 59, 301–11.

Simien, E. M. (2007), 'Doing intersectionality research: from conceptual issues to practical examples', *Politics and Gender* 3:2, 264–71.

World Health Organization (2012), *Women and Health: Today's Evidence Tomorrow's Agenda*. [Online: World Health Organization] Available at: http://www.who.int/gender/documents/9789241563857/en/index.html [accessed: 11 December 2012].

Index